OTOLARYNGOLOGY
A Case Study Approach

OTOLARYNGOLOGY
A Case Study Approach

Edited by

THOMAS A. TAMI, M.D.
Associate Professor
Department of Otolaryngology—
Head and Neck Surgery
University of Cincinnati Medical Center
Cincinnati, Ohio

ALLEN M. SEIDEN, M.D.
Associate Professor
Department of Otolaryngology—
Head and Neck Surgery
University of Cincinnati Medical Center
Cincinnati, Ohio

MYLES L. PENSAK, M.D.
Professor
Department of Otolaryngology—
Head and Neck Surgery
University of Cincinnati Medical Center
Cincinnati, Ohio

JACK L. GLUCKMAN, M.D.
Professor and Chairman
Department of Otolaryngology—
Head and Neck Surgery
Children's Hospital Medical Center
Cincinnati, Ohio

ROBIN T. COTTON, M.D.
Professor
Department of Otolaryngology—
Head and Neck Surgery
University of Cincinnati College of Medicine; and
Director
Department of Pediatric Otolaryngology & Maxillofacial Surgery
Children's Hospital Medical Center
Cincinnati, Ohio

1998
Thieme
New York • Stuttgart

Thieme Medical Publishers, Inc.
333 Seventh Avenue
New York, NY 10001

Otolaryngology: A Case Study Approach
Thomas A. Tami
Allen M. Seiden
Myles L. Pensak
Jack L. Gluckman
Robin T. Cotton

Library of Congress Cataloging-in-Publication Data

Otolaryngology : a case study approach / edited by Thomas A. Tami ...
    [et al.].
        p. cm.
    Includes index.
    ISBN 0-86577-773-X (TNY).—ISBN 3-13-111541-6 (GTV)
    1. Otolaryngology—Case studies.   I. Tami, Thomas A.
    [DNLM: 1. Otorhinolaryngologic Diseases—diagnosis case studies.
    2. Otorhinolaryngologic Diseases—therapy case studies.
    3. Otorhinolaryngologic Diseases examination questions.
    4. Diagnosis, Differential.   WV 140 0878 1998]
    RF69.086   1998
    617.5'1—dc21
    DNLM/DLC
    for Library of Congress   97-51988
                                                                  CIP

Important note: Medical knowledge is ever-changing. As new research and clinical experience broaden our knowledge, changes in treatment and drug therapy may be required. The authors and the editors of the material herein have consulted sources believed to be reliable in their efforts to provide information that is complete and in
accord with the standards accepted at the time of publication. However, in view of the
possibility of human error by the authors, editors, or publisher of the work herein, or
changes in medical knowledge, neither the authors, editors, publisher, nor any other
party who has been involved in the preparation of this work, warrants that the information contained herein is in every respect accurate or complete, and they are not responsible for any errors or omissions or for the results obtained from use of such information.
Readers are encouraged to confirm the information contained herein with other sources.
For example, readers are advised to check the product information sheet included in the
package of each drug they plan to administer to be certain that the information contained in this publication is accurate and that changes have not been made in the recommended dose or in the contraindications for administration. This recommendation is of
particular importance in connection with new or infrequently used drugs.

Some of the product names, patents, and registered designs referred to in this book are
in fact registered trademarks or proprietary names even though specific reference to
this fact is not always made in the text. Therefore, the appearance of a name without
designation as proprietary is not to be construed as a representation by the publisher
that it is in the public domain.

Printed in the United States of America

5 4 3 2

To my daughter Leigh and my son Aaron.
—T.T.

To my family.
—R.C.

To our present and former residents who continue to enrich us.
—M.P.

To the patients who over the years have provided the clinical material for this book, and therefore have afforded us an educational opportunity that we hope will result in better patient care.
—A.S.

Contents

viii • CONTENTS

Contributors

Mark J. Abrams, MD
Chief Resident
Department of Otolaryngology—
Head and Neck Surgery
University of Cincinnati Medical Center
Cincinnati, Ohio

Glenn O. Bratcher, MD
Assistant Professor
Department of Otolaryngology—
Head and Neck Surgery
University of Cincinnati Medical Center
Cincinnati, Ohio

James Clemens, MD
Chief Resident
Department of Otolaryngology—
Head and Neck Surgery
University of Cincinnati Medical Center
Cincinnati, Ohio

Eve Cornell, DDS
Chief Resident
Division of Oral and Maxillofacial Surgery
Department of Surgery
University of Cincinnati College of Medicine
Cincinnati, Ohio

Robin T. Cotton, MD
Professor
Department of Otolaryngology—
Head and Neck Surgery
University of Cincinnati College of Medicine;
and Director, Department of Pediatric
Otolaryngology & Maxillofacial Surgery
Children's Hospital Medical Center
Cincinnati, Ohio

Michelle M. Cullen, MD
Chief Resident
Department of Otolaryngology—
Head and Neck Surgery
University of Cincinnati Medical Center
Cincinnati, Ohio

Judith M. Czaja, MD
Head and Neck Fellow

Department of Otolaryngology—
Head and Neck Surgery
University of Cincinnati Medical Center
Cincinnati, Ohio

Rick A. Friedman, MD
Assistant Professor
Department of Otolaryngology—
Head and Neck Surgery
University of Cincinnati Medical Center
Cincinnati, Ohio

Mark E. Gerber, MD
Pediatric Ear, Nose, and Throat of Atlanta
Atlanta, Georgia; formerly Pediatric Fellow
Department of Otolaryngology—
Head and Neck Surgery
University of Cincinnati College of Medicine
Cincinnati, Ohio

Lyon L. Gleich, MD
Assistant Professor
Department of Otolaryngology—
Head and Neck Surgery
University of Cincinnati College of Medicine
Cincinnati, Ohio

Jack L. Gluckman, MD
Professor and Chairman
Department of Otolaryngology—
Head and Neck Surgery
Children's Hospital Medical Center
Cincinnati, Ohio

Robert C. Kersten, MD
Associate Professor
Department of Ophthalmology
University of Cincinnati College of Medicine
Cincinnati, Ohio

Dana Thompson Link, MD, MS
Pediatric Fellow
Department of Otolaryngology—
Head and Neck Surgery
University of Cincinnati College of Medicine
Cincinnati, Ohio

J. Scott McMurray, MD
Pediatric Fellow
Department of Otolaryngology—
Head and Neck Surgery
University of Cincinnati College of Medicine
Cincinnati, Ohio

Charles M. Myer, III, MD
Professor
Department of Otolaryngology—
Head and Neck Surgery
University of Cincinnati College of Medicine;
    and Department of Pediatric Otolaryn-
    gology & Maxillofacial Surgery
Children's Hospital Medical Center
Cincinnati, Ohio

Myles L. Pensak, MD
Professor
Department of Otolaryngology—
Head and Neck Surgery
University of Cincinnati Medical Center
Cincinnati, Ohio

Allen M. Seiden, MD
Associate Professor
Department of Otolaryngology—
Head and Neck Surgery
University of Cincinnati Medical Center
Cincinnati, Ohio

Sally R. Shott, MD
Assistant Professor
Department of Otolaryngology—
Head and Neck Surgery
University of Cincinnati College of Medicine;
    and Department of Pediatric Otolaryn-
    gology & Maxillofacial Surgery
Children's Hospital Medical Center
Cincinnati, Ohio

Kevin A. Shumrick, MD
Associate Professor
Department of Otolaryngology—
Head and Neck Surgery
University of Cincinnati Medical Center
Cincinnati, Ohio

Yoram Stern, MD
Pediatric Fellow
Department of Otolaryngology—
Head and Neck Surgery
University of Cincinnati College of Medicine
Cincinnati, Ohio

Thomas A. Tami, MD
Associate Professor
Department of Otolaryngology—
Head and Neck Surgery
University of Cincinnati Medical Center
Cincinnati, Ohio

Douglas B. Villaret, MD
Chief Resident
Department of Otolaryngology—
Head and Neck Surgery
University of Cincinnati Medical Center
Cincinnati, Ohio

David L. Walner, MD
Assistant Professor
Department of Otolaryngology
Rush-Presbyterian-St. Lukes
Chicago, Illinois; formerly
Pediatric Fellow
Department of Otolaryngology—
Head and Neck Surgery
University of Cincinnati College of Medicine
Cincinnati, Ohio

J. Paul Willging, MD
Associate Professor
Department of Otolaryngology—
Head and Neck Surgery
University of Cincinnati College of Medicine;
    and Department of Pediatric Otolaryn-
    gology & Maxillofacial Surgery
Children's Hospital Medical Center
Cincinnati, Ohio

Keith M. Wilson, MD
Assistant Professor
Department of Otolaryngology—
Head and Neck Surgery
University of Cincinnati Medical Center
Cincinnati, Ohio

Preface

Most traditional textbooks of otolaryngology contain basic clinical and scientific facts that form the foundation of the specialty. While these texts can provide an essential cornerstone for the practice of otolaryngology, applying this information to a clinical setting relies on sound judgment, clear presence of mind, and clinical experience. Systematically evaluating a clinical scenario, identifying key data elements, interpreting clinical information, arriving at a differential diagnosis, and deciding on an appropriate treatment plan are essential elements of the clinical practice of otolaryngology, yet are exceptionally difficult processes to learn and to teach.

This compendium of clinical cases was assembled to provide the reader with an opportunity to focus on clinical problem solving in otolaryngology. These cases focus on the four principal subspecialty areas of otolaryngology—general otolaryngology, head and neck surgery, otology, and facial plastic and reconstructive surgery—and provide insight into many of the diagnostic, treatment, rehabilitative, and emergency issues that face otolaryngologists on a daily basis. Although not meant to be comprehensive in its design, this well-illustrated collection should be a valuable educational tool for medical students exploring the specialty of otolaryngology; residents seeking a basic foundation in clinical judgment and problem solving; practicing otolaryngologists looking for a contemporary approach to the specialty; and primary care physicians who are often faced with clinical problems related to the head and neck region. A series of multiple choice questions based on information contained in individual cases adds yet another opportunity for the reader to assimilate and reinforce many of the clinical pearls offered in each case.

In preparing this manuscript, the editors have drawn upon the extensive clinical expertise of the faculty of the Department of Otolaryngology–Head and Neck Surgery at the University of Cincinnati. The end result has been the creation of a clinical compendium in otolaryngology that reflects the rich clinical experience of this highly respected group. As editors of this compendium, we have found its preparation to be both informative and rewarding. We hope that the reader will agree that this book will be a valuable tool for developing clinical problem solving skills in otolaryngology–head and neck surgery.

Thomas A. Tami, MD
Allen M. Seiden, MD
Myles L. Pensak, MD
Jack L. Gluckman, MD
Robin T. Cotton, MD

OTOLOGY

Pediatric
1. Congenital hearing loss
2. External auditory canal atresia
3. Otitis media
4. Congenital facial paralysis

Adult
5. Cholesteatoma
6. Otosclerosis
7. Temporal bone fracture

Neurotology
8. CSF otorrhea
9. Unilateral hearing loss
10. Pulsatile tinnitus
11. Meniere's disease
12. Benign paroxysmal positional vertigo
13. Perilymphatic fistula

Facial Nerve
14. Facial nerve neuroma
15. Bell's palsy
16. Iatrogenic facial palsy

Case I

CONGENITAL HEARING LOSS

David L. Walner, M.D.
Robin T. Cotton, M.D.

HISTORY

A 2 1/2-year-old boy presented to the otolaryngology clinic with a 2-month history of left-sided hearing loss. This was noted by the child's mother as her son was using the telephone. She noted that her son continually favored his right ear. The parents described no hearing problems previous to that time, and his speech development was appropriate for his age. However, the child had experienced two episodes of acute otitis media in the past, both of which resolved with antibiotic therapy.

The prenatal history was unremarkable, and the mother did not use drugs or medications during her pregnancy. The child was delivered by cesarean section without complications. The child had a transient episode of hypotonia shortly after birth, which resolved. The boy underwent strabismus surgery to repair an estropia at 18 months of age, but he was otherwise healthy.

Furthermore, the child was taking no medications and had no drug allergies. The head and neck examination was completely normal. The tympanic membranes were normal bilaterally, as were the external auditory canals and pinnae. The family history did, however, reveal a paternal cousin with an unknown hearing loss.

DIFFERENTIAL DIAGNOSIS—KEY POINTS

1. The incidence of permanent, moderate to severe sensorineural hearing loss (SNHL) is between 0.5 and 1.0 per 1000 live births. Neonatal audiometric screening plays an important role in detecting hearing loss at an early age. This can be in the form of evoked otoacoustic emissions (EOAEs) or, more commonly, auditory brain stem response (ABR). Legislation is moving in the direction of universal screening but at this time has been instituted in only a few states. It is well established that children with specific risk factors must be tested. Such risk factors include
   - Family history of hearing loss
   - Hyperbilirubinemia requiring exchange
   - Congenital infections (TORCHES)
   - Craniofacial anomalies
   - Birth weight <1500 g
   - Bacterial meningitis
   - Asphyxia (Apgar score of 04 at 1 minute or 06 at 5 minutes)
   - Ototoxic medication
   - Mechanical ventilation for 5 days or longer
   - Syndromes that include hearing loss

   These factors emphasize how necessary it is to conduct a complete and thorough history of the patient.

2. Terminology regarding childhood hearing impairment can be confusing. In children diagnosed with sensorineural hearing impairment, 75% of cases are due to noncongenital and 25% to congenital causes. Noncongenital causes include the following:
   - Meningitis
   - Ototoxicity
   - Trauma
   - Noise-induced hearing loss

- Mumps/measles

- Recurrent otitis/mastoiditis

- Unknown etiology

  Congenital causes of childhood SNHL by definition are present at birth and can be non-hereditary or hereditary. Approximately 50% of cases of congenital hearing impairment is due to nonhereditary causes. For example,

- TORCHES (toxoplasmosis, rubella, CMV, herpes, syphilis)

- Teratogenic drugs (thalidomide, isotretinoin)

- Neonatal sepsis

- Prematurity/low birth weight

The other 50% of cases of congenital hearing impairment is due to hereditary (genetic) causes. Of all children with hereditary hearing loss, one-third is associated with other abnormalities, termed *syndromic*, and two-thirds is not associated with any other abnormalities and is therefore termed *nonsyndromic*. More than 200 syndromes are associated with hearing loss. Most authors attribute about 75 to 80% of genetic deafness to autosomal recessive genes, 18 to 20% to autosomal dominant genes, and less than 5% to X-linked or chromosomal disorders.

Hereditary hearing impairments associated with abnormalities (syndromic) include the following:

- **Autosomal dominant syndromes**
  Teacher-Collins (mandibulofacial dysostosis): antimongoloid slant of eyes; coloboma; malar and mandibular hypoplasia; normal intelligence

  Goldenhar (hemifacial microsomia; oculoauriculovertebral dysplasia): facial asymmetry; underdeveloped mandible; cervical vertebral dysplasia; microtia

  Waardenburg: hypertelorism/dystopia canthorum; synophrys (growing together of eyebrows medially); white forelock; blue iridis/heterochomia

  Branchio-oto-renal: branchial abnormalities (clefts, fistulas, cyst); malformed pinnae, preauricular pits; renal anomalies

Stickler (arthro-opthalmopathy): flattening of facial profile; cleft palate; ocular changs; arthropathy

- **Autosomal recessive syndromes**
  Usher: retinitis pigmentosa; possible vestibular dysfunction

  Pendred: goiter (usually euthyroid); perchlorate discharge test is diagnostic

  Jervell and Lange–Nielsen: prolonged Q-T interval on cardiogram; can develop ventricular fibrillation

- **Sex-linked syndromes**
  Alport: Nephritis

  Hereditary hearing impairments not associated with abnormalities (nonsyndromic) include

- Autosomal dominant progressive SNHL

- Autosomal recessive SNHL: 200 or more genes may be responsible

- Sex-linked SNHL: may be associated with stapes fixation or perilymph gusher

  Hereditary hearing impairments sometimes associated with abnormalities (semi-syndromic) include

- **Inner ear structural malformations** (65% bilateral; 35% unilateral)
  Michel aplasia (autosomal dominant): complete agenesis of temporal bone; associated with Klippel–Feil syndrome

  Mondini aplasia (autosomal dominant): decreased number of cochlear turns; dilated endolymphatic sac and duct; associated with Klippel–Feil, Pendred's, DiGeorge, and Down syndromes

  Scheibe aplasia (autosomal recessive): Cochleosaccular dysplasia; Organ of corti poorly differentiated

  Alexander aplasia: Aplasia of the cochlear duct

  enlarged vestibular aqueduct

3. A multidisciplinary team evaluation is essential in all these patients. This team should include an otolaryngologist with pediatric experience, an audiologist with pediatric experience, a pediatrician, a geneticist, an ophthalmologist with pediatric experience, a deaf

education specialist, and a speech pathologist with pediatric experience.

TEST INTERPRETATION

Any child with a suspected hearing loss requires an audiologic evaluation. Behavioral assessment of hearing is performed differently based on the patient's age. Behavioral observational audiometry (BOA) is used for assessing auditory function in infants younger than 5 months of age. Visual reinforcement audiometry (VRA) is most successful for assessing infants who are 6 to 24 months of age. For children between the ages of 2 and 3 years, the technique of tangible reinforcement operant conditioning audiometry (TROCA) is effective. Play audiometry works well for children in the 2- to 5-year-old age group. Conventional audiometry is generally used in children ages 5 years or older. Play audiometry was used for the patient discussed in this case (Fig. 1–1).

The ABR is used to evaluate the auditory system of young or uncooperative patients. Infants who should be referred for ABR include the following:

- Postmeningitic infants
- Infants with recurrent acute otitis media
- Persistent otitis media with effusion

- Children with significant mental retardation or emotional disturbance (if they cannot be tested by behavioral techniques)
- Children with suspected eighth nerve or brain stem disorders
- Children with sudden-onset, fluctuating, progressive, or unilateral SNHL
- Difficult-to-test patients.

The patient presented in this case had an ABR performed (Fig. 1–2).

Computed tomography (CT) of the temporal bone is used to compile information with regard to the status of the facial nerve, ossicles, internal auditory canal, semicircular canals, and cochlea. This information assists with the counseling of patients and families on the etiology of the hearing loss. The CT scan of the case presented is shown in Figure 1–3.

Additional tests are also required. For example, blood testing should include a complete blood cell count, chemistry panel, thyroid function tests, and fluorescent treponemal antibody test (fTA-ABS). A urinalysis should be performed to search for proteinuria, hematuria, or signs of kidney dysfunction. Electrocardiography will detect cardiac conduction abnormalities. Intrauterine testing is available in at-risk mothers for congenital rubella, (cytomegalovirus (CMV), and syphilis.

DIAGNOSIS

1. Left-sided SNHL
2. Mondini malformation, bilateral

MEDICAL MANAGEMENT

Federal law now mandates that states provide comprehensive, family-oriented intervention programs for hearing-impaired infants and children. The management of children with congenital hearing loss focuses on appropriate audiologic intervention. The primary intervention is usually the fitting of hearing aids and should begin in infancy or as soon as the hearing loss is identified. Children with bilateral hearing loss are fitted binaurally. The use of hearing aids in children with unilateral hearing loss is

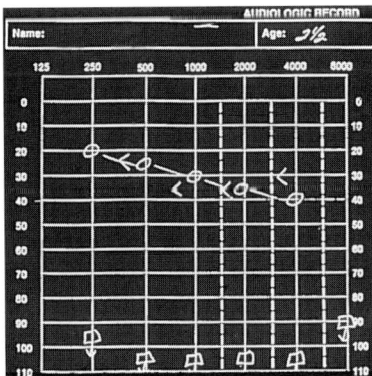

FIGURE 1–1 This audiogram reveals no measurable hearing in the left ear and normal to mild SNHL in the right ear. The tympanograms were normal.

A   B

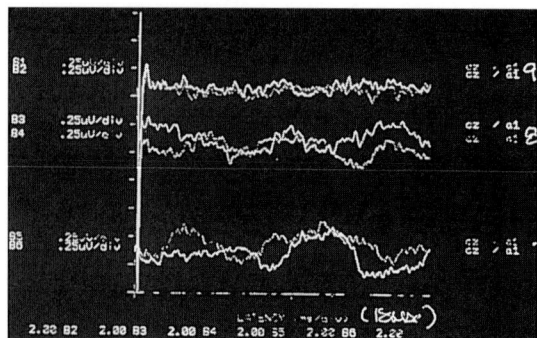

FIGURE 1–2 (A) The left side had no wave 5 response at maximum output, which is suggestive of a severe degree of hearing loss. (B) The right side had normal responses in the 2- to 4-kHz range. The 500-Hz stimulus confirmed a low-frequency hearing loss.

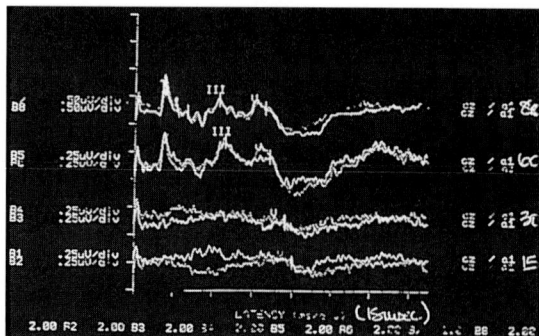

controversial and must be decided on an individual basis.

Genetic counseling should be arranged to address parental questions regarding the possible etiologies for the child's hearing loss and what implication this may have for siblings or future offspring.

SURGICAL MANAGEMENT

Identification of a perilymphatic fistula would be an indication for surgery with some clinicians.

Congenital malformations of the cochlea are not contraindications to cochlear implants. Implantation has been successfully performed in patients with Mondini deformities.

Patients must fit the standard criteria for cochlear implants and be evaluated by the implant team to establish their candidacy.

REHABILITATION AND FOLLOW-UP

Although habilitation is ongoing, a monitoring program for children with SNHL is essential. Some advocate audiometric testing four times in the first year following identification of the

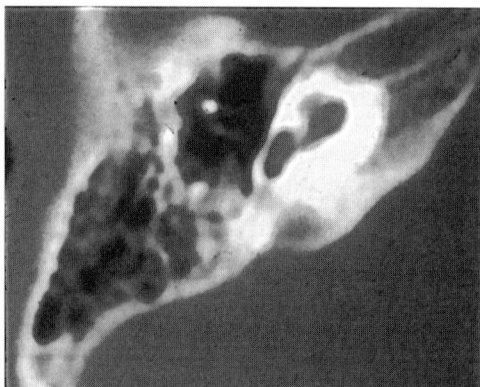

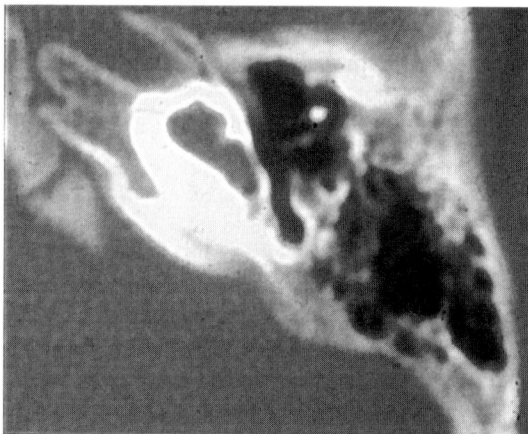

FIGURE 1–3 The axial image of the temporal bone (left and right) showed a malformed cochlea, enlarged vestibule, and a shortened wide horizontal semicircular canal.

hearing loss. This testing is done to exclude a progressive or fluctuating type of loss that may be associated with a perilymphatic fistula, autoimmune hearing loss, ototoxic hearing loss, or otitis media with effusion. At the minimum, an annual physical examination with audiologic assessment should be done.

SUGGESTED READINGS

BROOKHOUSER PE. Genetic hearing loss. In: Bailey BJ, ed. *Head and Neck Surgery—Otolaryngology.* Philadelphia, PA: Lippincott; 1993:Chapter 133.

CHAN KH. Sensorineural hearing loss in children—classification and evaluation. *Otolaryngol Clin North Am.* 1994;27(3)473–486.

GRUNDFAST KM, LAIWANI AK. Practical approach to diagnosis and management of hereditary hearing impairment. *ENT J.* 1992;71(10):479–493.

Joint Committee on Infant Hearing. 1994 position statement. *ASHA.* 1994;36:38.

NOZZA RJ. The assessment of hearing and middle-ear function in children. In: Bluestone CD, Stool SE, Kenna MA, eds. *Pediatric Otolaryngology.* Philadelphia, PA: WB Saunders, 1996:Chapter 11.

SCHUKNECHT HF. Mondini dysplasia—a clinical and pathological study. *Ann Otol Rhinol Laryngol.* 1980;89(1-part 2):1–23.

EXTERNAL AUDITORY CANAL ATRESIA

David L. Walner, M.D.
Robin T. Cotton, M.D.

HISTORY

A 5-year-old female was referred from her primary care provider for a right ear deformity, which her mother stated had been present since birth. The patient also reported diminished hearing from the right ear. The mother described no history of infections or trauma to the ear.

The prenatal history was unremarkable, and the mother used no drugs or medications during her pregnancy. The delivery and neonatal periods were unremarkable. The family history included an uncle with hearing loss but no external ear deformities.

The physical examination revealed a malformed pinna on the right side with accessory cartilage in the region of the tragus. A blind pit was present in the region of the external auditory canal (Fig. 2–1). The left pinna, external auditory canal, and tympanic membrane were normal in appearance. The remainder of the head and neck examination was normal.

DIFFERENTIAL DIAGNOSIS — KEY POINTS

1. A thorough history and physical examination are essential when evaluating children with external ear deformities. The history should include any history of drug use or toxic exposures during pregnancy and a family history of ear deformities, craniofacial deformities, or hearing loss. The physical examination should focus on any facial asymmetry due to bony abnormalities or facial nerve paralysis. As many as 45% of patients with aural atresia can have another systemic anomaly.

2. The frequency of moderate to severe forms of congenital aural atresia has been estimated as 1 to 5 in 20,000 live births. Unilateral atresia is approximately six times more common than bilateral, and boys are affected more commonly than girls.

3. These children should be evaluated by a multidisciplinary team consisting of a geneticist, a pediatrician, an otolaryngologist familiar with pediatric disorders, a plastic/reconstructive surgeon familiar with pediatric disorders, an audiologist, and a speech-language specialist.

4. A classification system (Weerda, 1988) can be used to assist with surgical guidance of the auricular deformity:

   I. First-degree dysplasia
      A. Definition: Most structures of a normal auricle are recognizable (minor deformities).
      B. Surgery: Reconstruction normally does not require the use of additional skin or cartilage.
   II. Second-degree dysplasia
      A. Definition: Some structures of a normal auricle are recognizable.
      B. Surgery: Partial reconstruction requires the use of some additional skin and cartilage.
   III. Third-degree dysplasia
      A. Definition: None of the structures of a normal auricle is recognizable.
      B. Surgery: Total reconstruction requires the use of skin and large amounts of cartilage.

(The patient presented in this case had a first-degree auricular dysplasia.)

TEST INTERPRETATION

An audiologic assessment is necessary in these patients. In younger or uncooperative children an auditory brain stem response (ABR) may be appropriate. If bilateral atresia is present, a masking dilemma may exist and require brain

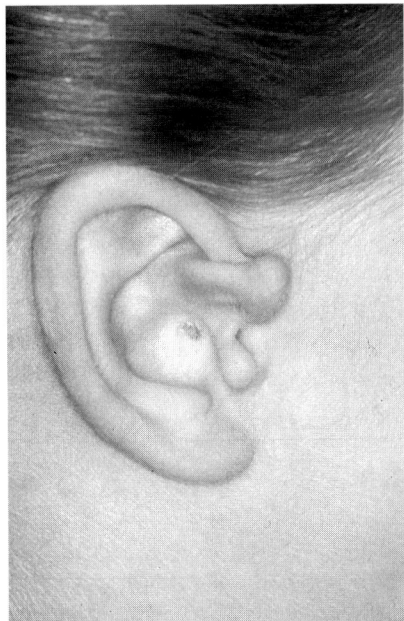

FIGURE 2–1 A photograph of the right ear.

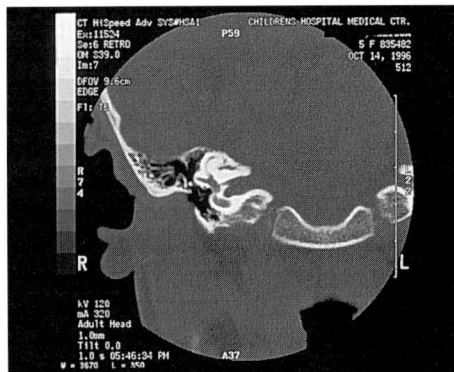

FIGURE 2–2 CT of right temporal bone (coronal image) showing a soft tissue obliteration of the external auditory canal, with absence of an inferior bony canal wall and an apparent ossicular malformation. Also seen were normal labyrinthine structures and facial nerve course.

stem testing. Most commonly children with canal atresia will have a 50- to 60-dB conductive hearing loss with normal nerve function. With cases of unilateral atresia, audiometric evaluation of the opposite ear is extremely important in surgical planning. In the child presented in this case, pure-tone audiometry revealed moderate conductive hearing loss in the right ear and normal hearing in the left ear.

Computed tomography (CT) of the temporal bone is necessary for preoperative planning. This should be of high resolution using thin-cut (1.5-mm) axial and coronal sections. It may be performed at any time prior to surgical repair. Waiting until the age of 4 or 5 years may obviate the need for sedation. The CT is used to assess the integrity of the tympanic bone, the extent of mastoid pneumatization, the presence and location of the ossicles, course of the facial nerve, and any inner ear malformations. Figure 2–2 shows the CT scan of the patient presented in this case.

DIAGNOSIS

1. Deformity of the right pinna
2. Right external auditory canal atresia

MEDICAL MANAGEMENT

Adequate auditory stimulation should be provided to the infant as soon as possible. In cases of bilateral atresia, this can be accomplished with bone conduction hearing aids when the child is 4 to 6 months of age. Implantable bone conduction aids are generally not recommended prior to 2½ or 3 years of age.

Poor surgical candidates and patients unwilling to undergo surgery should be maintained with bone conducting hearing aids.

SURGICAL MANAGEMENT

Preoperative assessment is important to determine surgical candidacy. A functioning and normal inner ear should be present. A grading system was developed by Jahrsdoerfer based on preoperative temporal bone CT scans and auricular appearance to aid in patient selection for surgical repair. The maximum score is 10 points, and a higher score reflects an improved chance for hearing improvement following surgery. The presence of a stapes receives 2 points; the presence of a open oval window, middle ear space, facial nerve, malleus–incus complex, mastoid pneumatization, incus–stapes connection, and round window receives 1 point each. Auricular appearance is also considered.

The timing of surgery and the expectations of surgery are key. Bilateral atresia cases should be operated on by the age of 4 or 5 years. The better hearing or more normal radiographically appearing ear should undergo repair first to optimize the chances for hearing improvement. Surgery for hearing improvement in cases of unilateral atresia is usually scheduled for the teenage or adult years unless chronic drainage has occurred and cholesteatoma is suspected. This delay allows the patient to mature such that he or she can understand the risks and benefits of the procedure. The cosmetic portion of the procedure in patients with unilateral atresia can occur at an earlier age to avoid ridicule from peers.

The surgical repair must be tailored to the specific anatomic problem. Canal atresia may be present with or without microtia or other pinna deformities. In general, microtia repair should precede atresia repair. The first stage involves construction and implantation of the auricular framework created from autogenous rib cartilage. The second stage involves transposing preexisting auricular remnants to form a lobule. The third stage involves correction of the aural atresia as well as alignment of the auricle to the newly created meatus of the external auditory canal. The fourth and fifth stages involve tragal construction and elevation of the auricle off the postauricular region. Four to 6 months should elapse between each stage.

The aural atresia repair must be carefully thought out due to the possible anomalous position of the facial nerve in patients needing this type of surgery. Intraoperative facial nerve monitoring is advocated. The repair involves creating an auditory canal, removing the atretic plate, restoring the sound-conducting mechanism, creating a new external auditory meatus, and skin grafting the newly created external auditory canal. The approach can be transmastoid or anterior. Intraoperative complications are unusual but can include facial nerve injury,

fenestration of the labyrinth, and acoustic trauma.

Hearing results in mild and moderate atresias are good, within 20 to 25 dB of the cochlear reserve in 80 to 90% of patients. In more severe atresias, a hearing result this good is only obtained in 60 to 75% of patients.

A 30% revision rate is required for restenosis, graft failure or migration, and persisting conductive hearing loss.

REHABILITATION AND FOLLOW-UP

Continued aural rehabilitation is essential for all hearing-impaired children. Regular otologic examinations should be performed twice annually. In addition, regular visits with a speech therapist and, in select cases, a psychologist may be beneficial.

SUGGESTED READINGS

AGUILAR EA. Major congenital malformation of the auricle. In: Bailey BJ, ed. *Head and Neck Surgery—Otolaryngology.* Philadelphia, PA: Lippincott; 1993:Chapter 116.

AGUILAR EA, JAHRSDOERFER RA. The surgical repair of congenital microtia and atresia. *Otolaryngol Head Neck Surg.* 1988;98:600.

CRESSMAN WR, PENSAK ML. Surgical aspects of congenital aural atresia. *Otolaryngol Clin North Am.* 1994;27(3):621–633.

JAHRSDOERFER RA, YEAKLEY JW, AGUILAR EA, et al. Grading system for the selection of patients with congenital aural atresia. *Am J Otol.* 1992;13:6.

MACERI DR. Congenital aural atresia. In: Gates GA, ed. *Current Therapy in Otolaryngology—Head and Neck Surgery.* St. Louis, MO: Mosby-Year Book; 1994:4–8.

SCHUKNECHT HF. Congenital aural atresia. *Laryngoscope.* 1989;99:908.

WEERDA H. Classification of auricular congenital deformities of the auricle. *Facial Plast Surg.* 1988;5:385.

Case 3

OTITIS MEDIA

Mark E. Gerber, M.D.
Robin T. Cotton, M.D.

HISTORY

A 5-year-old male presented to an emergency room with a 1-week history of left ear pain. He had been seen by his primary care physician the day before and started on amoxicillin (40 mg/kg/day) for acute otitis media. Later that evening he began to have increasing swelling behind the ear accompanied by fever. He has a history of recurrent otitis requiring three or four courses of antibiotics per year during the past 2 years.

Physicial examination revealed an alert boy with mild torticollis and a temperature of 39°C. Auricular examination was significant for loss of the left postauricular crease with erythema, tenderness, and fluctuance over the mastoid (Figure 3–1). Bilateral tympanic membranes were bulging with middle ear suppuration present (Figure 3–2). Cranial nerve examination was not significant for any weakness or asymmetry.

DIFFERENTIAL DIAGNOSIS—KEY POINTS

1. The differential diagnosis of extracranial complications of acute otitis media can be divided into two groups, intratemporal and extratemporal (Table 3–1). An accurate history, complete otolaryngologic and neurologic examination, and radiographic imaging is needed to differentiate the various complications (see Table 3–1). Essentially all cases of acute otitis media involve inflammation of the mastoid air cells. However, clinically significant acute mastoiditis is a clinical diagnosis based on the findings of suppurative otitis media, postauricular swelling with loss of postauricular crease, and protrusion of the auricle. Coalescent mastoiditis is a radiographic diagnosis based on computed tomography (CT) and is differentiated from acute mastoiditis by radiographic evidence of loss of the bony septations.

2. Suppurative labyrinthitis occurs when bacterial invasion penetrates the otic capsule, usually via the round window or oval window. The classic presentation is rapid onset of vertigo, sensorineural hearing loss, nausea, and vomiting during an episode of acute otitis media. In the absence of associated meningitis, the cerebrospinal fluid pressure and analysis are normal. Suppurative, acute petrositis occurs when there is extension of the middle ear infection into the petrous apex, resulting in symptoms of retro-orbital pain, persistent otorrhea, and sixth cranial nerve palsy. Facial paralysis, usually unilateral, can occur during an episode of acute otitis media either secondary to direct inflammation through a bony dehiscence in the tympanic segment of the facial nerve or secondary to osteitis involving the bony fallopian canal.

3. Extratemporal complications occur when infection progresses to involve the cortical bone surrounding the mastoid air cells. Osteitis of the lateral cortex can result in the development of a subperiosteal abscess. The patient usually presents with more pronounced auricular protrusion, loss of the postauricular crease, and fluctuance over the mastoid. Osteitis of the medial or inferior mastoid cortex can result in the development of a deep neck space infection known as Bezold's abscess.

4. Acute mastoiditis can be accompanied by a significant amount of inflammation of the cartilaginous external auditory canal, making visualization of the tympanic membrane difficult or impossible in the awake child. This can clinically mimic acute external otitis without middle ear or mastoid involvement. The physical examination can help differentiate the two entities. Manipulation of the external auditory canal by pulling on the tragus is extremely painful in acute external otitis, but not in mastoiditis. Occasionally, initial response to intravenous and ototopical treatments is needed to make an accurate diagnosis.

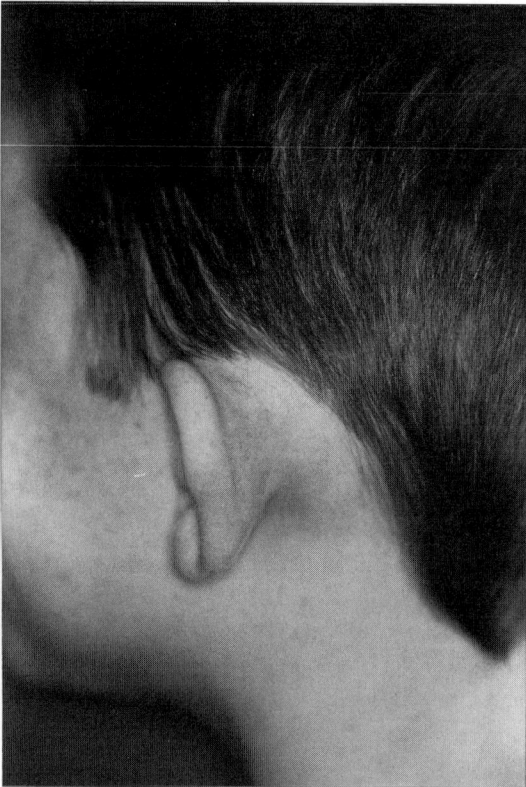

FIGURE 3–1 Auricular examination demonstrates loss of the left postauricular crease with erythema and fluctuance over the mastoid.

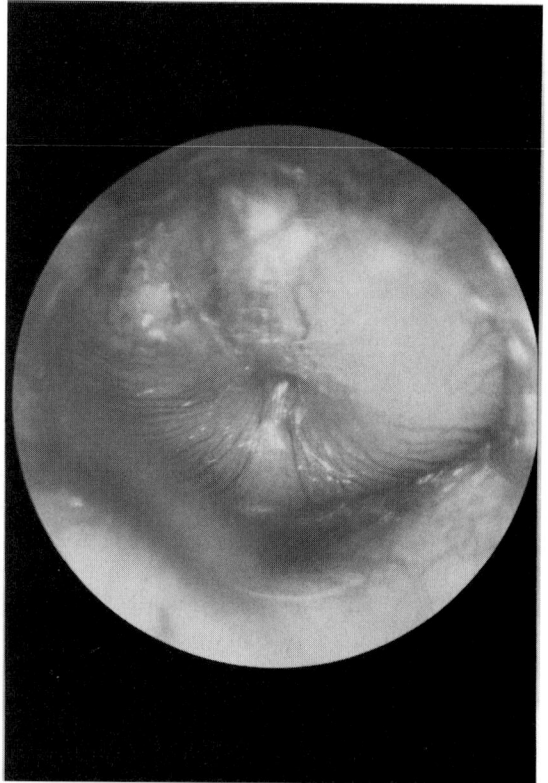

FIGURE 3–2 Endoscopy demonstrates bilateral tympanic membranes, bulging with middle ear suppuration.

TEST INTERPRETATION

CT scan revealed opacification of the left middle ear and mastoid without obvious loss of mastoid septations. However, the lateral mastoid cortex exhibited a break with an associated low-density collection in the periosteal space consistent with a subperiosteal abscess (Figure 3–3).

DIAGNOSIS

Acute mastoiditis with subperiosteal abscess.

MEDICAL MANAGEMENT

Empirical antimicrobial coverage should include coverage for the most common organisms that cause acute otitis media including *Streptococcus pneumoniae* and *Hemophilus influenzae*. Once culture results are obtained, coverage can be narrowed. Although initial therapy is nearly always intravenous, once adequate surgical drainage has been completed, symptoms usually dissipate quickly, and oral therapy can be instituted.

TABLE 3–1 Extracranial Complications of Acute Otitis Media

Intratemporal
    Acute mastoiditis
    Coalescent mastoiditis
    Suppurative labyrinthitis
    Petrositis
    Facial nerve dysfunction
    Tympanic membrane perforation
Extratemporal
    Subperiosteal abscess
    Bezold's abscess

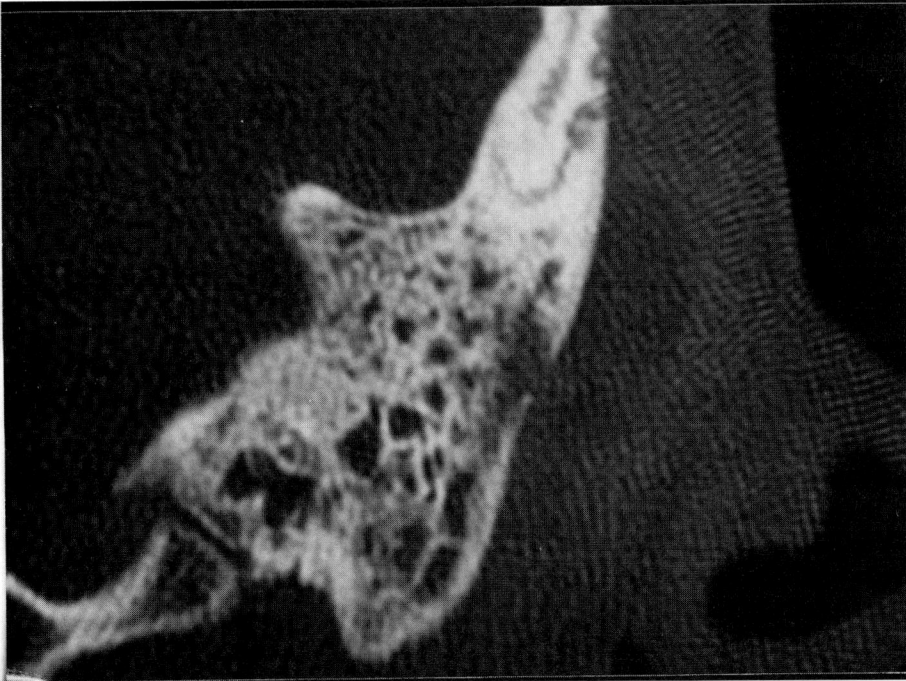

FIGURE 3-3 Collection in the periosteal space consistent with subperiosteal abscess.

SURGICAL MANAGEMENT

On the day of presentation, this child underwent myringotomy and pressure-equalizing tube placement, as well as a left cortical mastoidectomy with drainage of the subperiosteal abscess. He was started on intravenous cefuroxime at the time of surgery. Cultures taken at the time of surgery grew penicillin-sensitive *S. pneumoniae*. The postauricular drain was removed on postoperative day 2, and the patient was sent home on amoxicillin on postoperative day 3.

Most surgeons believe that a subperiosteal abscess complicating acute otitis media requires urgent surgical drainage of the middle ear space, mastoid, and abscess cavity. The middle ear can be drained using a wide-field myringotomy or pressure-equalizing tube. The mastoid and perimastoid abscess is drained with a cortical mastoidectomy that includes removing any obstruction at the aditus ad antrum that may have contributed to the development of the complication.

REHABILITATION AND FOLLOW-UP

At his last follow-up appointment 6 months after surgery, this child's pressure-equalizing tube had extruded, the tympanic membrane was intact, and hearing was normal. He has had one episode of otitis media since this complication.

SUGGESTED READINGS

BLUESTONE CD, KLEIN JO. Intratemporal complications and sequelae of otitis media. In: Bluestone CD, Stool SE, Kenna MA, eds. *Pediatric Otolaryngology*, 3rd ed. Philadelphia, PA: WB Saunders; 1996:583–635.

GLIKLICH RE, EAVEY RD, IANNUZZI RA, CAMACHO AE. A contemporary analysis of acute mastoiditis. *Arch Otolaryngol Head Neck Surg.* 1996;122:135–139.

HUGHES GB. Complications of otitis media. In: Hughes GB, Pensak ML, eds. *Clinical Otology.* 2nd ed. New York: Thieme; 1997:233–240.

NADOL JB Jr, EAVEY RD. Acute and chronic mastoiditis: clinical presentation, diagnosis, and management. *Curr Clin Top Infect Dis.* 1995;15:204–229.

CONGENITAL FACIAL PARALYSIS

Mark E. Gerber, M.D.
Robin T. Cotton, M.D.

HISTORY

A 3-day-old male presented to the outpatient office with a left facial paralysis that was noted immediately at birth. Maternal history was not significant for any illness during this first pregnancy, labor was less than 24 hours, and spontaneous vaginal delivery was obtained without forceps assistance. Birth weight was 3625 g. There was no family history of congenital facial paralysis. Mild facial assymetry was noted at rest, with complete absence of volitional movement of the left face, and mild left lagophthalmos. Otherwise, physical examination did not reveal any evidence of craniofacial, otologic, ophthalmologic, neurologic, or systemic abnormalities.

DIFFERENTIAL DIAGNOSIS— KEY POINTS

1. Determining whether the etiology is traumatic (secondary to intrauterine positioning or delivery) or developmental is the primary diagnostic dilemma in the evaluation.

2. Traumatic deformities usually present at birth with associated signs of lateral facial trauma including ecchymosis, lacerations, or hemotympanum. Forceps delivery, birth weight of 3500 g or more, and primaparity have been shown to be significant risk factors for development of acquired congenital facial paralysis. In most cases, the facial nerve appears to be injured by indentation of the bony fallopian canal. However, the site of injury can be anywhere along the course of the facial nerve: intracranial, intratemporal, or extratemporal. Prognosis in cases of congenital facial paralysis of traumatic origin is excellent with complete recovery in close to 90%.

3. Facial paralysis secondary to development defects usually presents at birth with associated craniofacial anomalies and / or other cranial nerve deficits. A history of maternal illness is often seen in the first trimester and, occasionally, a family history of congenital facial paralysis. The most common associated anomalies involve the first and second branchial arches, with resultant defects including cleft palate, hypoplastic maxilla, and auriclar atresia / microtia. Sensorineural hearing loss is also associated. Syndromes that involve congenital facial paralysis include Möbius' and oculoauriculovertebral syndromes. The prognosis for recovery in congenital facial paralysis secondary to developmental abnormalities is poor, with a nearly uniform need for suspension / animation later in life.

TEST INTERPRETATION

Initial testing included normal hearing bilaterally on brain stem auditory evoked response (BAER) testing and a normal computed tomography (CT) scan of the temporal bones. Observation of the child while crying revealed normal tear production bilaterally. Evoked electromyography (EEMG) done on the third day after birth revealed 30% degeneration compared with the normal right side.

Although the history is consistent with a developmental etiology, the birth weight of over 3500 g, the lack of any associated abnormalities, and only partial degeneration on EEMG testing suggest a traumatic etiology.

DIAGNOSIS

Congenital unilateral facial paralysis of traumatic etiology.

MEDICAL MANAGEMENT

Expectant care included ensuring (1) adequate eye protection and (2) adequate feeding ability. This child did not require specific eye care because of an adequate Bell's phenomenon and tear production that protected the cornea. In addition, feeding did not appear to be significantly impaired. When necessary, ophthalmic ointments can be used to help lubricate the eye; speech and swallowing therapy can assist with feeding an infant with complete facial paralysis.

Repeat EEMGs 3 days, 1 week, 2 weeks, and 1 month later revealed 65, 75, 70, and 50% degeneration, respectively. Clinical improvement became apparent at 2 months, and recovery was complete by 6 months.

In children with traumatic facial paralysis, EEMG testing in the first 2 to 3 days after birth will be normal, but can decrease with repeat testing. However, in developmental facial paralysis, EEMG responses in the first 2 to 3 days after birth will be decreased or absent and without change on repeat testing. Infants with congenital complete facial paralysis are divided into four groups on the basis of when they present and the results of electrophysiologic testing:

- Group 1 patients are seen within 3 days of birth and are stimulatable by EEMG. These children require close follow-up and repeat testing every 3 to 5 days until there is evidence of clinical return of function

- Group 2 patients are seen within 3 days and are initially stimulatable by EEMG, but subsequently become unstimulatable on repeat testing

- Group 3 patients are seen within 3 days of birth but are not stimulatable by EEMG. Both groups 2 and 3 children require EMG testing (after 2 to 3 weeks). If voluntary action potentials or polyphasic potentials are present, neural innervation is intact. However, if fibrillation potentials are present, then denervated muscle is present. If there is complete electrical silence, absence of facial muscles is suggested.

- Group 4 patients are not seen until more than 3 days after birth. The same test battery is undertaken, but the separation into traumatic and developmental etiologies is more difficult.

SURGICAL MANAGEMENT

Complete facial paralysis of traumatic origin has a spontaneous recovery rate of close to 90%. Therefore, surgical exploration of the facial nerve would have been considered only if there had been evidence of temporal bone trauma on radiographic evaluation, electrophysiologic tests demonstrated complete loss of facial nerve function by 5 days after birth, and there was no clinical or electrophysiologic evidence of functional return at 5 weeks of age.

Exploration of the facial nerve is not indicated in cases secondary to abnormal embryogenesis (developmental). When exploration has been done, the nerve was generally found to taper to a fibrous strand or strands in the vertical segment after the chorda tympani nerve take-off. Interposition grafting is futile because it is speculated that only the sensory and parasympathetic fibers are present proximally.

REHABILITATION AND FOLLOW-UP

In this case, full recovery was spontaneous; therefore, no rehabilitation was necessary. With persistent congenital facial nerve paralysis (usually developmental), rehabilitation of the facial function includes animation or suspension. Debate arises as to when surgical rehabilitation should be considered, either in the preschool years to try to avoid peer ridicule or in the teenage years when the patient is better able to participate in the decision-making process.

SUGGESTED READINGS

BERGSTROM L, BAKER BB. Syndromes associated with congenital facial paralysis. *Otolaryngol Head Neck Surg.* 1981;89:336–342.

COTE DN, GUARISCO JL. Facial paralysis in children [letter]. *Am J Otol.* 1994;15:818–819.

CRUMLEY RL. Neonatal facial paralysis [letter; comment]. *Plast Reconstr Surg.* 1990;86:609.

Goin DW. Case of differential diagnosis of facial paralysis noted at birth [letter]. *Am J Otol.* 1986;7:395.

Grundfast KM, Guarisco JL, Thomsen JR, Koch B. Diverse etiologies of facial paralysis in children. *Int J Pediatr Otorhinolaryngol.* 1990;19:223–39.

Harris JP, Davidson TM, May M, Fria T. Evaluation and treatment of congenital facial paralysis. *Arch Otolaryngol.* 1983;109:145–51.

May M. Facial paralysis at birth: medicolegal and clinical implications [editorial]. *Am J Otol.* 1995; 16:711–712.

May M, Fria TJ, Blumenthal F, Curtin H. Facial paralysis in children: differential diagnosis. *Otolaryngol Head Neck Surg.* 1981;89:841–848.

Shapiro AM, Schaitken BM, May M. Facial paralysis in children. In: Bluestone CD, Stool SE, Kenna MA, eds. *Pediatric Otolaryngology.* Philadelphia, PA: WB Saunders; 1996:312–331.

Shapiro NL, Cunningham MJ, Parikh SR, Eavey RD, Cheney ML. Congenital unilateral facial paralysis. *Pediatrics.* 1996;97:261–264.

Smith, JD, Crumley RL, Harker LA. Facial paralysis in the newborn. *Otolaryngol Head Neck Surg.* 1981;89:1021–1024.

Case 5

CHOLESTEATOMA
Myles L. Pensak, M.D.

HISTORY

A 45-year-old while female presented to the office with a 6-year antedating history of progressive hearing loss and intermittent episodes of otalgia with aural suppuration. She had been treated with topical antibiotics, and with an aural antibiotic for her otologic infection. Twenty-four hours before presentation she became cognizant of a marked degradation in auditory acuity associated with aural fullness and subjective nonpulsatile tinnitus. The patient had been aware of mild unsteadiness, but she now acknowledges true vertigo.

There is no antedating history of otologic or neurotologic trauma and the patient denies a familial history of hearing loss. Otomicroscopic assessment of the left ear reveals a normal external auditory canal and tympanic membrane. The right ear canal demonstrates soft cerumen with masserated skin. Following debridement, a large attic retraction pocket cholesteatoma is noted. The drum is somewhat inflamed and palpation in the region of the scutum reveals intense pain. Horizontal rotary right beating nystagmus is noted, especially when the canal is occluded by placing pressure on the tragus.

DIFFERENTIAL DIAGNOSIS— KEY POINTS

1. Aural cholesteatoma is the presence of keratinizing squamous epithelium that invades the spaces of the temporal bone. Although it

may be localized to the epitympanum, cholesteatoma can follow a preformed pathway to invade the mastoid, middle ear, or accessory region of the temporal bone including the petrous apex. The cholesteatoma may be primarily acquired due to chronic eustachian tube dysfunction resulting in retraction of the tympanic membrane.

2. Secondary cholesteatoma occurs when squamous epithelium is noted to ingrow into the middle ear through a membrane perforation resulting from either infection or trauma.

3. Congenital cholesteatomas are felt to arise from epithelial rests that are ultimately enveloped by the developing pneumatic spaces of the temporal bone.

4. Iatrogenic cholesteatomas can occur from surgical procedures that result in the deposition of skin medial to the tympanic membrane.

5. The differential diagnosis of cholesteatoma is limited. Included among the pathologies would be chronic otitis media with or without active suppuration, tuberculous otitis, osteoradionecrosis, squamous cell or basal cell carcinoma, foreign body reaction, and granulomatous disease such as Wegener's granulomatosis.

TEST INTERPRETATION

Diagnostic tests employed in the assessment of cholesteatoma would include a baseline audiogram, and selective utilization of electronystagmography in cases of acute vertigo. In addition, computed tomography (CT) scanning with 1.5-mm high-density bone window cuts provides for both the axial and coronal planes a satisfactory visualization of both the cholesteatoma and attendant osseous destruction. Furthermore, soft tissue invasion and its relationship to the labyrinth and fallopian canal can be ascertained. Figure 5–1 demonstrates typical findings of an acquired attic cholesteatoma in the soft tissue extending into Prussak's space.

In this case because of the paroxysmal onset of symptomatic change, a high degree of suspicion must point toward the presence of a labyrinthine fistula. CT scanning will provide optimal visualization although it is possible to fenestrate the labyrinth without clear demonstration on scanning.

An audiogram (Fig. 5–2) reveals the typical conductive hearing loss associated with cholesteatoma.

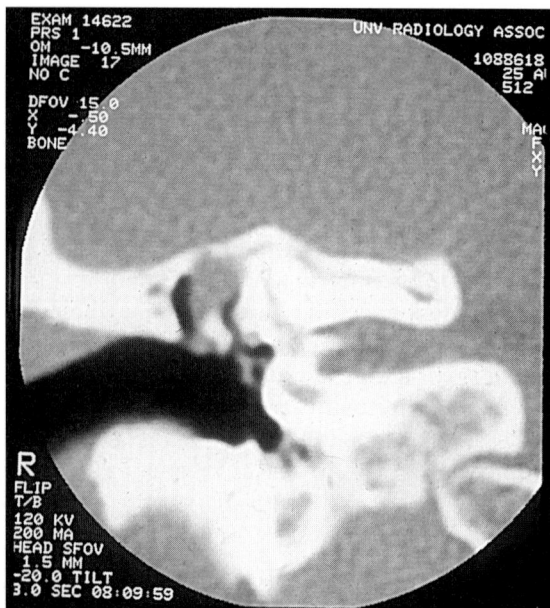

FIGURE 5-1 Typical findings of an acquired attic cholesteatoma in the soft tissue extending into Prussak's space.

DIAGNOSIS

Acquired cholesteatoma.

MEDICAL MANAGEMENT

The medical management of cholesteatoma centers around satisfactory debridement and the quieting of acute inflammatory changes. Commonly employed are acetic acid or vinegar and water douches with or without topical steroid-containing drops. The presence of active infection would warrant utilization of systemic antibiotics. The key to office management of cholesteatoma centers around regular cleansings and debridement of the ear. When cholesteatoma fails to respond to this therapy surgical intervention is indicated.

SURGICAL MANAGEMENT

A long-standing debate has surrounded the efficacy of canal wall-up versus canal wall-down surgical procedures. The options for management of cholesteatoma include (1) a canal wall-up tympanomastoidectomy with or without facial recess approach, (2) a staged procedure wherein the surgeon mandates a second look most often accompanied by ossiculoplasty, (3) a canal wall-down tympanomastoidectomy and, finally, (4) a radical mastoidectomy. Among the first three, the location of the cholesteatoma, its extent of bone destruction, and amount of mucosal inflammation will dictate whether reconstruction at the inaugural procedure is possible. Radical mastoidectomy for cholesteatoma is rarely performed today; however, diffuse gross invasion of the petrous bone wherein total extirpation is not anticipated, or mitigating circumstances including an only hearing ear, cholesteatoma enveloping the facial nerve, violation and invasion into the round or oval window niches, and finally extensive growth into the protympanic space warrant an open-cavity procedure.

Although controversy surrounds the management of labyrinthine fistulae, generally matrix can be removed from small (<2-mm) fistulae with safety. If a larger fistula exists, an open-cavity technique is recommended.

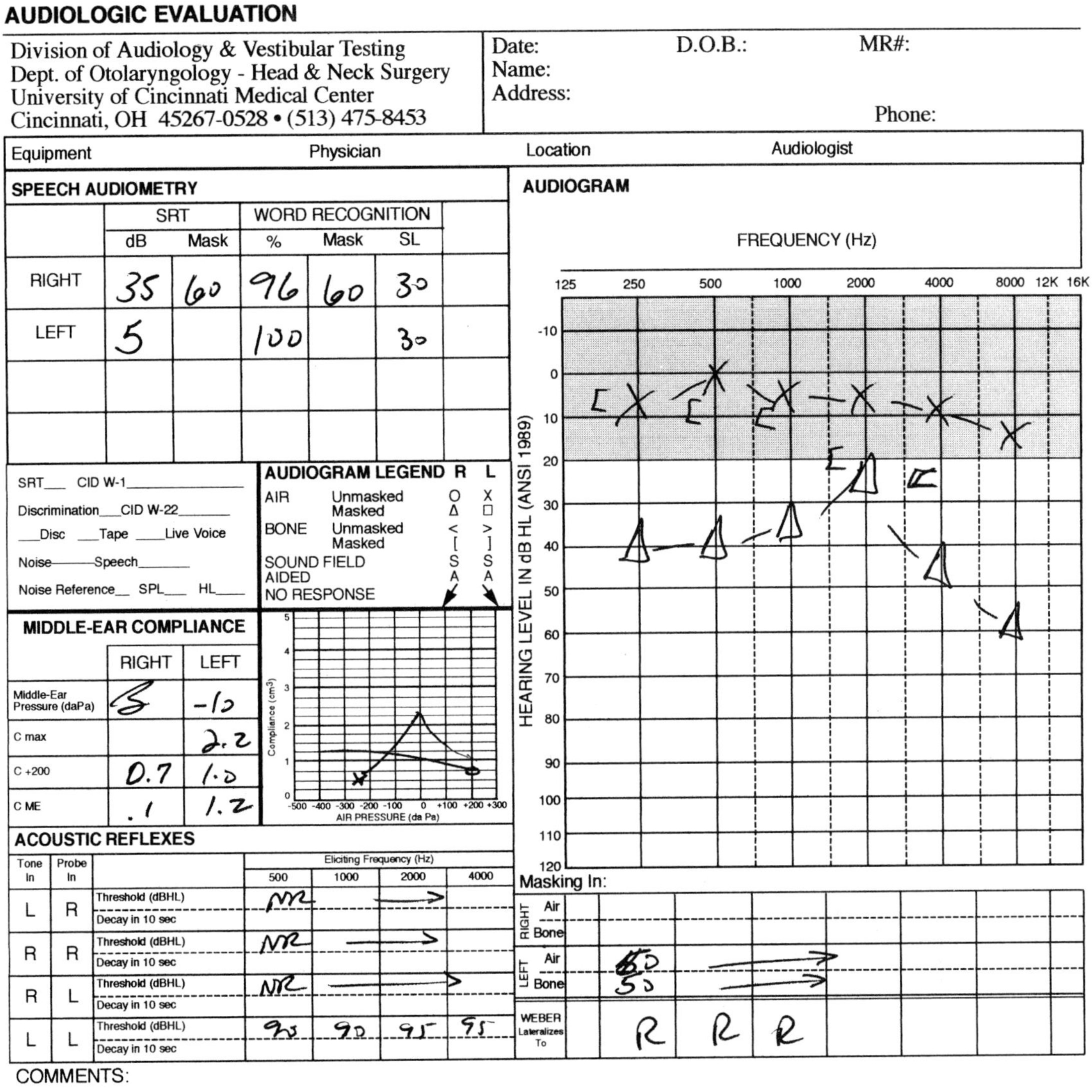

AUDIOLOGIC EVALUATION

Division of Audiology & Vestibular Testing Dept. of Otolaryngology - Head & Neck Surgery University of Cincinnati Medical Center Cincinnati, OH 45267-0528 • (513) 475-8453	Date: Name: Address:	D.O.B.:	MR#: Phone:

Equipment	Physician	Location	Audiologist

SPEECH AUDIOMETRY

	SRT dB	SRT Mask	WORD RECOGNITION %	WORD RECOGNITION Mask	WORD RECOGNITION SL
RIGHT	35	60	96	60	30
LEFT	5		100		30

SRT___ CID W-1_____

Discrimination___CID W-22_____

___Disc ___Tape ___Live Voice

Noise———Speech_____

Noise Reference__ SPL___ HL___

AUDIOGRAM LEGEND

		R	L
AIR	Unmasked	O	X
	Masked	Δ	□
BONE	Unmasked	<	>
	Masked	[	]
SOUND FIELD		S	S
AIDED		A	A
NO RESPONSE		S	S

AUDIOGRAM

MIDDLE-EAR COMPLIANCE

	RIGHT	LEFT
Middle-Ear Pressure (daPa)	5	-10
C max		2.2
C +200	0.7	1.0
C ME	.1	1.2

ACOUSTIC REFLEXES

Tone In	Probe In		Eliciting Frequency (Hz) 500	1000	2000	4000
L	R	Threshold (dBHL)	NR		→	
		Decay in 10 sec				
R	R	Threshold (dBHL)	NR		→	
		Decay in 10 sec				
R	L	Threshold (dBHL)	NR		→	
		Decay in 10 sec				
L	L	Threshold (dBHL)	90	90	95	95
		Decay in 10 sec				

Masking In:

	RIGHT Air	RIGHT Bone	LEFT Air	LEFT Bone	WEBER Lateralizes To
			60 50 →		R R R

COMMENTS:

FIGURE 5-2 An audiogram demonstrates the typical conductive hearing loss associated with cholesteatoma.

REHABILITATION AND FOLLOW-UP

During the first 6 months to 1 year, close follow-up for possible recurrence is important. While a second look procedure is often recommended in canal wall-up procedures, some authors advocate CT imaging or aural endoscopy as diagnostic alternatives.

When successful ossicular reconstruction cannot be achieved, referral for hearing aid evaluation is usually indicated.

SUGGESTED READINGS

ABEELE DV, OFFECIERS FE. Management of labyrinthine fistulae in cholesteatoma. *Acta Otolaryngol.* 1993; 47:311 321.

DAVES JDK, WATSON RT. Labyrinthine fistulae. *J. Laryngol Otol.* 1978;92:83–98.

GACEK RR. The surgical management of labyrinthine fistulae in chronic otitis media with cholesteatoma. *Am J Otol Rhinol Laryngol.* 1974;83:1–19.

HERZOG JA, SMITH PG, METZKER GR, et al. Management of labyrinthine fistulae secondary to cholesteatoma. *Am J Otol.* 1996;17(3):410–415.

McCabe BF. The incidence, STG, treatment and fate of labyrinthine fistulae. *Clin Otol.* 1978;3:239–242.

Parisier SC, Edelstein DR, et al. Management of labyrinthine fistulae caused by cholesteatoma. *Otol Head Neck Surg.* 1991;104:110–115.

Sanna M, Zini C, et al. Closed versus open technique in the management of labyrinthine fistulae. *Am J Otol.* 1998;9:470–475.

Sheehy JL, Brackmann DE. Cholesteatoma surgery: management of labyrinthine fistulae—a report of 97 cases. *Laryngoscope.* 1979;89:78–87.

OTOSCLEROSIS

Myles L. Pensak, M.D.

HISTORY

A 42-year-old white female presented with a 15-year history of auditory degradation. The patient was cognizant of hearing loss beginning after her first pregnancy at age 21. Subsequently, she became aware by her early 30s that her hearing was markedly diminished in her left ear. There is no antedating history of otologic or neurotologic infection or trauma.

Physical examination revealed the external auditory canals and tympanic membranes to be benign. The Weber lateralized to the left side at 512 Hz, the Rinne was negative at 512 Hz on the left and positive on the right. The remaining portion of the otoneurotologic examination was entirely within normal limits.

DIFFERENTIAL DIAGNOSIS— KEY POINTS

1. Based on the physical examination, this patient appears to have a conductive hearing loss in the left ear. Audiometric studies will be important to confirm this finding.

2. The differential diagnosis for a conductive hearing loss is extensive and includes osteogenesis imperfecta, Padget's disease, or concomitant ossicular fixation, in particular, the head of the malleus. The absence of an antedating history of otologic infection and a normal physical examination would make ossicular discontinuity highly unlikely.

3. Otosclerosis is probably the most common etiology of slowly progressive hearing loss. Otosclerosis occurs typically in Caucasian women and appears to be accelerated during pregnancy.

4. The conductive hearing loss associated with otosclerosis can be associated with a neurosensory loss, usually attributed to cochlear involvement. Audiometric evaluation would be important to delineate this possibility.

TEST INTERPRETATION

The audiometric evaluation reveals the right ear to have a Speech Reception Threshold (SRT) of 10 dB with 100% discrimination. The left ear has an SRT of 45 dB (Fig. 6–1). There is a shallow sensorineural hearing loss noted at 2000 Hz compatible with that of a Carhart's notch. Tympanometry demonstrates a shallow tympanogram (As). Acoustic reflexes are noted to be absent with ipsilateral stimulation to the left ear. The good discrimination score in the left ear and a lack of a high-frequency sloping neurosensory hearing loss argue against any cochlear component in this case.

DIAGNOSIS

Otosclerosis.

MEDICAL MANAGEMENT

Nonsurgical management of otosclerosis can usually be very effectively provided with amplification. Otolaryngologists generally agree that most patients should be offered amplification prior to undergoing surgery because this is a safe and usually effective therapeutic modality.

A small percentage of patients will have cochlear otosclerosis. High-density computed tomography (CT) scanning of the temporal bone will reveal a halo or ring sign due to demineralization of the otic capsule. Oral doses of sodium fluoride are recommended in an attempt to stabilize sensorineural thresholds.

SURGICAL MANAGEMENT

Surgery for otosclerosis is usually a very effective technique for managing this problem. Although the risks are minimal, they can, at times, be severe. These risks include anacusis, vertigo, dysgeusia, facial paralysis, infection, and perfo-

AUDIOLOGIC EVALUATION

Division of Audiology & Vestibular Testing Dept. of Otolaryngology - Head & Neck Surgery University of Cincinnati Medical Center Cincinnati, OH 45267-0528 • (513) 475-8453	Date: D.O.B.: MR#: Name: Address: Phone:

Equipment	Physician	Location	Audiologist

SPEECH AUDIOMETRY

	SRT		WORD RECOGNITION		
	dB	Mask	%	Mask	SL
RIGHT	10		100		
LEFT	45		96	60	30

SRT___ CID W-1_____

Discrimination ✔ CID W-22_____

✔ Disc ___Tape ___Live Voice

Noise_____Speech ✔___

Noise Reference__ SPL___ HL___

AUDIOGRAM LEGEND

		R	L
AIR	Unmasked	O	X
	Masked	Δ	□
BONE	Unmasked	<	>
	Masked	[	]
SOUND FIELD		S	S
AIDED		A	A
NO RESPONSE			

AUDIOGRAM

MIDDLE-EAR COMPLIANCE

	RIGHT	LEFT
Middle-Ear Pressure (daPa)	-5	-10
C max	1.9	1.3
C +200	1.0	.9
C ME	.90	.4

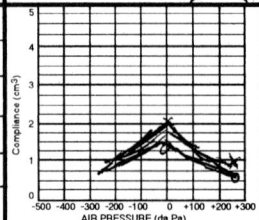

ACOUSTIC REFLEXES

Tone In	Probe In		Eliciting Frequency (Hz)			
			500	1000	2000	4000
L	R	Threshold (dBHL)				
		Decay in 10 sec				
R	R	Threshold (dBHL)	90	95	90	
		Decay in 10 sec				
R	L	Threshold (dBHL)				
		Decay in 10 sec				
L	L	Threshold (dBHL)	ABS	ABS	ABS	
		Decay in 10 sec				

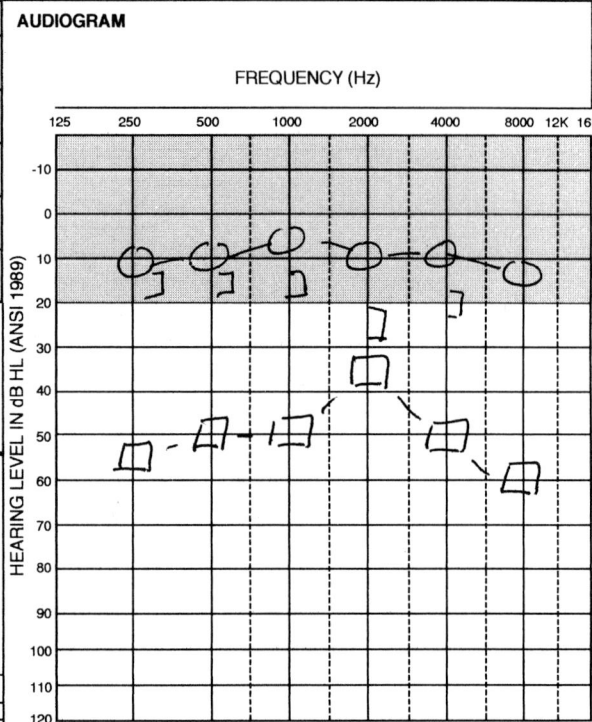

Masking In:

RIGHT	Air	60				
	Bone	60				
LEFT	Air					
	Bone					
WEBER Lateralizes To		L	L	L		

COMMENTS:

FIGURE 6–1 Audiogram demonstrates an SRT of 45 dB and shallow sensorineural hearing loss.

ration of the tympanic membrane. Current strategies include both stapedectomy, stapedotomy technique with direct microsurgical dissection, or the employment of an argon or CO_2 laser. Many surgeons employ a tissue seal around the prosthesis to prevent perilymphatic fistulae. Absolute contraindications to surgery in patients with otosclerosis would include individuals with an only hearing ear or those with a familial history of stapes footplate fixation wherein the possibility of a stapes gusher syndrome is raised. From a surgical perspective stapedotomy is an elective procedure.

Complications of stapes surgery include cerebrospinal fluid leak, vertigo, hearing loss, and injury to the facial nerve. Delayed complications include perilymphatic fistulae, erosion of the incus, lateralization of the prosthesis, or the formation of a reparative granuloma.

REHABILITATION AND FOLLOW-UP

In the immediate postoperative period, as the fenestration into the vestibule is sealing, patients should avoid straining, heavy lifting, sneezing, or barometric changes that may result in trauma and subsequent hearing loss. Although it is not clear that long-term (beyond 6 months) problems can result in patients who have undergone stapes surgery, doctors often recommend that these patients avoid situations associated with high, rapid changes in barometric pressure such as scuba diving. Long-term follow-up is probably worthwhile with serial audiograms to try to detect early changes consistent with cochlear otosclerosis so that they can be treated appropriately when they occur.

SUGGESTED READINGS

BAILEY HAT, PAPPAS JJ, GRAHAM SS. Small fenestra stapedectomy technique: reducing risk and improving hearing. *Otol Head Neck Surg.* 1983;91:516–522.

BELLUCI RJ. Trends and profiles in stapes surgery. *Am J Otol.* 1979;88:108.

GHERINI SG, HORN KL, BOWMAN C, et al. Small fenestra stapedotomy using a fiber optic hand-held Argon laser in obliterative otosclerosis. *Laryngoscope.* 1990;100:1276–1282.

GLASSCOCK ME. Revision stapedectomy surgery. *Otol Head Neck Surg.* 1987;96:141–148.

HOUGH JVD. Longterm results in partial stapedectomy. *Arch Otol.* 1989;89:230.

LESINSKI SG, STEIN J. CO_2 laser stapedotomy. *Laryngoscope.* 1989;99(suppl 46):20–23.

SILVERSTEIN H, ROSENBERG S, JONES R. Small fenestra stapedotomies with and without KTP laser. A comparison. *Laryngoscope.* 1989;99:485–488.

WIET RJ, CAUSSE JB, SHAMBAUGH GE. *Monograph on Otosclerosis.* Washington, DC: AAO-HNS Foundation; 1991.

WIET RJ, HARVEY SA, BAUER GP. Complications in stapes surgery in otosclerosis. *Otol Clin North Am.* 1993;26(3):471–490.

TEMPORAL BONE FRACTURE

Myles L. Pensak, M.D.

HISTORY

A 21-year-old unrestrained male driver is involved in a motor vehicle accident. At the time of presentation to the emergency room the patient is alert, although complaining of violent vertigo. Physical examination reveals the right external auditory canal to be excoriated with debris and blood. The tympanic membrane cannot be fully visualized but there appears to be a laceration extending across the roof of the ear canal. The contralateral external auditory canal is benign. A hemotympanum, however, is noted. Tuning forks demonstrate the Weber, which lateralizes to the right ear, the Rinne is negative in the right and the patient reports hearing sound only directed to the right side. The mastoid area is discolored bilaterally, and brisk right-beating horizontal rotary nystagmus is noted. With any change in head position the patient complains of severe waves of nausea. Subjective nonpulsatile tinnitus is reported. The patient has no evidence of asymmetry on facial examination. The remaining portion of his head and neck examination is unremarkable, as is his neurologic examination.

DIFFERENTIAL DIAGNOSIS— KEY POINTS

1. Temporal bone trauma may manifest in a multiplicity of fashions. Classically, temporal bone fractures are described as longitudinal, transverse, or mixed. In a classic longitudinal fracture, the site of initial trauma occurs along the temporal or parietal aspects of the cranium. Patients will present with conductive hearing loss and bloody otorrhea. Longitudinal fractures may be bilateral and are the most common source of facial nerve paralysis

due to the fact that longitudinal temporal bone fractures occur with a greater frequency than transverse temporal bone fractures.

2. Longitudinal fractures extend from the squamous portion of the temporal bone along the anterior portion of the petrous apex to the region of foramen lacerum and foramen ovale, passing through the posterior/superior aspect of the external auditory canal, which is often torn. The ossicular chain is frequently disrupted. Because of its laterality and direction, the otic capsule is preserved as is the internal auditory canal. In longitudinal temporal bone fractures, sensorineural hearing loss is rare.

3. In contradistinction, transverse temporal bone fractures are much less common. The injury usually extends across the petrous ridge from the foramen spinosum to the posterior fossa dura. Fractures across the internal auditory canal and/or labyrinth result in profound anacusis and immediate debilitating vertigo. The incidence of facial paralysis in transverse fracture may be as high as 50%.

4. Assessment of patients with temporal bone fracture begins with a thorough otologic and neurotologic examination. The external auditory canals are assessed under sterile conditions. Examination is made for the possibility of identification of cerebrospinal fluid (CSF) otorrhea. Concomitantly, the patient is assessed for CSF rhinorrhea. Ocular motility is noted, and the function of the facial nerve appreciated.

5. Following full neurologic assessment, an audiometric profile should be obtained to establish bone conduction threshold levels. Again, sterility is of considerable importance and in-set earphones should be avoided in cases of contamination. Electronystagmography and

rotation chair assessment may give information relative to the functioning of the labyrinthine. In acute labyrinthine injury, however, these tests are of no clinical relevance.

TEST INTERPRETATION

The computed tomography (CT) scan (Fig. 7–1) reveals a longitudinal temporal bone fracture. Blood and soft tissue are seen in the mastoid and epitympanum.

The audiogram (Fig. 7–2) shows complete anacusis in the left ear, probably reflecting injury to the labyrinth. The conductive loss in the right ear may be due to the hemotympanum. Ossicular chain abnormalities can only be ruled out following resolution of the hemotympanum.

High-resolution CT scanning of the temporal bone in both the axial and coronal planes will provide optimal visualization of the pathway of the noted fracture.

DIAGNOSIS

Longitudinal temporal bone fracture.

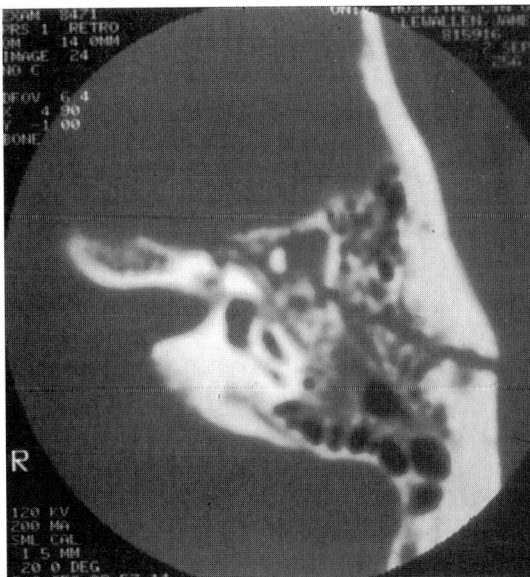

FIGURE 7–1 CT scan demonstrates a longitudinal temporal bone fracture. Note the bone and soft tissue in the mastoid and epitympanum.

MEDICAL MANAGEMENT

Conservative management is the hallmark for most patients with temporal bone fracture. Head elevation, stool softeners, and bed rest will often see the spontaneous resolution of CSF otorrhea or rhinorrhea. Acute vestibulopathy may be treated with vestibular suppressant medications; however, within a short period of time (usually within 72 hours), the whirling debilitating vertigo is replaced by a sense of unbalanced lightheadedness that will generally be compensated for over a 6-month period of time.

Hemotympanum generally will resolve within 30 to 90 days and the middle ear requires no evacuation. In contradistinction, in longitudinal temporal bone fracture it is important to assess early on whether the fracture line transversing the tympanic ring has, in fact, resulted in a perforation with the introduction of squame into the middle ear. Early therapy will obviate the possibility of cholesteatoma development.

SURGICAL MANAGEMENT

If the patient evidences trauma to the ossicular chain with associated vertigo, the possibility of subluxation of the stapes with or without an active perilymphatic fistula must be entertained and prompt surgical intervention undertaken.

In general, patients who have facial nerve injuries, either delayed or immediate in onset, should be managed according to protocols established elsewhere in this text.

Neurologic complications associated with temporal bone fractures need to be addressed. These would include epidural and subdural hematomas, hydrocephalus, and/or intracranial bleeding.

REHABILITATION AND FOLLOW-UP

Rehabilitation may be directed at resultant hearing loss with amplification. For gait and postural instability, balance rehabilitation is quite frequently beneficial.

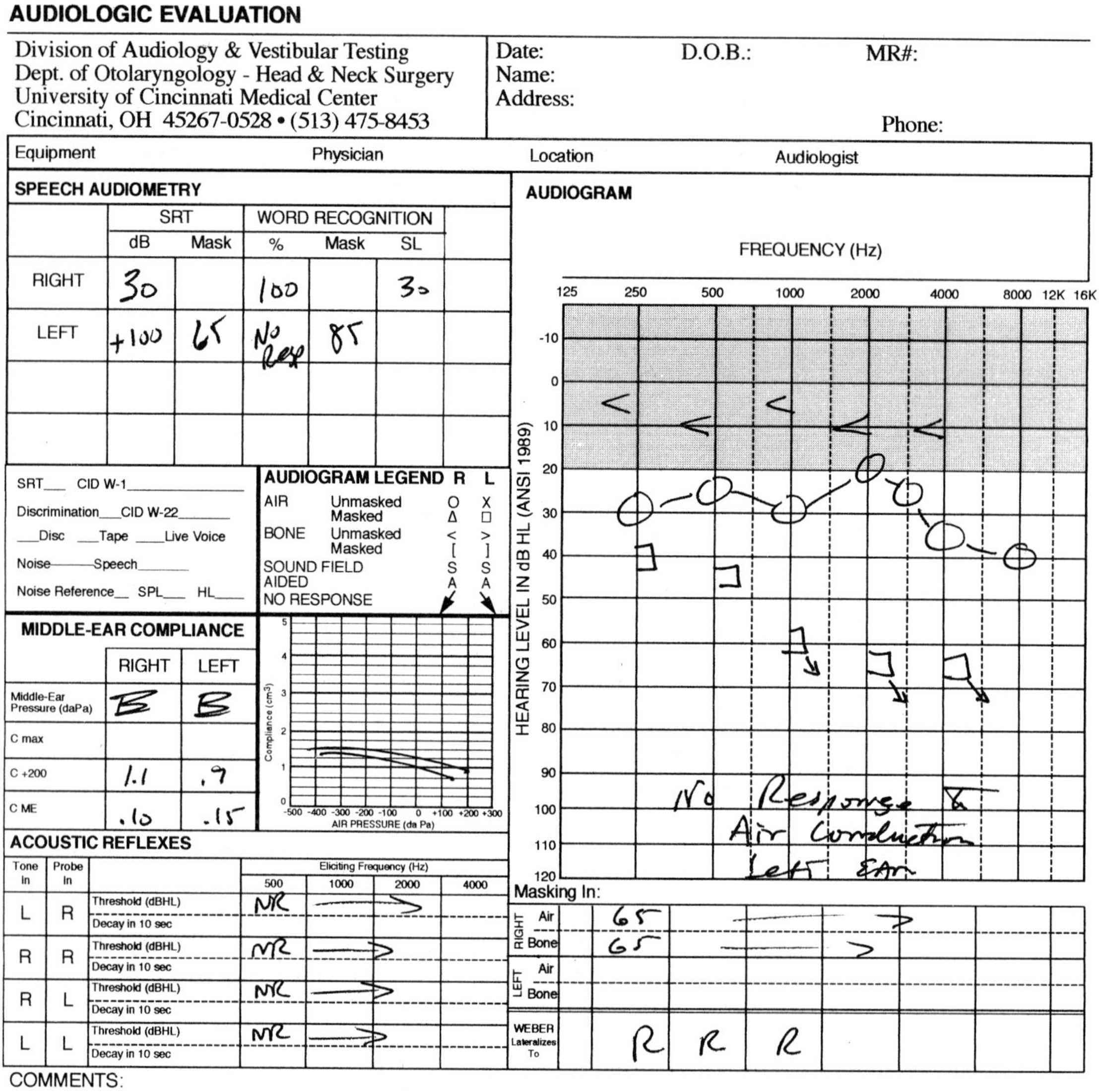

AUDIOLOGIC EVALUATION

Division of Audiology & Vestibular Testing Dept. of Otolaryngology - Head & Neck Surgery University of Cincinnati Medical Center Cincinnati, OH 45267-0528 • (513) 475-8453	Date: D.O.B.: MR#: Name: Address: Phone:

Equipment	Physician	Location	Audiologist

SPEECH AUDIOMETRY

	SRT		WORD RECOGNITION		
	dB	Mask	%	Mask	SL
RIGHT	30		100		30
LEFT	+100	65	No Rep	85	

SRT___ CID W-1_____

Discrimination___CID W-22_____

___Disc ___Tape ___Live Voice

Noise_____Speech_____

Noise Reference__ SPL___ HL___

AUDIOGRAM LEGEND

		R	L
AIR	Unmasked	O	X
	Masked	Δ	□
BONE	Unmasked	<	>
	Masked	[	]
SOUND FIELD		S	S
AIDED		A	A
NO RESPONSE		↙	↘

MIDDLE-EAR COMPLIANCE

	RIGHT	LEFT
Middle-Ear Pressure (daPa)	B	B
C max		
C +200	1.1	.7
C ME	.10	.15

ACOUSTIC REFLEXES

Tone in	Probe in		Eliciting Frequency (Hz)			
			500	1000	2000	4000
L	R	Threshold (dBHL)	NR			
		Decay in 10 sec				
R	R	Threshold (dBHL)	NR			
		Decay in 10 sec				
R	L	Threshold (dBHL)	NR			
		Decay in 10 sec				
L	L	Threshold (dBHL)	NR			
		Decay in 10 sec				

AUDIOGRAM

FREQUENCY (Hz)

HEARING LEVEL IN dB HL (ANSI 1989)

No Response to Air Conduction Left Ear

Compliance (cm³) — AIR PRESSURE (da Pa) -500 -400 -300 -200 -100 0 +100 +200 +300

Masking In:

		500	1000	2000	4000
RIGHT	Air	65			➝
	Bone	65			➝
LEFT	Air				
	Bone				
WEBER Lateralizes To		R	R	R	

COMMENTS:

FIGURE 7–2 Audiogram demonstrates complete anacusis in the left, reflective of injury to the labyrinth.

SUGGESTED READINGS

Duncan NO III, Coker NJ, Jenkins HA, et al. Gunshot injuries of the temporal bone. *Otolaryngol Head Neck Surg.* 1986;94:47–55.

Fee GA. Traumatic perilymphatic fistulas. *Arch Otol.* 1968;88:477–480.

Freeman J. Temporal bone fractures and cholesteatoma. *Ann Otol Rhinol Laryngol.* 1983;92:558–560.

Harker L, McCabe BF. Temporal bone fractures and facial nerve injury. *Otolaryngol Clin North Am.* 1974;7:425–431.

Herdman SJ Jr, Herdman SJ, eds. *Vestibular Rehabilitation.* Philadelphia, PA: FA Davis; 1994;68–79.

Lambert PR, Brackmann DE. Facial paralysis longitudinal temporal bone fractures: a review of 26 cases. *Laryngoscope.* 1984;94:1022–1026.

McGuirt WF Jr, Stool S. Temporal bone fractures in children: a review with emphasis on long-term sequelae. *Clin Pediatr.* 1992;31:12–18.

McKennan KX, Chole RA. Facial paralysis in temporal bone trauma. *Am J Otol.* 1992;13(2):167–172.

Schuknecht HF. Cupulolithiasis. *Arch Otol.* 1969; 90:765–778.

Spector G, Pratt LL, Randall G. A clinical study of delayed reconstruction in ossicular fractures. *Laryngoscope.* 1973;83:837–851.

Case 8

CEREBROSPINAL FLUID OTORRHEA

Rick A. Friedman, M.D.

HISTORY

A 17-year-old white male presents to the Emergency Department after falling from a fast-moving vehicle. Paramedics on the scene state that he had a Glascow coma score of 9, and he had what appeared to be blood emanating from his left external auditory canal. There was no further information on the report obtained at the scene. Upon admission to the Emergency Department, a computed tomography (CT) scan was emergently ordered, which revealed an epidural hematoma. The neurosurgical service intervened and took the patient emergently to the operating room for evacuation of the epidural hematoma. Postoperatively, the patient's mental status improved; however, the otolaryngology service was consulted because the patient had a persistent bloody drainage from his left ear that demonstrated a target sign on his pillow.

Physician examination of the patient revealed a left-sided incision from the previous craniotomy and abrasions of the scalp. His facial skeleton was intact. Examination of his ears revealed a normal pinna, external auditory canal, and tympanic membrane on the right. On the left, blood-tinged clear fluid was dripping from the ear. Microscopic examination at the bedside with sterile preparation of the ear canal revealed laceration of the posterosuperior external auditory canal with a laceration of the tympanic membrane through the pars flacida and part of the pars tensa. Pulsatile clear fluid was filling the middle ear and emanating from the laceration in the tympanic membrane and canal skin. A tuning fork examination was unobtainable as

the patient was arousable but not cooperative. Examination of the patient's eyes revealed no spontaneous nystagmus. His facial tone was symmetric. The remainder of his head and neck examination was unremarkable.

DIFFERENTIAL DIAGNOSIS— KEY POINTS

1. Bloody otorrhea without cerebrospinal fluid (CSF) could occur in this patient because he sustained lacerations of his external auditory canal and tympanic membrane. This injury, in addition to the mucosal injury of the middle ear from what is presumably a longitudinal or oblique temporal bone fracture, can lead to bloody otorrhea.

2. CSF otorrhea occurs in between 1 and 6% of all basalar skull fractures. Disruption of the floor of the middle cranial fossa with laceration of the dura, combined with a longitudinal fracture that traverses the external canal and tympanic membrane, allows the egress of CSF through the ear canal. Typically transverse temporal bone fractures, when associated with CSF leak, result in CSF rhinorrhea because the tympanic membrane is often intact.

TEST INTERPRETATION

Definitive diagnosis of CSF otorrhea can most typically be made by a careful history and physical examination. Clear fluid emanating from the ear canal is unlikely to be anything but CSF. When there is question about the source of fluid emanating from the external auditory canal, laboratory studies and radiographic tests can be performed.

Collection of the fluid from the external auditory canal for evaluation of total protein, glucose, and β_2-transferrin may be helpful in confirming the presence of CSF but is infrequently necessary.

High-resolution CT scan of the temporal bones will often aid in the diagnosis of temporal bone fracture and demonstrate the pathways for egress of CSF (Fig. 8–1). Distinguishing CSF from blood and/or soft tissue injury by CT scan is often not possible. Although metrizamide has been used in the past to identify the site of cerebrospinal leakage, it is rarely necessary in these cases. Although CT scan does aid in demonstrating the fracture line, it is not essential to the diagnosis of CSF otorrhea. High-resolution CT scans of the temporal bones are essential for surgical planning.

DIAGNOSIS

1. Longitudinal temporal bone fracture.
2. CSF otorrhea.

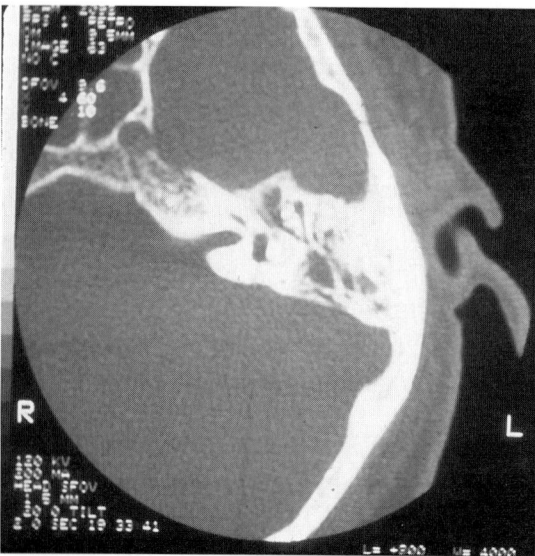

FIGURE 8–1 CT scan of the temporal bone demonstrating longitudinal fracture.

MEDICAL MANAGEMENT

There has been much debate in the literature about the use of prophylactic antibiotics for the prevention of meningitis in CSF otorrhea. Although the data are conflicting, most agree that the use of prophylactic antibiotics is not indicated and may in fact mask bacterial infection, resulting in delayed treatment of a serious infection complication.

Nonoperative management is the initial course taken in these patients. The majority of traumatic CSF leaks resolve within 10 to 14 days. A recent study in children demonstrated that leaks that did not resolve within 7 days after admission, with or without the institution of continuous lumbar spinal drainage, did not resolve without surgical intervention. Despite this, observation with head of bed elevation, institution of laxatives, and bed rest are recommended in these cases for at least 10 to 14 days. Generally, lumbar drainage is not required. The vast majority of cases of traumatic CSF otorrhea will resolve with this therapy.

SURGICAL MANAGEMENT

The choice of surgical approach depends largely on the size of the defect and the presence or absence of herniated brain tissue. The approaches available include the middle cranial fossa approach, the transmastoid approach, or a combination of these approaches. Repair of the defect requires tissue strong enough to withstand normal intracranial pressure and compliant enough to conform to the contours of the middle fossa floor. Although high-resolution CT scanning will often delineate the areas involved, other fracture sites or an appreciation for the overall size may not be obtained until the time of surgical intervention.

Small fractures in the region of the mastoid tegmen can be approached through the mastoid using a transmastoid approach. The fracture site can be identified and repaired usually with temporalis facia that is inserted through the defect into the epidural space.

Lesions in the region of the tegmen tympani can most easily be approached through the middle cranial fossa. Middle fossa craniotomy and temporal lobe retraction delineate the fractures well and provide ample exposure for complete repair.

Many times the best approach is a combined approach that allows complete delineation of fracture lines as well as the ability to reinforce the repair of the cranial defect from below.

Various materials and methods have been described for repair of fractures of the floor of the middle cranial fossa. The preferred approach is the use of a fascia–bone–fascia sandwich. Temporalis fascia or fascia lata can be harvested and used for this purpose. The inner table of the temporal craniotomy provides useful bone for the repair. Utilizing this method a large piece of fascia is cut to the appropriate size and laid down over the fracture line on the floor of the middle cranial fossa. Following this, a thin sheet of bone of equal size is used to reinforce this repair. The last layer is provided by a large piece of fascia that covers the previously placed fascia and bone. Fibrin glue may be used to reinforce the repair. Following this, the temporal lobe retraction is released and the craniotomy bone flap is replaced. The wound should be closed in layers, and the patient maintained at strict bed rest with the head of the bed elevated. Continuous spinal lumbar drainage can be used as an adjunct.

REHABILITATION AND FOLLOW-UP

During the early postoperative period, the patient should be observed closely for any evidence of recurrent CSF leak or intracranial infection such as meningitis. The patient should be instructed to decrease his or her physical activity for 1 to 2 months postrepair to ensure that there is no recurrent leak. No other long-term sequelae should be expected once the injury has resolved.

SUGGESTED READINGS

Brawley BW, Kelly WA. Treatment of basal skull fractures with and without cerebrospinal fluid fistulae. *J Neurosurg.* 1967;26:57–61.

Klastersky J, Sadeghi M, Brihiye J. Antimicrobial prophylaxis in patients with rhinorrhea or otorrhea: a double blind study. *Surg Neurol.* 1976;6:111–114.

Jones DT, Magill TJ, Healy GB. Cerebrospinal fistulas in children. *Laryngoscope.* 1992;102:443–446.

Lundy LB, Graham MD, Kartush JM, LaRouere MJ. Temporal bone encephalocele and cerebral spinal fluid leaks. *Am J Otol.* 1996;17:461–469.

Case 9

UNILATERAL HEARING LOSS

Rick A. Friedman, M.D.

HISTORY

A 32-year-old male presents with left-sided hearing loss that has been present for many years and has slowly progressed over time. He states that he first noted this in his late teens and early 20s when he used to have to ask people to repeat themselves. During college and medical school he noted that he would sit with his right ear facing his instructors. Being right handed, he had previously held the telephone to his left ear; however, during the past 2 years he has noted increasing difficulty with the telephone and has had to switch to his right ear. He has no other complaints currently, although he states he does have occasional tinnitus, but he has no aural fullness, fluctuation in his hearing, or vertigo. His medical history is significant for the usual childhood illnesses, although he does not specifically recall having mumps. He denies a history of trauma or ototoxic exposures. Although he had a few bouts of acute otitis media as a child, he has had no otitis as an adolescent or adult. There are no other medical problems. There is no family history of hearing loss.

Physical examination reveals no craniofacial abnormalities. His neuro-otologic examination is significant for a Weber that lateralizes to the right ear. His Rinne demonstrates air conduction greater than bone conduction on the right, with masking in the right ear; there is no response on the left. Microscopic examination of his ear canals and tympanic membranes reveals normal anatomy. Of note, there is no evidence of the sequelae of either acute or chronic otitis media. His cranial nerves are intact, and there is no evidence of spontaneous, gaze-evoked, or positional nystagmus. The cerebellar exam is unremarkable and he has a normal tandem Romberg.

DIFFERENTIAL DIAGNOSIS— KEY POINTS

The causes of unilateral hearing loss are numerous, but the number of potential entities can often be streamlined by the patient's history and physical examination. This patient's history and physical examination reveal a unilateral hearing loss but do not suggest a specific etiology. When considering unilateral hearing loss it is helpful to consider the possibilities in categories, such as infectious, inflammatory, neoplastic, traumatic, toxic, and idiopathic.

1. *Infectious.* Many infectious processes can affect the inner ear both unilaterally and bilaterally. In particular, early viral infections either *in utero* or in early childhood or adulthood can lead to hearing loss. One of the more common etiologies that would include unilateral hearing loss would be labyrinthitis from cytomegalovirus. Other viruses are associated with inner ear infection and include mumps, measles, varicella, and rubella. Mumps virus should be suspected in this patient, because mumps is often associated with unilateral hearing loss. Bacterial labyrinthitis can be tympanogenic or meningogenic and often results in bilateral disease. However, unilateral or asymmetric loss can occur. Certainly tuberculous and fungal infections of the ear can lead to unilateral hearing loss; however, this patient did not have evidence of an infectious process in the middle ear.

2. *Inflammatory.* A number of inflammatory processes can affect the inner ear. First, autoimmune inner ear disease, whether associated with other autoimmune phenomenon or isolated to the inner ear, can, uncommonly, result in unilateral hearing loss. These patients may demonstrate evidence of an inflamma-

tory process on serologic testing; however, many of them do not and are identified by their responses to steroids. Autoimmune diseases known to be associated with sensorineural hearing loss include Cogan's syndrome, Wegener's granulomatosis, rheumatoid arthritis, systemic lupus erythematosus, and several other rheumatologic disorders. Multiple sclerosis, although more commonly associated with vertigo, can be associated with a demyelinating plaque of the cochlear nucleus leading to unilateral hearing loss.

3. *Neoplastic.* There are several tumors that can directly or indirectly affect the inner ear. Facial neuroma, acoustic neuroma, squamous cell carcinoma of the external and middle ear, glomus tympanicum and jugulare, and Hefner tumor or papillary adenocarcinoma of the endolymphatic sac. All of these tumors, except for the acoustic neuroma and facial neuroma, will cause hearing loss by direct invasion of the inner ear. Acoustic neuroma and facial neuroma are difficult to distinguish clinically because they both present typically with a slowly progressive sensorineural loss with retrocochlear findings on site of lesion testing. In about 15 to 20% of patients with acoustic neuroma, sudden hearing loss is a presenting symptom. Certainly other lesions of the cerebellopontine angle, most commonly meningioma, can result in a unilateral hearing loss.

4. *Trauma.* Trauma to the inner ear is a frequent cause of unilateral hearing loss. Penetrating or blunt trauma to the temporal bone can result in either direct or indirect damage to the labyrinth. Penetrating trauma with disruption of the ossicular chain and possible subluxation of the stapes can result in sensorineural hearing loss. More commonly, temporal bone fracture is associated with hearing loss. The hearing loss associated with temporal bone fracture is not necessarily the result of violation of the labyrinth and can result from commotio labyrinthi. In transverse temporal bone fractures, either the labyrinth or the internal auditory canal is violated, resulting in complete hearing loss in the involved ear.

5. *Toxins.* There are a variety of ototoxins that can result in unilateral or bilateral hearing loss. Some of the more commonly clinically

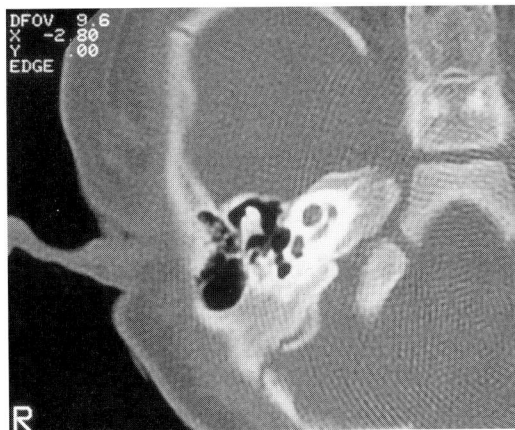

FIGURE 9–1 CT scan of the temporal bones demonstrates a Mondini's deformity.

encountered toxins include aminoglycoside antibiotics, loop diuretics including furosemide and ethacrynic acid, and several antineoplastic agents including cisplatin. Although these often cause bilateral hearing loss, unilateral hearing loss may occur.

6. *Miscellaneous.* Endolymphatic hydrops and otosclerosis can result in unilateral hearing loss. Endolymphatic hydrops typically presents as a fluctuating hearing loss associated with aural fullness, tinnitus, and vertigo. Otosclerosis is most often a mixed hearing loss; however, isolated involvement of the cochlea can rarely result in sensorineural hearing loss. Many patients demonstrate the characteristic abnormalities on a high-resolution computed tomography (CT) scan of the temporal bones. Congenital anomalies of the inner ear, such as Mondini's deformity, can result in unilateral hearing loss (Fig. 9–1). Cochlear hypoplasias often show some evidence of bilaterality; however, there is often asymmetry. The large vestibular aqueduct syndrome frequently presents with unilateral hearing loss, although it is bilateral in approximately 70%. A familial form of unilateral sensorineural loss has been described.

TEST INTERPRETATION

A search for the etiology of this hearing loss should include serologic testing with complete blood count, erythrocyte sedimentation rate, and chemistry panel including thyroid function and serum glucose. Further testing can include assays for rheumatoid factor and antinuclear antibody, the Raji cell assay, and lymphocyte transformation and migration inhibition tests. If autoimmune disease is highly suspect, then Western blot assays can be used to detect antibody to cochlear antigens. Audiometric testing in the form of pure tone thresholds, speech reception and discrimination, and acoustic reflexes is essential. Acoustic reflex decay or threshold evaluation and poor speech discrimination may assist in localizing the site of lesion to the retrocochlear pathways.

Auditory brain stem evoked response audiometry is more sensitive than acoustic reflex or speech discrimination testing in the identification of retrocochlear pathology. Its usefulness in the diagnosis of acoustic neuroma has recently been called into question because it is approximately 80% sensitive in the identification of small intracanilicular acoustic tumors. The definitive diagnostic test available for the identification of retrocochlear pathology is a gadolinium-enhanced T1-weighted magnetic resonance image. These studies are very helpful compared with enhanced views when identifying even the smallest lesions of the internal auditory canal and cerebellopontine angle. High-resolution CT scan of the temporal bone is often useful for identifying inner ear anomalies. Although struc-

tural anomalies of the cochlea only appear in between 10 and 25% of affected patients, high-resolution CT scan is useful for the identification of the enlarged vestibular aqueduct, as in this case, and provides a basis for patient counseling (Fig. 9–2).

DIAGNOSIS

Unilateral enlarged vestibular aqueduct.

MEDICAL MANAGEMENT

A hearing aid evaluation would be useful in this patient. This patient would be a candidate for a CROS hearing aid or a conventional CIC hearing aid with maximum amplification. The patient should be instructed to avoid head trauma due to the possibility of further hearing loss.

SURGICAL MANAGEMENT

There is currently no surgical therapy for unilateral hearing loss.

REHABILITATION AND FOLLOW-UP

This patient will require yearly follow-up with audiometric testing to ensure no disease is present in the normal ear. The patient should

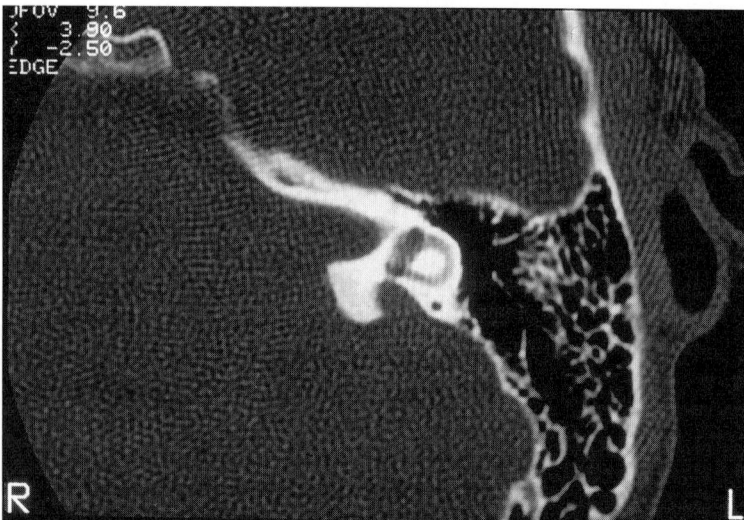

FIGURE 9–2 CT scan demonstrates enlarged vestibular aqueduct.

be instructed to protect his good ear and avoid noise exposure. He should be advised to consult his otolaryngologist in the event that potential ototoxic exposure might ensue. In addition, a hearing aid evaluation, as previously mentioned, is essential as the patient may derive significant benefit from either CROS or maximum output CIC in the diseased ear.

SUGGESTED READINGS

Chandrasekhar SS, Brackmann DE, Devgan KK. Utility of auditory brainstem response audiometry in diagnosis of acoustic neuromas. *Am J Otol.* 1995;16:63–67.

Everberg G. Hereditary unilateral deafness. *Acta Otolaryngol (Stockh).* 1957;47:303–311.

Harris JP, Sharp PA. Inner ear autoantibodies in patients with rapidly progressive sensorineural hearing loss. *Laryngoscope.* 1990;100:516.

Jackler RK, DeLaCruz A. The large vestibular aqueduct syndrome. *Laryngoscope.* 1989;99:1238–1243.

Kelemen G, Linthicum F. Labyrinthine otosclerosis. *Acta Otolaryngol.* 1969;supplement 253.

Rockline RE. Production and assay of macrophage inhibitory factor. In: Rose NR, Friedman H, eds. *Manual of Clinical Immunology.* 2nd ed. Washington, DC: American Society for Microbiology; 1980:233.

Schuknecht HF. Mechanism of inner ear injury from blows to the head. *Ann Otol Rhinol Laryngol.* 1969a;78:253–262.

PULSATILE TINNITUS
Rick A. Friedman, M.D.

HISTORY

A 33-year-old black female presents with a complaint of right-sided pulsatile tinnitus that has been present for the past 6 or 7 months and has been getting worse during the past several weeks. She was initially seen by her family physician and on otoscopic examination was noted to have a discoloration of the tympanic membrane. In addition to her pulsatile tinnitus, she states that her hearing does sound a bit muffled on the right side. She denies fevers, chills, sweats, headaches, or other neurologic symptoms. She denies a history of otitis media or trauma to the temporal bone. Her medical history is unremarkable. On neuro-otologic examination, her Weber lateralizes to her right ear, and her Rinne reveals bone conduction greater than air conduction on the right and air conduction greater than bone conduction on the left. Examination of her pinnae and external auditory canals is unremarkable. Microscopic examination of the tympanic membranes reveals a normal mobile tympanic membrane on the left and right. There is evidence of a violatious mass medial to the tympanic membrane, abutting its medial surface. Pneumotoscopy reveals a blanching of the mass with positive pressure (Brown's sign). Auscultation with a Toynbee tube reveals audible pulsatile tinnitus. Examination of her cranial nerves, including indirect laryngoscopy, reveals normal function of cranial nerves II through XII. The remainder of the neurologic examination is unremarkable.

DIFFERENTIAL DIAGNOSIS— KEY POINTS

1. Vascular anomalies of the middle ear often present with pulsatile tinnitus. The principal anomalies include the aberrant or laterally displaced internal carotid artery, the dehisscent or high riding jugular bulb, and the congenital or acquired intratympanic carotid artery aneurysm. The aberrant internal carotid artery can be distinguished by high-resolution computed tomography (CT) scan. Four features typical of this anomaly include: enlargement of the inferior tympanic canaliculus by the aberrant vessel at its entry into the middle ear, an enhancing mass in the hypotympanum, absence of the vertical segment of the internal carotid canal, and absence of the bony covering of the internal carotid artery. These anomalies are most frequently identified in females (90%) and in right ears (75%).

The high riding jugular bulb is the most common vascular anomaly of the middle ear and is readily recognized on high-resolution CT scan. It is defined as a jugular bulb extending above the inferior tympanic annulus and is present in approximately 6% of patients. Intratympanic carotid aneurysms are quite rare. Two other less frequent abnormalities include petrous carotid dissection and carotid stenosis either from atherosclerosis or fibromuscular dysplasia.

2. Benign intercranial hypertension is often characterized by pulsatile tinnitus, papilledema, and elevated intercranial hypertension. This disorder is often found in obese middle-age females and can progress to visual field deficits and blindness. The etiology of the pulsatile tinnitus is felt to be turbulent flow in the transverse and sigmoid sinuses. The diagnosis is confirmed with radiographic imaging and lumbar puncture, which reveals elevated intracranial pressure.

3. Patients with either tortuous anatomy of the sigmoid sinus or prior history of sigmoid sinus thrombosis with recanalization can experience venous hum tinnitus. Venous hum tinnitus of this variety is characterized by its elimination with gentle compression over the jugular vein by or turning the patient's head to the side opposite the tinnitus.

4. Dural arterial venous malformations are one of the most common lesions identified in pulsatile tinnitus. Depending on the direction of

flow, these lesions can be life threatening and a complete evaluation of pulsatile tinnitus is warranted. There are often identified with a combination of magnetic resonance imaging (MRI) and magnetic resonance angiography (MRA).

5. Jugulotympanic paragangliomas are one of the most common causes of pulsatile tinnitus. Glomus bodies of the temporal bone reside in the area of the jugular bulb, along the course of Jacobson's and Arnold's nerves, and occasionally within the fallopian canal. Paragangliomas are felt to arise from the neural crest and migrate in close association with the ganglia of the sympathetic nervous system. These highly vascular masses are made up of chief cells and oxyphil cells and belong to the diffuse neuroendocrine system (DNES), the system of neuropeptide and catacholemine secreting cells.

Paragangliomas appear to be most common in Caucasians although there is no clear-cut racial predilection. They are found more often in women, and they have been described in patients as young as 6 months and as old as 88 years. These tumors may be multiple or synchronous in 3 to 10% of patients.

Paragangliomas typically demonstrate a slow and insidious pattern of growth. The signs and symptoms can generally be placed into three categories based on the tumor characteristics and location: (1) Those due to the presence of tumor in the middle ear can lead to conductive hearing loss, aural polyp, and aural discharge. (2) Those due to the vascular area of the tumor can lead to pulsatile tinnitus, aural bleeding, and a positive Brown's sign. (3) Those that suggest tumor extension to vital structures include sensorineural hearing loss, vertigo, aural pain, and cranial neuropathy.

TEST INTERPRETATION

A search for the underlying etiology of pulsatile tinnitus is often necessary because potentially life-threatening lesions may be present, which including jugulotympanic paragangliomas and intracranial venous malformations. Behavioral audiometry tests including pure tones, speech reception threshold and discrimination, and acoustic reflexes are useful. Tympanometry may demonstrate the pulsations. Audiometric testing most often yields a conductive hearing loss. Pulsatile tinnitus is often associated with a low-frequency sensorineural hearing loss that is thought to be artifactual. Certainly, invasion of the temporal bone and optic capsule by paraganglioma may lead to sensorineural loss. In these cases, assessment of 24-hour urine for catacholamines, metanephrines, and vanillyl mandelic acid (VMA) should be performed. It is felt that most paragangliomas secrete; however, only approximately 4% secrete at a clinically detectable and significant level. It is important to identify these tumors preoperatively because significant hypertension can result intraoperatively. Glomus tympanicum tumors rarely secrete.

• *Complete blood count with differential.* Anemia with an associated high-output cardiac state can result in pulsatile tinnitus in otherwise healthy individuals.

• *Thyroid function studies.* Hyperthyroidism often presents with multiple symptoms prior to pulsatile tinnitus; however, it is another state in which the cardiovascular system is hyperdynamic and can result in pulsatile tinnitus.

• *Radiographic evaluation.* High-resolution CT scanning and MRI provide useful information in the differential diagnosis of pulsatile tinnitus. High-resolution CT scan of the temporal bone is excellent for demonstrating involvement of the middle ear by glomus tympanicum or superiorly extended glomus jugulare. Furthermore, it provides excellent bone detail of the jugular foramen. The characteristic finding on high-resolution CT scan of a glomus jugulare is enlargement of the jugular foramen and erosion of the jugulocarotid spine (Fig. 10–1). This study will also delineate vascular anomalies of the middle ear and skull base.

MRI, with and without gadolinium, and MRA together provide a powerful tool in the differential diagnosis of pulsatile tinnitus. They are useful not only for identifying jugulotympanic paragangliomata, but are also useful for the identification of intracranial arterial venous malformations. When considering le-

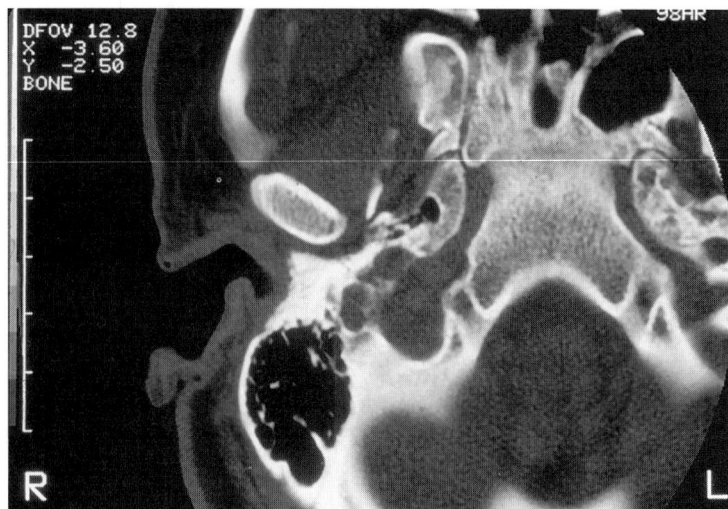

FIGURE 10–1 CT scan of a glomus jugulare demonstrates enlargement of the jugular foramen and erosion of the jugulocarotid spine.

sions of the jugular foramen, one must keep in mind the phenomenon of slow flow with what appears to be abnormal enhancement of the jugular foramen resulting from turbulent flow in the jugular bulb. These lesions can be distinguished from true tumors of the jugular foramen when combined with high-resolution CT scanning.

- *Four-Vessel Angiography.* Four-vessel angiography can usually be obviated in smaller jugulotympanic paraganglioma. This study is useful in cases that will undergo preoperative embolization.

- *Pathologic evaluation of tissue.* Jugulotympanic paragangliomas have characteristic histopathologic findings. The H&E-stained specimen often reveals clusters of chief cells surrounded by connective tissue stroma (zelballen) (Fig. 10–2).

- *Immunostaining.* Immunostaining for a variety of catacholemines and S100 is also useful in the differential diagnosis.

DIAGNOSIS

Jugulotympanic paraganglioma or glomus tympanicum.

MEDICAL MANAGEMENT

Perioperative management of jugulotympanic paragangliomas is essential. As stated previously, approximately 4% of these tumors can secrete catacholymines. Epinephrine is the most commonly secreted substance. Evidence of secretion preoperatively can be obtained from the patient's history. Patients often complain of headaches, pallor, excessive perspiration, palpitations, hypertension, and nausea, and demonstrate postural changes in blood pressure. Management of patients with secreting tumors includes perioperative blood pressure control with α-blocking agents including phentolamine and phenoxybenzamine and intraoperative invasive hemodynamic monitoring.

Therapy for jugulotympanic paraganglioma is primarily surgical; however, radiation therapy is useful in selected cases. Many reports have appeared in the literature reporting tumor control rates of 70 to 90% with radiation as primary, adjunctive, or salvage therapy. The doses given in these studies are between 3,500 and 5,000 cg. The primary effect of radiation therapy appears to be on the vascular and stromal elements of the tumor, with little effect on the tumor cells.

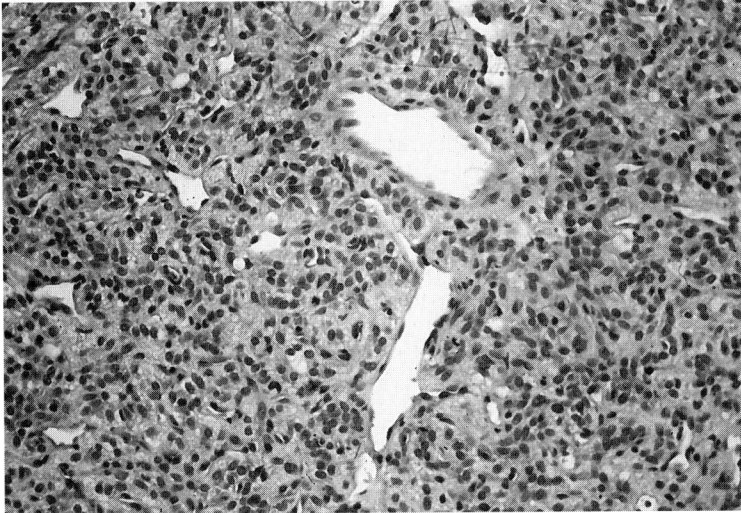

FIGURE 10–2 H&E-stained specimen reveals clusters of chief cells surrounded by connective tissue stroma.

SURGICAL MANAGEMENT

The surgical management of jugulotympanic paragangliomas is based on a classification scheme devised by Antonio De La Cruz, M.D. (Table 10–1). Those confined to the tympanic cavity and visualizable through the tympanic membrane in their entirety can be managed through the transcanal approach. Jugulotympanic paragangliomas that involve the tympanic cavity and mastoid are best approached through a mastoid-extended facial recess approach. Tumors involving the jugular bulb are managed with a mastoid neck approach (possible limited facial nerve rerouting). Tumors involving the ca-

rotid artery and those that are transdural are managed by the infratemporal fossa approach, which can be extended intracranially.

REHABILITATION AND FOLLOW-UP

Jugulotympanic paragangliomas are often associated with lower cranial nerve deficits either preoperatively or postoperatively. These patients will often benefit from eye care and cosmesis for facial nerve paresis and amplification with hearing aids for hearing loss. Lower cranial nerve palsies rarely require tracheotomy and either intraoperative or postoperative management of vocal cord palsy with vocal cord medialization procedures can be beneficial in the speech and swallowing rehabilitation of these patients. A speech and swallowing team is essential for their comprehensive management.

SUGGESTED READINGS

BRACKMANN DE, HOUSE WF, TERRY R, SCANLAN RL. Glomus jugulare tumors: effect of irradiation. *Proc Trans-Am Acad Ophthalmol Otolaryngol.* 1972;76:1423–1431.

DEJONG AL, COKER NJ, JENKINS HA, GOEPFERT H, ALFORD BR. Radiation therapy in the management of

TABLE 10–1 Classification Scheme Devised by Antonio De La Cruz, M.D.

Anatomic Classification	Surgical Approach
Tympanic	Transcanal
Tympanomastoid	Mastoid-extended facial recess
Jugular bulb	Mastoid-neck (possible limited facial nerve rerouting)
Carotid artery	Infratemporal fossa
Transdural	Infratemporal fossa / intracranial

paragangliomas of the temporal bone. *Am J Otol.* 1995;16:283–289.

Dietz RR, Davis WL, Harnsberger HR, et al. MR imaging and MT angiography in the evaluation of pulsatile tinnitus. *Am J Neuroradiol.* 1994;15:879–889.

Glasscock ME, Dickins JRE, Jackson CG, Wiet RJ. Vascular anomalies of the middle ear. *Laryngoscope.* 1980;90:77.

Gulya AJ. The glomous tumor and its biology. *Laryngoscope.* 1993;103(suppl 60):3.

McElveen JT, Lo WWM, El Gabri TH, Nigri P. Aberrant internal carotid artery: classic findings on computed tomography. *Otolaryngol Head Neck Surg.* 1986;94:616.

Sismanis A, Smoker WR. Pulsatile tinnitus: recent advances in diagnosis. *Laryngoscope.* 1994;104:681–688.

Spector GJ, Sobol S, Thawley SE, Maisel RH, Ogura JH. Glomus jugulare tumors of the temporal bone. Patterns of invasion in the temporal bone. *Laryngoscope.* 1979;89:1628.

MENIERE'S DISEASE

Rick A. Friedman, M.D.

HISTORY

A 32-year-old woman presents with complaints of left-sided fluctuating hearing loss, tinnitus, and aural fullness associated with episodic vertigo. She was in her usual state of health until approximately 1 month ago when she began experiencing aural fullness in her left ear. During the past several weeks, she has developed symptoms that she describes as aural fullness followed by roaring tinnitus with some impairment in her hearing. This coincides with sudden attacks of vertigo that last anywhere from several minutes to 2 to 3 hours. She states that between episodes she does have some occasional aural fullness; however, she is free of dizziness. Her left-sided hearing loss has remained despite resolution of the other symptoms. Her medical history is unremarkable, including no history of otologic disease, autoimmune related disease, trauma, or migraine headaches. Her family history is unremarkable. On neuro-otologic examination, her Weber lateralizes to her right ear and her Rinne demonstrates air conduction greater than bone conduction bilaterally. Diplacusis is noted using a 512-Hz tuning fork. During examination with the tuning fork she notes the sound to be uncomfortable in her left ear. Micro-otoscopic examination as well as neurologic examination are normal.

DIFFERENTIAL DIAGNOSIS— KEY POINTS

1. This patient's symptom complex of aural fullness, fluctuating hearing loss, tinnitus, and vertigo are classic for Meniere's disease. The pathophysiology of Meniere's disease appears to involve endolymphatic hydrops. Other diseases associated with endolymphatic hydrops fall into the differential diagnosis encompassing secondary Meniere's disease.

2. Otosyphilis may present as either congenital or acquired with either profound bilateral hearing loss or, more commonly, symptoms characteristic of Meniere's disease including aural fullness, fluctuating hearing loss, tinnitus, and vertigo. These patients often demonstrate poor discrimination scores. Otosyphilis often demonstrates some asymmetry.

3. Obstruction to the endolymphatic duct or sac has been associated with Meniere-like symptoms. Both normal anatomic structures as well as neoplastic and inflammatory diseases can lead to obstruction of the duct or the sac. A high riding jugular bulb has been shown to be ideologic in some cases of endolymphatic hydrops. Gummatous involvement of the temporal bone in syphilis has been associated with obstruction of the endolymphatic duct. Primary tumors of the endolymphatic sac or papillary adenocarcinomas can be associated with symptoms of endolymphatic hydrops. Posterior fossa or cerebellopontine angle tumors have been reported to be associated with Meniere-like symptoms and these include acoustic neuroma and meningioma. Other factors associated with endolymphatic hydrops include a history of chronic otitis media, trauma to the temporal bone, meningitis, or postviral labyrinthitis.

4. Delayed endolymphatic hydrops is often the result of a postinflammatory insult to the inner ear. Often patients present with a history of a hearing loss on one side from viral labyrinthitis. Presumably a subclinical infection in the contralateral ear results in impaired endolymphatic homeostasis and delayed endolymphatic hydrops.

5. Autoimmune inner ear disease can present with symptoms of endolymphatic hydrops. Many patients with Meniere's disease have been noted to have elevated levels of immune complexes in the serum. Most often these are female patients presenting with a bilaterally

symmetric rapidly progressive hearing loss; however, autoimmune inner ear disease can be associated with multiple auditory and vestibular symptoms including classic vestibular hydrops.

TEST INTERPRETATION

A search for the etiology of this patient's endolymphatic hydrops should include the following:

• A measure of the erythrocyte sedimentation rate.

• Presence of autoantibodies such as rheumatoid factor and antinuclear antibody.

• Other tests including lymphocyte migration inhibition and lymphocyte transformation tests and Western blot assays can be reserved for more complicated cases.

• Behavioral and speech audiometry with acoustic reflexes (Fig. 11–1). Note the characteristic low-frequency sensorineural hearing loss.

• Electronystagmography (ENG) provides useful information about the degree of vestibular impairment. Often in Meniere's disease, the

AUDIOLOGIC EVALUATION

| Division of Audiology & Vestibular Testing
Dept. of Otolaryngology - Head & Neck Surgery
University of Cincinnati Medical Center
Cincinnati, OH 45267-0528 • (513) 475-8453 | Date: D.O.B.: ·   MR#:
Name: F – R.
Address:
                                  Phone: |

| Equipment GSI – 16 | Physician | Location MAB | Audiologist RWK |

SPEECH AUDIOMETRY

	SRT		WORD RECOGNITION		
	dB	Mask	%	Mask	SL
RIGHT	40		80	60	30
LEFT	10		96		3ɔ

SRT___ CID W-1_____
Discrimination ✓CID W-22_____
___Disc ✓Tape ___Live Voice
Noise_____Speech ✓____
Noise Reference__ SPL___ HL ✓

AUDIOGRAM LEGEND

		R	L
AIR	Unmasked	O	X
	Masked	Δ	□
BONE	Unmasked	<	>
	Masked	[	]
SOUND FIELD		S	S
AIDED		A	A
NO RESPONSE		↙	↘

AUDIOGRAM

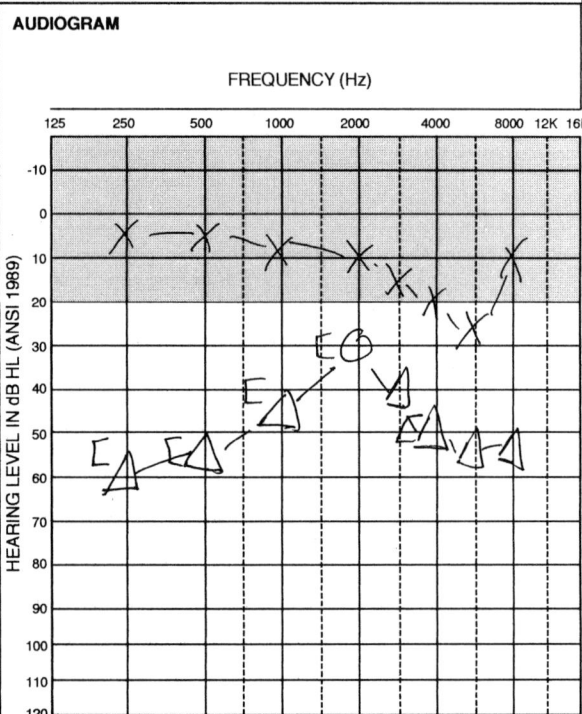

MIDDLE-EAR COMPLIANCE

	RIGHT	LEFT
Middle-Ear Pressure (daPa)	– 20	–(0
C max	2.5	2.3
C +200	0.9	0.8
C ME	1.6	1.5

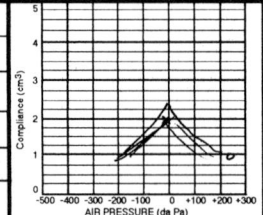

ACOUSTIC REFLEXES

Tone In	Probe In		Eliciting Frequency (Hz)			
			500	1000	2000	4000
L	R	Threshold (dBHL)				
		Decay in 10 sec				
R	R	Threshold (dBHL)	95	95	90	100
		Decay in 10 sec				
R	L	Threshold (dBHL)				
		Decay in 10 sec				
L	L	Threshold (dBHL)	90	90	95	95
		Decay in 10 sec				

Masking In:

		500	1000	2000	4000
RIGHT	Air				
	Bone				
LEFT	Air				
	Bone				
WEBER Lateralizes To		L	L	L	

COMMENTS:

FIGURE 11–1 Audiogram demonstrates characteristic low-frequency sensorineural hearing loss.

symptoms are episodic, as are the findings. Between episodes the ENG may very well be normal.

- A search for retrocochlear pathology in patients with unilateral hearing loss should always be instituted. Tumors of the cerebellopontine angle can present with symptoms mimicking Meniere's disease. There is much debate in the literature as to the appropriate method for screening for retrocochlear pathology. In patients with low suspicion for retrocochlear pathology, auditory brain stem evoked emissions can be used. In patients with suspicion of retrocochlear pathology, several recent reports have shown greater efficacy with magnetic resonance imaging studies. Historically, T1-weighted images with and without gadolinium have been used for the identification of acoustic neuroma. Newer methodologies including T2 fast spin echo have demonstrated excellent sensitivity and lower cost.

DIAGNOSIS

Idiopathic Meniere's disease.

MEDICAL MANAGEMENT

The goal of treatment in Meniere's disease is to control or eliminate the episodes of vertigo. A secondary goal is prevention of the progression of sensorineural hearing impairment. Preservation of hearing is important in Meniere's disease because the disease will develop in the contralateral lateral ear in 30 to 50% of patients who are followed for 10 or more years. The majority of patients with Meniere's disease can be controlled by medical and dietary measures.

Management of the acute attack of Meniere's disease often involves vestibular suppressants. A variety of medications are useful in this patient population. For patients who are not vomiting, meclizine 25 mg every 4 hours is useful for relief of vestibular symptoms. If the patient is vomiting and is unable to take oral medications, promethazine hydrochloride 25-mg suppositories every 6 hours are useful. For prolonged attacks associated with severe nausea and vomiting and poor oral intake, many patients will require admission and intra-

venous hydration. For resistant cases, Valium 2–5 mg orally or 5–10 mg intravenously is effective in relieving the acute symptoms. There are no medications that have been shown in prospective, randomly controlled trials to control the progression of endolymphatic hydrops. Nevertheless, most agree that a trial of medical management should be given before surgical therapy is instituted. A variety of medications have been used for Meniere's disease, including niacin, lipoflavinoid vitamins, diphenhydramine, and histamine by the sublingual, subcutaneous, and intravenous routes. The primary modes of therapy include a low-salt diet, diuretics, and vasodilators. Patients are instructed not to add salt to their food or to use salt when cooking their meals. Diuretic therapy is instituted with hydrochlorothiazide 50 mg, each morning; a potassium supplement is provided with this. Vasodilating medications such as papaverine hydrochloride 150 mg, twice daily, are also used in the management. There is currently no proof in the literature that systemic vasodilators improve inner ear circulation; however, many patients have demonstrated relief of symptoms on this therapy. In addition to the vestibular suppressants previously mentioned, Cawthorne positional exercises are useful. Patients are advised to avoid the use of caffeine, alcohol, tobacco, and stress because these have been shown to exacerbate Meniere's disease.

SURGICAL MANAGEMENT

Despite intensive medical therapy for patients with Meniere's disease, there are those who continue to experience attacks of vertigo that are frequent and severe enough to cause disability. Surgical management of Meniere's disease depends largely on the auditory function of the diseased ear and the age of the patient. Surgical procedures can be characterized as destructive and nondestructive of auditory function. For patients with useful hearing, an endolymphatic mastoid shunt is recommended. Although this operation is controversial, the long-term efficacy of this operation was demonstrated in a recent review. Young patients with no useful hearing are often managed with translabyrinthine vestibular nerve section.

Elderly patients with poor hearing and good vestibular function can be treated with cochleosacculotomy. For elderly patients with no useful hearing, a transcanal labyrinthectomy is performed. In those patients in whom endolymphatic mastoid shunt fails, although hearing remains useful, a retrolabyrinthine vestibular nerve section is recommended. This procedure has demonstrated success at alleviating the symptoms of vertigo in patients with Meniere's disease. The management of patients with no useful hearing who fail endolymphatic mastoid shunt is largely determined by their age. Younger patients are treated with translabyrinthine vestibular nerve section and elderly patients are treated with transcanal labyrinthectomy.

REHABILITATION AND FOLLOW-UP

Patients with Meniere's disease often develop long-term balance problems. Elderly patients who typically have limited central nervous system plasticity are at particular risk to develop chronic imbalance due to impaired central compensation. Referral to a physical therapy team for vestibular rehabilitation therapy can often help alleviate the chronic imbalance which can accompany this problem.

Due to the incidence of bilateral Meniere's disease, patients can experience recurrence of symptoms even after apparent successful medical and/or surgical therapy. Constant vigilance on the part of the patient as well as the physician can help detect the early occurrence of problems in the opposite ear so that early medical and/or surgical intervention can be considered.

SUGGESTED READINGS

Derebery MJ, Rao VS, Siglock TJ, Linthicum FH, Nelson RA. Meniere's disease: an immune complex-mediated illness? *Laryngoscope.* 1991;101(3):225–229.

Friedman RA, Nelson RA, Harris JP. Posterior fossa meningiomas intimately involved with the endolymphatic sac. *Am J Otol.* 1996;17:612–616.

Hallpike CS, Wright AJ. On the histological changes in the temporal bones of a case of Meniere's disease. *J. Laryngol Otol.* 1940;55:59–66.

Heffner DK. Low grade adenocarcinoma of probable endolymphatic sac origin. A clinicopathologic study of 20 cases. *Cancer.* 1989;64(11):2292–2302.

Hughes GB, Barna BP, Kinney SE, et al. Autoimmune endolymphatic hydrops: five year review. *Otolaryngol Head Neck Surg.* 1988;98(3):221–225.

Jahrsdoerfer RA, Cail WS, Cantrell RW. Endolymphatic duct obstruction from a jugular bulb diverticulum. *Ann Otol.* 1981;90:619–623.

Kinney WC, Nalepa N, Hugues GB, Kinney SE. Cochleosacculotomy for the treatment of Meniere's disease in the elderly patient. *Laryngoscope.* 1995;105(9, Part 1):934–937.

Linthicum FH, El-Rahman AGA. Hydrops due to syphilitic endolymphatic duct obliteration. *Laryngoscope.* 1987;97(5):568–574.

McElveen JT Jr, Shelton C, Hitselberger WE, Brackmann DE. Retrolabyrinthine vestibular neurectomy: a reevaluation. *Laryngoscope.* 1988;98(5):502–560.

Rockline RE. Production and assay of macrophage inhibitory factor. In: Rose NR, Friedman H, eds. *Manual of Clinical Immunology.* 2nd ed. Washington, DC: American Society for Microbiology; 1980;233.

Ruckenstein MJ, Cueva RA, Morrison DH, Press G. A prospective study of ABR and MRI screening for vestibular schwannomas. *Am J Otol.* 1996;17:317–320.

Shelton C, Harnsberger HR, Allen R, King B. Fast spin echo magnetic resonance imaging: clinical application in screening for acoustic neuroma. *Otolaryngol Head Neck Surg.* 1996;114(1):71–76.

Telischi FF, Luxford WM. Long term efficacy of endolymphatic sac surgery for vertigo in Meniere's disease. *Otolaryngol Head Surg.* 1993;109(1):83–87.

BENIGN PAROXYSMAL POSITIONAL VERTIGO

Rick A. Friedman, M.D.

HISTORY

A 45-year-old woman presents 3 months after a motor vehicle accident with complaints of dizziness. The dizziness was exacerbated when her head was turned to the right while lying in bed. It was also worsened by rising up from bed just prior to standing. Those symptoms have persisted, and now she feels unsteady with rapid head movement or while looking up or down. The episodes are described as true vertigo associated with nausea, vomiting, and diaphoresis, lasting approximately 2 to 3 minutes. She has no history of hearing loss or tinnitus. The remainder of her otologic history is unremarkable. Her review systems are unremarkable, including no other neurologic complaints.

Neurotologic examination included a normal microscopic exam of her ears and normal function of cranial nerves II through XII. There was no spontaneous nystagmus and her cerebellar examination was unremarkable. With the Frenzel glasses in place, a Dix–Hallpike maneuver was performed. The Dix–Hallpike maneuver with the left ear down revealed no symptoms or signs of vestibular dysfunction. The test was performed next with her head in the midline and again there were no symptoms or signs of vestibular dysfunction. Upon placement of the patient's head in the right ear down position, she developed geotropic rotatory nystagmus, which was delayed in onset. She displayed a crescendo/decrescendo pattern that resolved over a 20-second period. Upon repeat Dix–Hallpike testing with the right ear down, the symptoms recurred; however, the latency was longer and the duration of symptoms and signs was less (fatiguability).

DIFFERENTIAL DIAGNOSIS— KEY POINTS

The first step in the differential diagnosis of vestibular disorders is the delineation of a peripheral versus a central process, and this can often be done with physical examination and vestibular and auditory testing.

1. Benign paroxsysmal positional vertigo is characterized by the onset of disequilibrium in the supine position typically with the affected ear down. The pathophysiology is felt to be cupulolithiasis and/or canalithiasis. This patient's presentation is certainly consistent with this process.

2. Traumatic injury to the inner ear or commotio labyrinthi is a post-traumatic disorder thought to be associated with hemorrhage and membrane disruption of the inner ear that can be associated with dizziness and hearing loss.

3. Another possible etiology is vestibular neuritis from viral infection of the vestibular nerve. The dizziness, often true vertigo, is sudden and severe lasting for several days to weeks.

4. Toxic labyrinthitis often presents with auditory and vestibular symptoms usually in association with acute otitis media. Viral labyrinthitis can present in a similar manner and is differentiated from vestibular neuritis by the associated auditory symptoms and signs.

5. Suppurative labyrinthitis often presents with severe vestibular and auditory symptoms and in association with acute otitis media or meningitis.

6. Meniere's disease most typically presents with a history of fluctuating hearing loss,

roaring tinnitus, and episodic vertigo with associated aural fullness. There are, however, variants of Meniere's disease that can present with symptoms of the vestibular or auditory symptoms in isolation.

7. Perilymphatic fistula, a much debated entity in otolaryngology, is often associated with auditory and vestibular symptoms. Perilymphatic fistula should be suspected in patients with a clear history of physical trauma or barotrauma and the onset of symptoms immediately associated with those events.

8. Multiple sclerosis with demyelinating plaques of the vestibular nuclei can be associated with episodic vertigo.

9. Orthostatic hypotension is often described as a feeling of lightheadedness or giddiness associated with a change in posture. These patients rarely describe true vertigo.

10. Multisensory disequilibrium often found in the elderly is associated with peripheral neuropathy, visual failure, cerebellar degenerative disease, and vestibulopathy in any combination.

11. Acoustic neuroma most often presents with hearing loss and tinnitus; however, many patients present with vestibular complaints.

12. Inflammatory diseases of the inner ear including autoimmune and syphilitic labyrinthitis can present with auditory and vestibular symptoms.

13. Vertebrobasilar insufficiency or brain stem stroke often presents with symptoms of dizziness and vertigo.

14. Many commonly used prescription and nonprescription drugs can be associated with dizziness. These include alcohol, tranquilizers, antihypertensives, anticonvulsants, and aminoglycoside antibiotics.

15. Psychiatric illness is associated with a wide range of dizzy sensations. Acute anxiety, agoraphobia, and chronic anxiety may all be associated with complaints of dizziness.

16. Mal de debarquement syndrome is described as a persistent rocking sensation after disembarking from a boat, particularly after a long journey.

TEST INTERPRETATION

Behavioral and speech audiometry revealed normal behavioral thresholds and normal speech discrimination. Her acoustic reflexes were intact bilaterally.

Electronystagmogram revealed normal saccades, normal opticokinetic nystagmus, and no evidence of gaze nystagmus. Bithermal caloric testing revealed normal slow phase velocity in both ears. Dix–Hallpike testing revealed geotropic nystagmus in the right head down position and ageotropic nystagmus was noted upon rising to a sitting position.

DIAGNOSIS

Benign paroxsysmal position vertigo.

MEDICAL MANAGEMENT

fBy definition, this disease is paroxysmal and positional; hence, patients do not often require vestibular suppressant therapy. For those patients with severe disequilibrium, a variety of vestibular suppressants can be prescribed. Meclizine HCI, promethazine hydrochloride, and, if need be, diazepam are all useful medications for the suppression of vestibular symptoms in these patients. By and large, these patients respond to vestibular rehabilitation exercises. Cawthorne positional exercises have been proven effective in improving symptoms in patients with chronic vestibulopathy. Patients who do not respond to Cawthorne exercises or patients who desire immediate relief can be treated using a particle repositioning maneuver. Utilizing this maneuver, approximately 80 to 85% of patients are relieved of their symptoms after one treatment. When patients require a second treatment approximately 90% of patients are relieved of their positional vertigo. The vast majority of patients with benign positional vertigo will either resolve spontaneously or will resolve with conservative management. There are those patients, however, with persistent disease who require surgical intervention.

SURGICAL MANAGEMENT

Surgical management of benign paroxsysmal positional vertigo (BPV) involves deafferentation of the posterior semicircular canal while preserving hearing. Singular neurectomy, or disruption of the nerve to the posterior canal ampulla, has been demonstrated to be successful in treating patients with persistent BPV. More recently, a procedure of posterior canal occlusion has been described. This procedure involves exposure of the membranous posterior semicircular canal by a transmastoid approach. The membranous canal is then occluded by a variety of techniques, including obliteration of the perilymphatic space with materials including bone dust, fascia, or bone wax. The mechanical obliteration can be preceded by laser ablation of the endolymphatic space. Posterior canal occlusion has been shown to successfully relieve symptoms of BPV with little risk to auditory function.

REHABILITATION AND FOLLOW-UP

Although this condition is by definition a benign problem, even after successful management these symptoms can occasionally recur. In those instances where symptoms persist or recur it is important that the original diagnosis be reassessed and that the possibility of other underlying problems be excluded.

SUGGESTED READINGS

Gacek RR. Pathophysiology and management of cupulolithiasis. *Am J Otol.* 1985;6(2):66–74.

Parnes LS, McClure JA. Free floating endolymph particles: a new operative finding during posterior semicircular canal occlusion. *Laryngoscope.* 1992;102: 988–992.

Parnes LS, McClure JA. Posterior semicircular canal occlusion for intractable benign paroxysmal positional vertigo. *Ann Otol Rhinol Laryngol.* 1990;99(5, Part 1):330–334.

Semant A, Freyss G, Vitte E. Curing the BPPV with a liberatory maneuver. *Adv Otol Rhinol Laryngol.* 1988;42:290–293.

Shuknecht HF. Cupulolithiasis. *Arch Otol.* 1969;90: 113–126.

Shuknecht HF, Kitamura K. Second Louis H. Clerf lecture. Vestibular neuritis. *Ann Otol Rhinol Laryngol.* 1981;90(1, Part 2):1–19.

PERILYMPHATIC FISTULA

Rick A. Friedman, M.D.

HISTORY

The patient is a 14-year-old Caucasian female recently involved in a roll-over motor vehicle accident in which she was an unrestrained passenger. She was found on the scene with a Glasgow coma score of 13 and was noted to have bloody otorrhea emanating from her right ear. A complete workup by the trauma service revealed only a minor concussion with evidence of a temporal bone fracture identified on computed tomography (CT) scan of the head.

The otolaryngology service was consulted, and on the first day after the injury the patient was seen. She complained of hearing loss in the right ear and extreme dizziness. There was still obvious blood without cerebrospinal fluid (CSF) draining from the right ear. Inspection of her ear canal revealed a laceration of the canal and tympanic membrane. Her medical history, including history of otologic disease, was unremarkable.

Neuro-otologic examination revealed a Weber test that lateralized to the left ear. A Rinne test with a Barany masker in the contralateral ear revealed air conduction greater than bone conduction in the injured ear. Similar findings were found for the noninjured ear. Cranial nerve examination revealed intact cranial nerve function for cranial nerves I through XII except for cranial nerve VII due to the hearing loss. Of note also was a leftward beating nystagmus. Her Dix–Hallpike test was negative. She demonstrated normal cerebellar function. She had no long track signs on motor examination and her sensory function was intact to touch, pressure, pain, temperature, and joint position.

DIFFERENTIAL DIAGNOSIS

1. Temporal bone fracture is often associated with closed head injury. Blows to the side of the head often result in longitudinal fractures, whereas blows in the anterior-posterior direction often result in transverse fractures. The site of impact in this patient is unknown, so it is difficult from history to speculate as to the type of temporal bone fracture. Approximately 75% of temporal bone fractures are longitudinal. The other 25% are transverse. Longitudinal temporal bone fractures are often associated with visible laceration of the external canal and tympanic membrane and ossicular disruption. They are most often associated with conductive hearing loss. Secondary concussive forces can cause vertigo and sensorineural hearing loss on occasion. Transverse temporal bone fractures are more often associated with sensorineural hearing loss. Unilateral deafness and loss of vestibular function often result due to either a fracture through the internal auditory canal or directly through the otic capsule and inner ear.

2. Of all the topics in otology, perilymphatic fistula is one of the more controversial. Although no one disputes the existence of traumatic perilymphatic fistulae, there is much debate over the existence of spontaneous perilymphatic fistulae or sudden hearing loss associated with perilymphatic fistulae. Traumatic perilymphatic fistulae often result from subluxation of the stapedial footplate and appear to be more common in children. Subluxation of the stapes often results in mixed hearing loss, often with a severe to profound sensory loss. Patients with subluxation of the stapes footplate often experience intense vertigo. Perilymphatic fistulae have been described to occur either from an explosive phenomenon with increased intracranial pressure creating a communication between the inner and middle ears, or an implosive phenomenon, with elevated atmospheric pressure resulting in an inward displacement of the membranes of the inner ear and communication between the inner ear and the middle ear. The existence of spontaneous per-

ilymphatic fistulae resulting from anatomic defects of the inner ear leading to communication of the perilymphatic space with the middle ear has been described.

Many authors feel that the area of the fissula antefenestrum or a fissure identified between the ampula of the posterior canal and the round window niche provides routes for leakage of perilymph.

TEST INTERPRETATION

Further exploration for the cause of this patient's auditory and vestibular symptoms is warranted because on physical examination she was identified to have left beating nystagmus and a positive Rinne test.

- *Behavioral audiogram.* Behavioral audiometry revealed a high-frequency profound sensorineural hearing loss. There was some preservation of the lower frequencies up to approximately 1000 Hz. In the low-frequency region a mixed loss was noted. Her speech reception threshold was approximately 65 dB in the injured ear and her speech discrimination was 64%.
- *Electronystagmography (ENG).* ENG testing revealed spontaneous beating nystagmus; no calorics were obtained.
- *Radiography.* Fistula testing can be useful but may be difficult in patients with severe temporal bone trauma. High-resolution CT scan of the temporal bones, which included 1.5-mm sections, both coronal and axial, revealed a longitudinal fracture of the temporal bone extending anterior to the otic capsule. Of note was a small air bubble in the vestibule, called pneumolabyrinth. This was highly suggestive of stapes subluxation. The soft tissue of the middle ear obscured an adequate view of the oval window niche on CT.

DIAGNOSIS

Traumatic subluxation of the stapes.

MEDICAL MANAGEMENT

Although this patient's vertigo improved with intravenous diazepam, many feel that the sun should never rise or set on a subluxed stapes.

It was elected to take this patient to the operating room for exploratory tympanotomy and possible repair of perilymphatic fistula and tympanic membrane perforation.

SURGICAL MANAGEMENT

The procedure involved a postauricular tympanoplasty and repair of traumatic perilymphatic fistula. The postauricular approach with a lateral graft technique for repair of the eardrum was chosen as the operator's procedure of choice. Exploration of the middle ear revealed a posteriorly subluxed and dislocated incus with posterior subluxation of the stapedial footplate with a perilymphatic fistula in the region of the anterior footplate. The footplate was gently rocked into place and the annular ligament was covered with temporalis fascia cut into thin strips. Using the remaining temporalis fasciae, tympanic membrane was fashioned medial to the malleus and the incus was removed. Postoperatively, the patient demonstrated a maximum conductive hearing loss in the low tones with preservation of low-frequency hearing, but no resolution of the high-frequency profound loss. The patient's dizziness was resolved within days of surgery.

REHABILITATION AND FOLLOW-UP

This patient may benefit from the placement of an incus replacement prosthesis or a partial ossicular reconstructive prosthesis at a later date. Furthermore, this patient may benefit from some low-frequency amplification.

SUGGESTED READINGS

CANNON CR, JAHRSDOERFER RA. Temporal bone fractures. *Arch Otol.* 1983;109:285–288.

ELBROND I, HASTRUP JE. Isolated fractures of the stapedial arch. *Acta Otolaryngol.* 1973;75:357–358.

GOODHILL V. Leaking labyrinth lesions, deafness, tinnitus and dizziness. *Ann Otol.* 1981;90:99–106.

KOHUT RI, HINOJOSA R, THOMPSON JN, RYU JH. Idiopathic perilymphatic fistulas. *Arch Otolaryngol Head Neck Surg.* 1995;121:412–420.

Case 14

FACIAL NERVE NEUROMA

Myles L. Pensak, M.D.

HISTORY

A 47-year-old patient is referred with a 9-month antedating history of slowly progressive facial paresis. The patient denies a history of otologic/neuro-otologic infection or trauma. Concomitant to the aforementioned has been the sense of degradation in auditory acuity during the previous 2 years, and a mild sense of aural fullness. The remaining portion of the otorhinologic history is noncontributory.

Physical examination reveals a well-developed, well-nourished female in no acute distress. The external auditory canal on the right side is benign, the tympanic membrane normal. The contralateral ear suggests a pink soft tissue mass in the posterior/superior quadrant; the remaining portion of the mesotympanic space is unremarkable. The facial nerve examination on the right side demonstrates a House–Brackmann grade I/VI normal mimetic response, and on the left side a facial asymmetry is noted, House–Brackmann IV/VI. The remaining portion of the patient's neurologic examination is unremarkable.

DIFFERENTIAL DIAGNOSIS— KEY POINTS

1. The differential diagnosis of the aforementioned lesion would include meningioma, adenoma, adenocarcinoma, facial neuroma, glomus tumor, and trigeminal nerve schwannoma.

2. Bell's palsy or idiopathic facial paralysis is a diagnosis of exclusion. Not infrequently the patient will report an antedating history of viral upper respiratory infection. The paralysis is often paroxysmal in onset, with the patient reporting a sense of weakness in facial mimetic function or asymmetry one day only to awaken the next day with a facial paralysis. Most patients with Bell's palsy will have an uneventful recovery; however, a small number of individuals will have an unfavorable outcome. The management remains controversial. Steroids and acyclovir are popular medical regimens while surgery is recommended by some for patients demonstrating poor prognosis on electrophysiologic studies including electromyography (EMG) and EN_OG.

3. The House–Brackmann scale (Table 14–1) is often utilized in the description of facial mimetic dysfunction.

4. Electrophysiologic tests cannot distinguish among the various degrees of nerve injury, but aim to identify the degree of neural degeneration.

1°—neuropraxia	4°—perineural disruption
2°—axontemesis	5°—epineural disruption
3°—neurotemesis	6°—fascicle disruption

   Currently most neuro-otologists do not employ the MET (minimal nerve excitability test) or the MST (maximal stimulation test). Most recently, electromyography (EMG, EEMG, or EN_OG) have been advocated. The EMG will identify voluntary motor potentials even in a clinically paralyzed face. Second, the

TABLE 14-1   The House–Brackmann Scale

Grade	Description	Characteristics
I	Normal	Normal facial function in all areas

II	Mild dysfunction	*Gross:* slight weakness noticeable on close inspection; may have very slight synkinesis
		At rest: normal symmetry and tone
		Motion
		    Forehead: moderate to good
		    Eye: complete closure with minimum effort
		    Mouth: slight asymmetry

III	Moderate dysfunction	*Gross:* obvious but not disfiguring difference between two sides; noticeable but not severe synkinesis, contracture, and/or hemifacial spasm
		At rest: normal symmetry and tone
		Motion
		    Forehead: slight to moderate movement
		    Eye: complete closure with effort
		    Mouth: slightly weak and maximum effort

IV	Moderate severe dysfunction	*Gross:* obvious weakness and/or disfiguring asymmetry
		At rest: normal symmetry and tone
		Motion
		    Forehead: none
		    Eye: incomplete closure
		    Mouth: asymmetric with maximum effort

V	Severe dysfunction	*Gross:* only barely perceptible motion
		At rest: asymmetry
		Motion
		    Forehead: none
		    Eye: incomplete closure
		    Mouth: slight movement

VI	Total paralysis	No movement

Adapted from House JW, Brackmann DE. Facial nerve grading system. *Otolaryngol Head Neck Surg.* 1985;93:146–147.

EMG will demonstrate findings consistent with denervation potentials between days 10 and 21 following the onset of paralysis.

EEMG or EN_oG loss of potential reflects the degree of degeneration when compared to the normal side. The test is most reliable when performed within the first 2 weeks following paralysis. Repeat EN_oG degeneration loss of greater than 95% portends the possibility of a poor prognosis.

TEST INTERPRETATION

An audiogram is performed and magnetic resonance imaging (MRI) ordered. The patient undergoes audiometric studies that demonstrate normal hearing in the right ear and a 50-dB conductive hearing loss in the left (Fig. 14–1). Acoustic reflexes are absent on the left side; they are present on the right with ipsilateral and stimulation. Gadolinium-enhanced MRI scanning is undertaken (Fig. 14–2). A large tumor mass is noted on the floor of the middle cranial fossa, extending in continuity into the epitympanum and mesotympanic space. The mass is enhancing, and assessment reveals no evidence of enhancement in the labyrinthine segment of the facial nerve, nor in the mastoid segment.

DIAGNOSIS

Facial nerve neuroma.

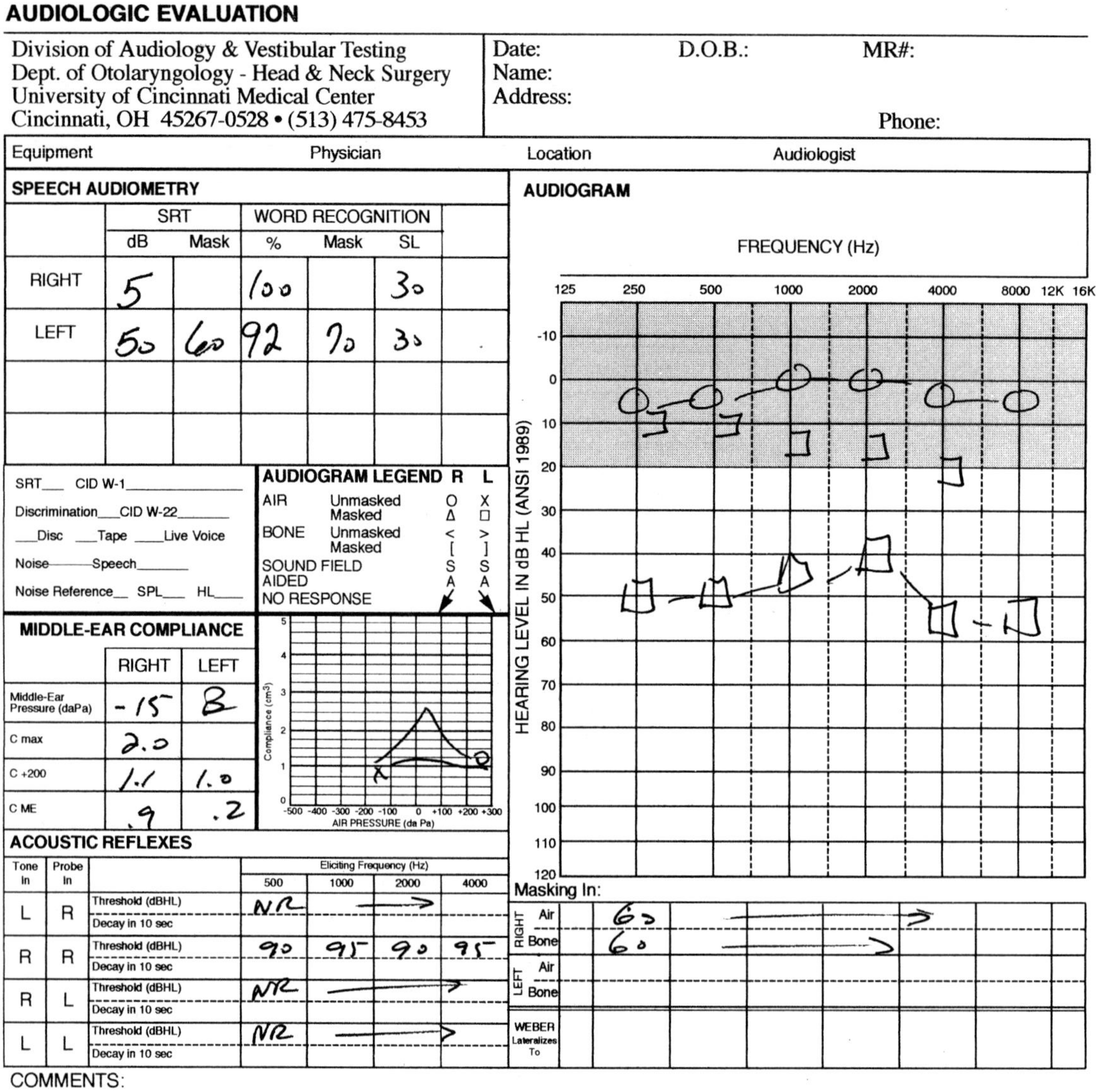

AUDIOLOGIC EVALUATION

Division of Audiology & Vestibular Testing Dept. of Otolaryngology - Head & Neck Surgery University of Cincinnati Medical Center Cincinnati, OH 45267-0528 • (513) 475-8453	Date: Name: Address:	D.O.B.:	MR#: Phone:

Equipment	Physician	Location	Audiologist

SPEECH AUDIOMETRY

	SRT		WORD RECOGNITION		
	dB	Mask	%	Mask	SL
RIGHT	5		100		30
LEFT	50	60	92	70	30

SRT___ CID W-1_____

Discrimination___CID W-22_____

___Disc ___Tape ___Live Voice

Noise_____Speech_____

Noise Reference__ SPL___ HL___

AUDIOGRAM LEGEND

		R	L
AIR	Unmasked	O	X
	Masked	Δ	□
BONE	Unmasked	<	>
	Masked	[	]
SOUND FIELD		S	S
AIDED		A	A
NO RESPONSE		↘	↙

AUDIOGRAM

FREQUENCY (Hz)

MIDDLE-EAR COMPLIANCE

	RIGHT	LEFT
Middle-Ear Pressure (daPa)	-15	B
C max	2.0	
C +200	1.1	1.0
C ME	.9	.2

ACOUSTIC REFLEXES

Tone in	Probe in		Eliciting Frequency (Hz)			
			500	1000	2000	4000
L	R	Threshold (dBHL)	NR	→		
		Decay in 10 sec				
R	R	Threshold (dBHL)	90	95	90	95
		Decay in 10 sec				
R	L	Threshold (dBHL)	NR	→		
		Decay in 10 sec				
L	L	Threshold (dBHL)	NR	→		
		Decay in 10 sec				

Masking In:

RIGHT	Air	65				→	
	Bone	60				→	
LEFT	Air						
	Bone						
WEBER Lateralizes To							

COMMENTS:

FIGURE 14–1 Audiogram demonstrates normal hearing in the right ear and a 50 dB conductive hearing loss in the left.

MEDICAL MANAGEMENT

In discussing management options with the patient, gamma knife radiosurgery should be considered, as well as surgical extirpation. It is important that the patient be counseled to the fact that, while it is possible for the tumor to be excised without sacrifice of the facial nerve, should there be marked tumor infiltration and/or a skip lesion identified with a facial nerve tumor, the nerve would need to be sacrificed and a graft required.

Should the patient opt not to undergo surgical intervention and undergo radiation or elect for surgery, eye protection is very important. The patient should be counseled to wear sunglasses when outside or a protective bubble or patch to avoid corneal trauma. Moreover, natural tears and lubricant should keep the eye moist.

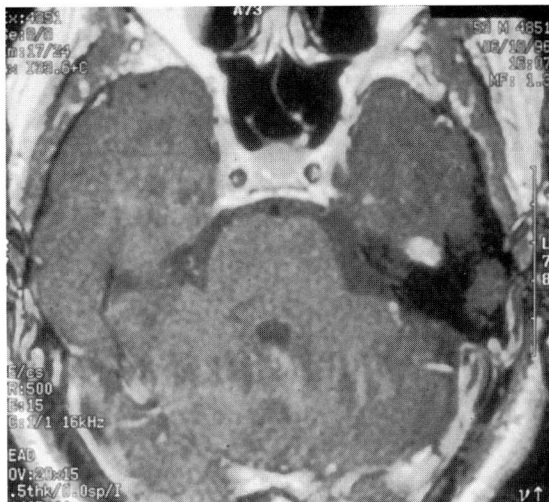

FIGURE 14-2 Gadolinium-enhanced MRI demonstrates a large tumor mass on the floor of the middle cranial fossa, extending into the epitympanum and mesotympanic space.

craniotomy is performed, and the tumor mass is mobilized from the floor of the middle fossa. The geniculate ganglion region is dissected, the labyrinthine segment of the facial nerve is intact, and the nerve is now followed through the first genu with tumor being mobilized from the epitympanic region where it has enveloped and destroyed the ossicular head across the semicanal into the proximal portion of the protympanic space. Total tumor removal is accomplished, and the facial nerve is preserved.

Preparation during the course of this case would require that the patient be prepared for either a greater auricular or sural cable graft. Other options would include a delayed VII–XII anastomosis if the proximal stump of the nerve could not be satisfactorily prepared for receiving a graft, as would be the case if the tumor extended into the cerebellopontine angle through the root entry zone of the facial nerve at the brain stem.

SURGICAL MANAGEMENT

Should the patient elect for surgical intervention, while she does have a substantial conductive hearing loss, the sensorineural thresholds are normal and, therefore, a combined transmastoid middle fossa approach is warranted to optimize the preservation of sensorineural thresholds.

An extended postauricular middle fossa dissection is undertaken, transmastoid exploration identifies the facial nerve in its vertical segment, the facial recess is opened and an extended facial recess is performed. The tumor encountered fills the mesotympanic space, and the posterior canal wall is removed. Dissection in the middle ear reveals that the incudostapedial joint and suprastructure of the stapes have been eroded, the tumor mass is separated and the drum and remaining portions of canal skin are likewise removed as a two-layered canal closure is undertaken. For smaller tumors reconstruction of the ossicular chain would be most appropriate. The facial nerve is identified in the mesotympanic space and is noted to be uncovered by bone from the second genu to the cochleariformis process. Active stimulation with the facial nerve probe demonstrates good response. A temporal

REHABILITATION AND FOLLOW-UP

Temporizing measures in cases wherein the facial nerve is taken would include the placement of a gold weight and the possible use of early static reanimation with a Gortex® sling. Important to the overall strategy and management of this patient would be the protection of the eye. From a rehabilitative perspective a regimen course of facial mimetic exercises should be undertaken early in the perioperative period.

SUGGESTED READINGS

BRADFORD C. Facial reanimation. *Curr Opin Otolaryngol Head Neck Surg.* 1994;2:369–374.

HOUSE JW, BRACKMANN DE. Facial nerve grading system. *Otolaryngol Head Neck Surg.* 1985;93:146–147.

JANECKA IP, CONLEY J. Primary neoplasms of the facial nerve. *Plast Reconstr Surg.* 1987;79:177–183.

JUNG TTK, JON B, SHEA D, et al. Primary and secondary tumors of the facial nerve. A temporal bone study. *Arch Otolaryngol Head Neck Surg.* 1986;112:1269–1273.

KARTUSH JM, LINSTROM CJ. Early gold weight eyelid implantation for facial paralysis. *Arch Otolaryngol Head Neck Surg.* 1990;103:1016–1023.

MAY M. Surgical rehabilitation of facial palsy total approach. In: May M, ed. *The Facial Nerve.* New York: Thieme; 1986:695–777.

O'DONOGHUE GM, BRACKMANN DE, HOUSE JW, et al. Neuromas of the facial nerve. *Am J Otol.* 1989;10: 49–54.

O'DONOGHUE GM. Tumors of the facial nerve. In: Jackler RK, Brackmann DE eds. *Neurotology.* St. Louis, MO: Mosby-Year Book; 1994:1321–1331.

PARNES LS et al. Magnetic resonance imaging of facial neuromas. *Laryngoscope.* 1991;101:31–35.

SHUMRICK KA. Facial reanimation. In: Hughes GB, Pensak ML, eds. *Clinical Otology.* 2nd ed. New York, Thieme; 1997:417–433.

BELL'S PALSY

Myles L. Pensak, M.D.

HISTORY

A 26-year-old male presents with a 48-hour history of rapidly progressive loss of function of the right side of his face. The patient reports an antedating history of URI and viral associated rhinosinusitis and sinonasal tract congestion. In addition, the patient states that several coworkers have been out with flu-like symptoms.

The patient denies an antedating history of otologic or neurotologic infection or trauma.

Physical examination reveals a well-developed male in no acute distress. The facial nerve on the right side is paralyzed, demonstrating a House–Brackmann grade VI/VI absence of mimetic function. Contralateral facial response is normal. The external auditory canals and tympanic membranes are clear. In particular, there is no evidence of auricular vesicular eruption. The head and neck examination is, likewise, unremarkable and the remaining portions of the patient's exam are benign.

Pertinent history reveals that the patient has not been exposed to toxins, nor has he been traveling recently, in particular, to tick-infested locales.

DIFFERENTIAL DIAGNOSIS— KEY POINTS

Without an antedating history of otologic or neuro-otologic infection or trauma, paroxysmal onset of facial paralysis is uncommon. Included among the entities that need to be differentiated from Bell's palsy are (1) herpes zoster oticus and (2) facial neuroma or other cerebellopontine angle lesions including acoustic neuroma, meningioma, lipoma, or unusually large lesions associated with either the trigeminal nerve or the lower cranial nerves of the jugular foramen. Paragangliomas, including glomus tympanicum and jugulare tumors, while known to cause facial paralysis rarely do so in the absence of concomitant pathology.

In a pediatric population, congenital disorders such as hemifacial mycrosomia, Mobius syndrome, and virally induced paresis need to be considered. Other disorders that have been associated with facial paralysis include osteopetrosus (Albers–Shoenberg's disease and Mechelson–Rosenthal syndrome). Inflammatory processes including, but not limited to, acute and chronic otitis media with and without cholesteatoma uncommonly manifest with facial palsy. Lyme disease has also been associated with facial paralysis.

TEST INTERPRETATION

The utilization of facial nerve testing has been controversial. Earlier enthusiastic utilization of the minimal nerve excitability test (MET) employing the Hilger® nerve stimulator, as well as that of the maximal stimulation test (MST), have not been uniformly accepted. Most recently, evoked electromyography (EEMG) or electroneuronograpy (EN_0G) has gained increased favor. Currently, in many practices, EN_0G beginning 72 hours after the initial onset of facial palsy has been employed to follow serially the degree of degeneration manifesting. In general, denervation of less than 90% has been uniformly accepted as indicative of anticipating an excellent recovery. When the degeneration occurs at a degree greater than 95%, the degree of recovery is unpredictable. Concomitant use of EMG, wherein motor unit potentials may be demonstrated, should correlate with good recovery. The opposite, however, is a poor prognostic indicator. EEMG or EN_0G employed at greater than 3 weeks period of time appears to be of little value. The utilization of gadolinium-enhanced magnetic response imaging (MRI) for Bell's palsy appears to play little role in the overall clinical management of the patient with a facial paralysis. Although an MRI scan can differentiate between Bell's palsy and facial neuroma, the clinical history should obviate the need for this costly study. In cases of Bell's palsy, enhancement along the course of the nerve has been demonstrated to a variable degree.

DIAGNOSIS

Bell's palsy.

MEDICAL MANAGEMENT

Bell's palsy is an idiopathic facial paralysis presumed to be due to viral inflammation of the facial nerve. Although a series of studies has been performed over the years regarding the efficacy of a variety of modalities for treatment, statistically based evidence is currently unavailable to indicate whether any particular form of treatment is truly efficacious.

It is generally felt that the utilization of prednisone early in the treatment with the concomitant employment of acyclovir will minimize virally induced edema, in particular, when dealing with a palsy due to herpes zoster oticus.

During the course of management of the patient with Bell's palsy, it is imperative that the patient be instructed in the utilization of eye care. An ocular lubricant and natural tears are applied on a regular basis, the eye should be patched and covered at nighttime, and during the daytime when the patient is out in the ambient environment, protection with either a sealed bubble pack or glasses will minimize the possibility of dust or wind causing corneal irritation.

Although to date no studies have demonstrated the efficacy and validity of the utilization of a formal facial mimetic exercise program, this has been employed with great satisfaction by a number of patients.

SURGICAL MANAGEMENT

The utilization of surgery for Bell's palsy remains controversial. Several centers perform serial electroneuronography. In patients in whom there is a degeneration of nerve action potentials greater than 95% or absence of EMG response, surgical decompression is offered. To date, there are no statistically based, blinded studies that demonstrate the efficacy of surgical intervention. The vast majority of patients with Bell's palsy improve. A small percentage, while improved, will maintain a poor return of mimetic function.

For patients electing to undergo facial nerve decompression, a total facial nerve decompression is advocated. Although it has, in fact, been demonstrated that the area of the labyrinthine segment reflects the region of most physical limitation within the fallopian canal, enhancement of the nerve can be found at all levels. A transmastoid facial recess approach is employed to follow the nerve from the stylomastoid foramen to its tympanic segment. To optimize visualization of the nerve in a contracted space, the incus may be removed, the fossa incudes taken down, and the facial nerve followed to the level of the cochleariformis process. At the conclusion of the procedure interposition ossiculoplasty is to be performed. At this point a middle fossa approach is employed wherein the facial nerve is identified at the first genu followed cephalically to the geniculate ganglion through the labyrinthine segment and into the distal portion of the internal auditory canal. At the conclusion of the procedure, if the dura of the canal has been violated, a small muscle plug is employed to control cerebrospinal fluid leakage.

REHABILITATION AND FOLLOW-UP

A patient who has a Bell's palsy that shows no evidence of resolution in a month to 6 weeks should undergo gadolinium-enhanced MRI scanning to rule out the possibility of tumor as the etiology. Note, however, that cerebellopontine angle lesions, in particular, meningiomas and acoustic neuromas, rarely cause the paroxysmal loss of facial mimetic function.

SELECTED READINGS

Adour KK. Bell's palsy treatment with acyclovir and prednisone compared with prednisone alone. *Ann Otol Rhinol Laryngol.* 1996;105:(5)371–378.

Adour KK. Medical management of idiopathic (Bell's) palsy. *Otolaryngol Clin North Am.* 1991;24(3): 663–673.

ADOUR KK et al. The true nature of Bell's palsy. Analysis of 1,000 conservative patients. *Laryngoscope.* 1978; 88:787–811.

DICKENS JRE, SMITH JT, GRAHAM S. Herpes zoster oticus: treatment with intravenous acyclovir. *Laryngoscope.* 1988;98:776–779.

FISCH U. Surgery for Bell's palsy. *Arch Otol.* 1981; 107:1–11.

GANTZ BJ. Idiopathic facial paralysis. *Curr Ther Otolaryngol Head Neck Surg.* 1987;3:62–66.

HOUSE JW, BRACKMANN DE. Facial nerve grading system. *Otolaryngol Head Neck Surg.* 1985;93:146–147.

MAY M. Facial nerve disorders: update 1982. *Am J Otol.* 1982;4:77–88.

MAY M, KLEIN SR, TAYLOR FH. Idiopathic (Bell's) facial palsy: natural history defies steroid or surgical treatment. *Laryngoscope.* 1985;95:406–409.

OROBELLO P. Congenital and acquired facial nerve paralysis with children. *Otolaryngol Clin North Am.* 1991;24(3):647–652.

IATROGENIC FACIAL PALSY

Myles L. Pensak, M.D.

HISTORY

A 17-year-old student is brought to the operating room for the surgical management of chronic otitis with cholesteatoma. During the course of surgery, the patient is found to have dense cholesteatoma matrix enveloping the mesotympanic space. The incudostapedial joint has been destroyed and a marked scutal erosion is encountered. The surgeon performs a canal wall-up tympanomastoidectomy and reports scraping the cholesteatoma from the middle ear space. No note is made as to whether the facial nerve is dehiscent in the middle ear; however, the surgeon reports that he did not directly visualize the nerve. Upon awakening from surgery, the patient is noted to have a dense facial paralysis.

DIFFERENTIAL DIAGNOSIS– KEY POINTS

1. Iatrogenic facial palsy is an uncommon but serious complication of otologic surgery. Immediate possibilities would include the persistence of topical anesthetic, which may have affected the nerve at the onset of surgery when canal injections were made, and/or packing, which may be occluding the region around the facial nerve. Removal of the mastoid dressing and evacuation of the packing should be done promptly.

2. Following several hours, if there has been no return of facial function, the patient should be brought to the operating room for immediate exploration of the facial nerve.

3. The injury sites most commonly encountered in iatrogenic facial palsy because of chronic ear surgery (not related to tumor extirpation of cerebellopontine angle lesions) are well described. Because the direction of the nerve is changing from the vertical to the horizontal plane, the region of the second genu of the nerve is bound to be disrupted prior to completing the turn into the middle ear. A secondary location for injury is in the tympanic segment. The nerve may be naturally dehiscent, or due to chronic ear disease and cholesteatoma the fallopian canal may have been eroded with the nerve exposed. Finally, disease that lies in the anterior epitympanic space may put the facial nerve at risk in the region of the first genu distal to the geniculate ganglion. Optimal exposure by removing the incus and the malleolar head, as well as taking down the cog, may lessen the likelihood of injury.

TEST INTERPRETATION

None.

DIAGNOSIS

Postoperative facial nerve paralysis. The diagnosis of postoperative facial paralysis is made by observation; a complete facial palsy requires no neuroradiographic or electrophysiologic studies. A partial weakness or a delayed-onset lesion should be followed as would a Bell's palsy.

MEDICAL MANAGEMENT

Steroids are employed to mollify edema and swelling and should the paresis go on to a full paralysis (delayed) serial electroneuronography (EN_OG) is followed. If the nerve degenerates to greater than 95%, surgical reexploration should be considered.

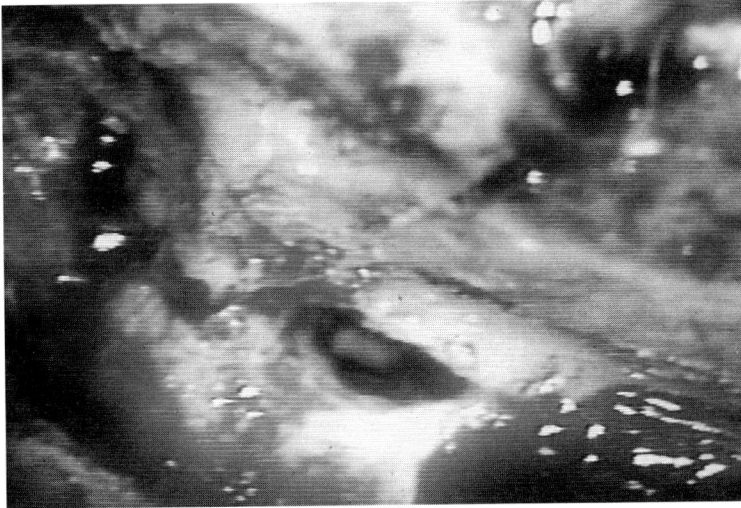

FIGURE 16-1 The facial nerve is noted to be violated in the horizontal (tympanic) segment.

SURGICAL MANAGEMENT

Upon return to the operating room, with a bone conduction audiogram done to ensure preservation of sensorineural thresholds, the field should be prepared for possible exploration to the geniculate region. This would imply a middle fossa exposure although it is possible to reach the region in a well-pneumatized bone via the mastoid route.

The dissection would include identification of the facial nerve in its vertical segment, opening up of the facial recess, and full tympanic exposure of the facial nerve (Fig. 16-1). If the nerve is noted to be intact and hyperemic, a decompression both proximally and distally should be done. If the nerve has been partially severed, but remains intact for the majority of its diameter, the edges should be freshened and the nerve coapted. If the nerve has been transected, the nerve should be mobilized from the fallopian canal, the edges freshened and the nerve approximated. If approximation cannot be done in a tension-free fashion, then a short cable graft should be placed.

REHABILITATION AND FOLLOW-UP

As with Bell's palsy, ocular care is important, and facial mimetic exercises should be instituted in the postoperative period.

Facial paralysis is a recognized potential complication of otic surgery. The single most important caveat when operating in the temporal bone with regards to the facial nerve is that the patient and family are well versed and informed prior to any surgical procedure regarding the potential for injury to the nerve. Should an untoward event occur, it is imperative that the surgeon discuss with the patient and/or responsible family member the nature of the injury and the need for immediate management. Under no circumstances should the surgeon provide any information to the family that is not direct, clear, and forthright. Reexploration is often attended to with a high degree of anxiety and stress, not only on the part of the patient and family, but by the operating surgeon. If the circumstances allow, a colleague with more experience should either perform the surgery or accompany the operating surgeon during the reexploration. If circumstances do not allow this to take place, the surgeon is certainly at liberty to refer the patient to a regional or national expert for care.

SUGGESTED READINGS

BEAUCHAMP ML, KEMINK JL. Facial paralysis complicating iontophoresis of the tympanic membrane. *Am J Otol.* 1982;4:93–94.

COKER N, KENDALL K, JENKINS A, et al. Traumatic intratemporal facial nerve injury: management rationale for preservation of function. *Otolaryngol Head Neck Surg.* 1987;97:262.

GLASSCOCK ME, SHAMBAUGH GE JR. *Surgery of the Ear.* 4th ed. Philadelphia, PA: WB Saunders; 1990.

MAY M. *The Facial Nerve.* New York: Thieme-Stratton; 1986.

MCCABE B. Facial nerve grafting. *Plast Reconstr Surg.* 1975;45:70.

NADOL JB JR, SCHUKNECHT HF. *Surgery of the Ear and Temporal Bone.* New York: Raven Press; 1993.

SHUMRICK KA. Facial reanimation. In: Hughes GB, Pensak ML, eds. *Clinical Otology.* 2nd ed. New York: Thieme;1997:417–433.

SUNDERLAND S, ed. *Nerve and Nerve Injuries.* Edinburgh: E&S Livingstone; 1968:31–60, 263–273.

HEAD AND NECK

Case 17

STOMAL RECURRENCE Jack L. Gluckman, M.D.

HISTORY

A 52-year-old male recites a history of having undergone a total laryngectomy and left modified radical neck dissection for a T_3N_1 left transglottic squamous cell cancer. This was followed by postoperative radiation. He did extremely well; however, 14 months later he presents with a noticeable decrease in size of the lumen of the tracheostoma and peristomal granulation tissue. He is otherwise generally well and specifically there is no history of dyspnea and dysphagia. Other than a long-standing history of smoking, there is no medical history of note.

Examination revealed a generally fit patient with evidence of a total laryngectomy and neck dissection. The stoma was narrowed and surrounded by proliferative tissue, which bled easily to the touch. There was a significant subcutaneous mass present in the left parastomal area (Fig. 17–1).

DIFFERENTIAL DIAGNOSIS— KEY POINTS

1. Crusting and granulations at the tracheostoma can occur particularly if there is exposed cartilage or the patient is not diligent regarding stoma care. However, the *new* development of these findings is highly suggestive of stomal recurrence of the cancer.

2. Knowledge of the site and size of the original cancer and the manner in which it was treated may give a clue as to why the patient developed a stomal recurrence. Subglottic extension and involvement of the cervical esophagus may predispose to inadequate excision or the development of paratracheal nodal me-

tastases, which increase the incidence of stomal recurrence.

A preoperative emergency tracheostomy in the past was thought to be a predisposing factor, probably due to seeding; however, today the belief is that the advanced nature of the laryngeal cancer needing the tracheostomy is more likely to be the causative factor.

TEST INTERPRETATION

- First, a biopsy needs to be taken to confirm the diagnosis. If the lesion is subcutaneous, a fine-needle aspiration biopsy or open biopsy should be obtained.

- Once the stomal recurrence has been diagnosed, the extent of the recurrence needs to be determined because this will dictate the therapeutic options available to the patient.

- A computed tomography (CT) scan of neck and chest will delineate the gross extent plus whether there are any associated superior mediastinal nodal metastases. In this case, a significant subcutaneous mass confined to the left lateral aspect of the stoma was noted (Fig. 17–2).

- A full metastatic workup should always be performed as a prelude to further investigation. Ideally this should consist of a CT scan of the chest and abdomen, and a bone scan. The reason is that if there are distant metastases, further workup designed to determine whether resection is feasible is moot. In this case it was negative.

- At this stage the patient should undergo endoscopy. Esophagoscopy will reveal whether the esophagus is involved and the extent of this

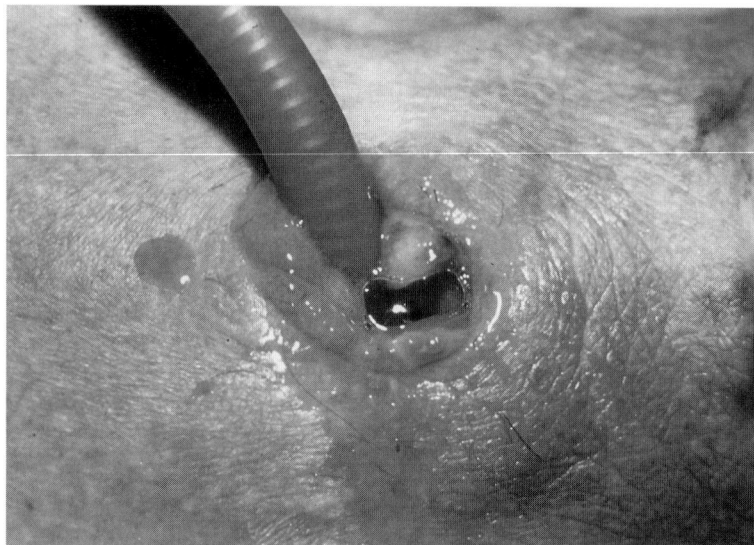

FIGURE 17-1 Stoma with surrounding proliferative tissue.

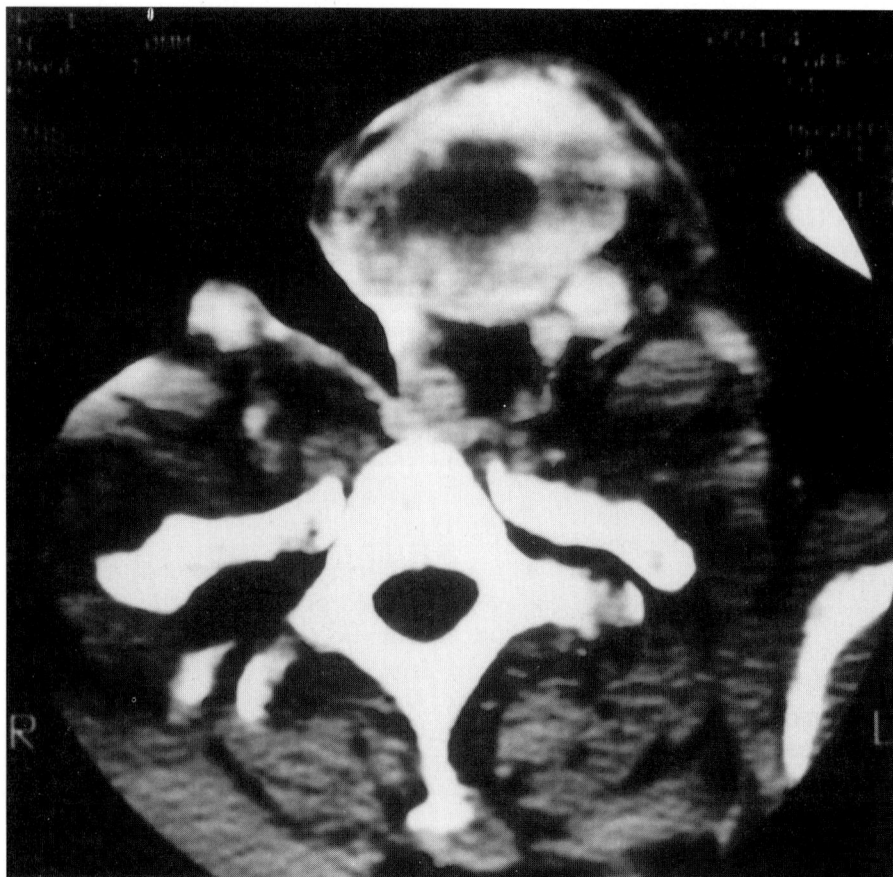

FIGURE 17-2 CT scan delineating parastomal recurrence.

involvement. This will determine how much esophagus to resect and the reconstructive approach. Bronchoscopy will determine the mucosal involvement of the trachea, which is not obvious on CT scan. In this case the esophagus appeared free but the tracheal involvement extended to almost 2 cm from the carina.

DIAGNOSIS

Type III, stomal recurrence.

MEDICAL MANAGEMENT

Because these patients' situations are often complicated by numerous underlying medical conditions including pulmonary disease, coronary vascular disease, and malnutrition, optimization of medical status is very important prior to instituting definitive therapy. Adjuvant therapy with a head and neck cancer chemotherapy protocol or radiation therapy can often provide palliation for patients with unresectable disease.

SURGICAL MANAGEMENT

Stomal recurrence is classified into four types:

I. Localized to superior aspect of stoma. No esophageal involvement.

II. Localized to superior aspect of stoma with esophageal involvement.

III. Originates from inferior aspect of stoma and involves upper portion of superior mediastinum.

IV. Extensive superior mediastinal involvement

The only treatment with any success is wide excision. This usually consists of resection of the tracheastoma, cervical esophagus, skin, manubrium, and clavicular heads. Reconstruction usually consists of using jejunum or gastric pull-up and coverage of the exposed superior mediastinal vessels with muscle and a regional flap for skin coverage. Types I and II can be resected

with minimal morbidity and a fair chance of success (20–30%). Type III can only be resected under ideal circumstances, and type IV is incurable with an unacceptable surgical morbidity in the perioperative period.

For these reasons, careful delineation of the extent of the lesion is necessary before offering the patient the option of surgery. If doubt exists, as to the extent intraoperative exploration may be needed with the procedure aborted if involvement of prevertebral musculature, great vessels, etc., is encountered.

Palliative treatment including placement of a G-tube, tracheostomy tube, and analgesics is a reasonable alternative. Death is usually from vessel rupture.

This patient is not a candidate for surgical resection because of extensive tracheal involvement, which would not permit mobilization of the residual trachea to the skin.

REHABILITATION AND FOLLOW-UP

In cases that are unresectable (most type III and all type IV lesions), long-term management should include psychosocial support and palliative measures to maintain the comfort of the patient as much as possible. In those cases where surgical therapy has been undertaken, long-term surveillance for a local, as well as distant and regional, recurrence of carcinoma is very important. Because the trachea is often very short and the stoma difficult to maintain, particular care is often required postoperatively for adequate humidification, cleaning, and maintenance of stomal patency.

SUGGESTED READINGS

GLUCKMAN JL, HAMAKER R, SCHULLER DE, et al. Surgical salvage for stomal recurrence: a multi-institutional experience. *Laryngoscope.* 1987;97:1025–1029.

KRESPI YP, WURSTER C, SISSION GA. Immediate reconstruction after total laryngopharyngoesophagectomy and mediastinal dissection. *Laryngoscope.* 1985;95: 156–161.

FIELD CANCERIZATION

Jack L. Gluckman, M.D.

HISTORY

A 62-year-old female presents with a 40-year history of tobacco abuse and a long-standing sore mouth that has increased in severity during the past year. She denies any significant alcohol abuse, and other than hypertension, has been well.

Examination revealed a generally fit, well-nourished individual with evidence of marked leukoplakia and erythroplakia involving the soft palate (Fig. 18–1) and left lateral aspect of the anterior tongue (Fig. 18–2). The rest of the mucosa of the upper aerodigestive tract was normal in appearance and palpation of the neck was negative. X-ray of the chest was normal.

Biopsy of the tongue lesion revealed microinvasive cancer and biopsies of the soft palate erythroplakia demonstrated carcinoma *in situ* in multiple areas.

DIFFERENTIAL DIAGNOSIS— KEY POINTS

1. Leukoplakia and erythroplakia are both premalignant although the incidence of malignant transformation differs in each group. Leukoplakia rarely transforms—approximately 1% of cases—although leukoplakia of the lip and ventral surface of the tongue, particularly if associated with erythroplakia ("speckled leukoplakia"), renders it more likely to become malignant. Erythroplakia, however, has a greater than 90% incidence of being malignant or undergoing malignant transformation.

2. These lesions need to be differentiated from white and red patches secondary to trauma, for example, bite leukoplakia, chemical irritation, and various stomatitides. An adequate history will usually eliminate these causes.

3. Field cancerization ("condemned mucosa") due to smoking and alcohol abuse is likely to involve to some degree all the mucosa of the upper aerodigestive tract (excluding nose, sinuses, and nasopharynx) and is responsible for the phenomenon of multiple primary cancers.

TEST INTERPRETATION

- The greatest dilemma when confronted with field cancerization is deciding which areas are suspicioius for malignancy. As already stated, site and appearance of the leukoplakia are important; however, all erythroplakia should be viewed with suspicion and biopsied.

- Supravital staining (e.g., toluidine blue) can be most useful in deciding which areas should be biopsied. This can be used as an oral rinse or local application to the affected area. It is important to ensure that all mucus has been removed from the surface of the mucosa before applying the stain.

- Biopsy can be of selected areas that appear suspicious or may consist of excision biopsy of the whole affected area if feasible.

- Patients with multiple areas of premalignancy and a strong smoking history should undergo panendoscopy including laryngoscopy, bronchoscopy, and esophagoscopy to ensure that an asymptomatic second cancer does not exist elsewhere in the upper aerodigestive tract.

MEDICAL/SURGICAL MANAGEMENT

No ideal technique exists for treating "condemned mucosa"; however, the following therapeutic options exist:

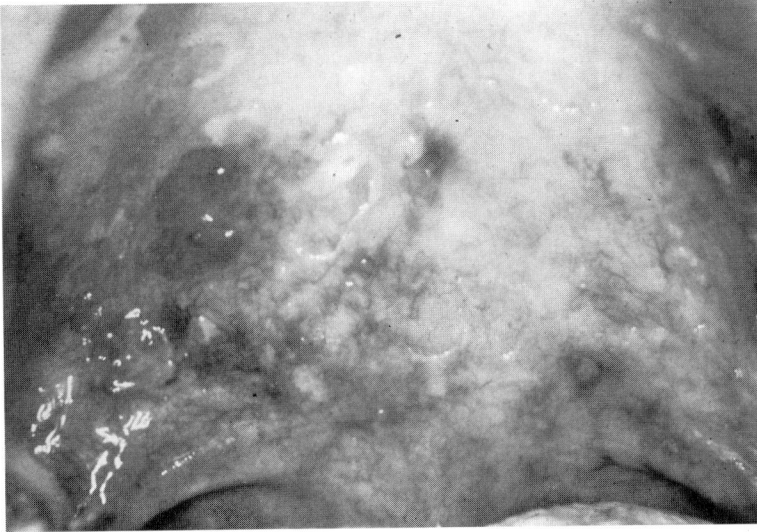

FIGURE 18-1 Areas of leukoplakia and erythroplakia involving the soft palate.

1. Ablation of the premalignant and overt malignant areas with a CO_2 laser. This may be repeated as often as needed. Extent of the ablation can be determined by using toluidine blue intraoperatively. The problem with this approach is the lack of definitive histology.

2. Excision of the affected area using a knife or CO_2 laser, which allows a biopsy specimen to be available for evaluation.

3. Radiotherapy to the affected area. This is usually not desirable because of the diffuse area that requires therapy. However, if a focal area of condemned mucosa recurs and all else fails, local radiotherapy can be administered.

REHABILITATION AND FOLLOW-UP

In all cases careful follow-up and possibly the use of chemoprevention agents are indicated

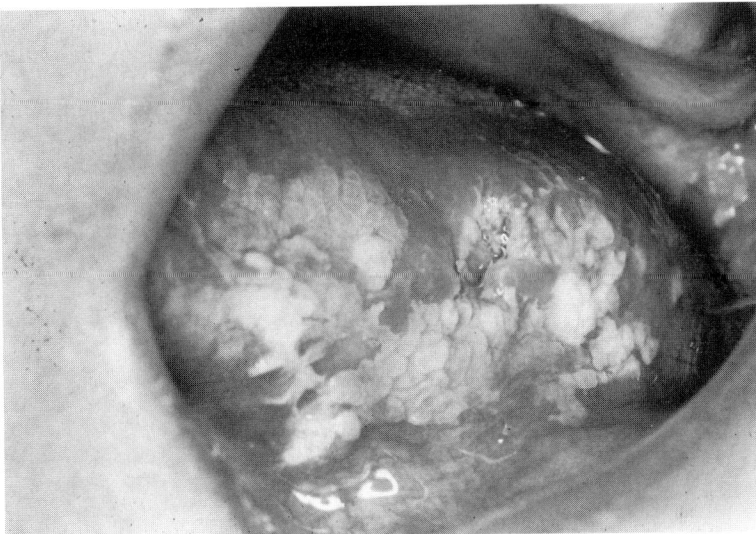

FIGURE 18-2 Area of leukoplakia of tongue with early malignancy.

to try and prevent the development of future multicentric cancers. In this case, excision of the overt cancer of the tongue was performed and the soft palate lesions were treated with CO_2 laser ablation. During the ensuing years, multiple further resections were required for recurrences and new cancers. The patient ultimately demised from a lung cancer.

SUGGESTED READINGS

DeVries N, Gluckman JL, eds. *Multiple Primary Tumors of the Head and Neck.* New York: Thieme; 1990.

Mashberg A. Re-evaluation of toluidine blue application as diagnostic adjunct in the detection of asymptomatic oral cavity cancer. *Cancer.* 1980;46: 758–763.

NASOPHARYNGEAL CARCINOMA

Judith M. Czaja, M.D.
Jack L. Gluckman, M.D.

HISTORY

A 52-year-old white male presents with a 4-week history of right-sided ear pressure, some decrease in hearing, and a complaint that sounds are "muffled." He was placed on antibiotics 2 weeks ago by his family physician for acute right otitis media, which has not resolved. He comes in for evaluation of his refractory otitis media. He denies otorrhea, otalgia, facial nerve weakness, vertigo, or tinnitus. He has never had ear surgery and wears ear protection on the job at the canning factory where he has been employed for 20 years. On further questioning, he admits to mild nasal obstruction for 2 months, however has had "allergies" for years. He denies headaches, dysphagia, voice changes, aspiration, or weight loss. During the past several weeks he has begun to experience almost constant diplopia. He smokes one pack per day and admits to drinking 4 to 6 beers on the weekends only. His medical history is not significant.

On physical exam, the right tympanic membrane is retracted against amber-colored fluid that fills the middle ear space. Anterior rhinoscopy after topical decongestion reveals a lesion in the posterior right nasal cavity, obstructing the choana. A mirror is used to examine the nasopharynx and a large friable mass is easily seen on the right, obstructing the eustachian tube orifice. The remainder of the nasopharynx is normal. Neck palpation reveals one 4- × 4-cm firm mobile node in the right posterior triangle with multiple smaller nodes in the spinal accessory chain. A 1- × 1-cm node is palpable in the left posterior triangle. The remainder of the upper aerodigestive tract examination is normal. Extraocular movements reveal a right abducens nerve palsy (Fig. 19–1).

DIFFERENTIAL DIAGNOSIS— KEY POINTS

1. The onset of unilateral serous otitis media in an adult should make the clinician suspicious for a nasopharyngeal abnormality, especially with palpable cervical adenopathy. These subtle signs may lead the primary care physician astray, therefore a presumptive diagnosis of acute otitis media is made and antibiotics given without thorough evaluation of the nasopharynx. This delay allows tumors to become very advanced before diagnosis is made. Extraocular muscle weakness suggests skull base invasion.

2. Specific queries regarding nasal obstruction or epistaxis must be made to the patient. Often, a patient will admit to mild obstruction, some mild epistaxis, and head pressure—often passed off as "history of allergies" or "sinus trouble."

3. Fevers and night sweats are constitutional type B symptoms associated with lymphoma. Because lymphoma is the second most common tumor to arise in the nasopharynx, questions regarding these symptoms must be specifically asked.

4. The differential diagnosis of an obstructing nasopharyngeal mass with evidence of adenopathy in the neck is a malignancy until proven otherwise. A brief list of possible malignancies include squamous cell carcinoma, lymphoma, adenocarcinoma, adenoid cystic carcinoma, mucoepidermoid carcinoma, plasma cell myeloma, rhabdomyosarcoma, malignant melanoma, fibrosarcoma, chondrosarcoma, and clivus chordoma. The most important next step in the diagnosis of the mass is a biopsy and histopathologic examination. In cooperative patients, a large ob-

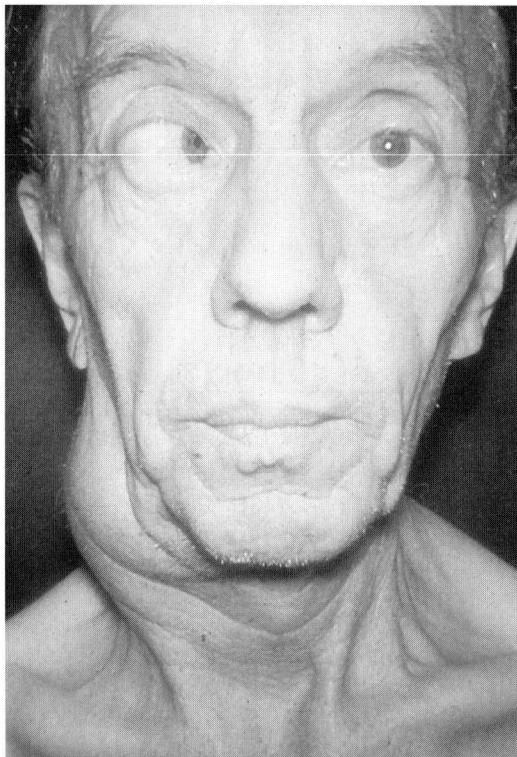

FIGURE 19–1 Extraocular movements reveal a right abducens nerve palsy.

structing nasopharyngeal mass may be easily biopsied transnasally in the office after adequate topical anesthesia. This is done under endoscopic guidance. Minimal bleeding occurs that is easily controlled with a light pack of a hemostatic agent. Tumor biopsy specimens suspected to be lymphoma should be placed in saline for fresh specimen preparation. Often, the tissue obtained by transnasal biopsy is enough for pathologists to diagnose lymphoma with special stains and immunotyping. In the case where the biopsy specimens are of questionable quality or if the patient is reluctant or unable (secondary to significant septal pathology) to undergo transnasal biopsy, a formal transoral nasopharyngeal biopsy is performed under general anesthesia in the operating room. Transoral biopsy is also needed in cases where a lesion appears to be completely submucosal. Deeper biopsies are often difficult in the office setting.

TEST INTERPRETATION

A patient with an obstructing nasopharyngeal mass, bilateral cervical adenopathy, and a unilateral serous otitis media must undergo several tests in order to establish a diagnosis and be staged appropriately before treatment is selected.

1. *Computed tomography (CT) scan.* CT scan with contrast from the skull base to the clavicles will delineate the extent of the primary tumor and cervical metastases. Some surgeons advocate the importance of obtaining imaging prior to biopsy of the tumor. If it is convenient for the patient to undergo biopsy with minimum morbidity at the initial visit, it should be done. Imaging is obtained subsequently. Skull base invasion occurs in approximately 25% of cases. This typically presents as cranial neuropathy. Tumor extension occurs through the petrosphenoidal route in the region between the foramen rotundum and foramen lacerum to involve the anterior group of cranial nerves (II through VI). Posterior extension into the posterior cranial fossa will affect the lower cranial nerves (VII through XII), especially those in the region of the jugular foramen.

2. *Magnetic resonance imaging (MRI) scan.* In patients with obvious signs of intracranial extension, including cranial neuropathies or other signs suggestive of central nervous system invasion, MRI should be obtained to evaluate the extent of disease.

3. *Biopsy.* The technical aspects of nasopharyngeal biopsy have been discussed. Histopathologically, there are three distinct forms of nasopharyngeal carcinoma (NPC). An accurate diagnosis of the subtype is critical as prognosis may differ. The WHO classification is used herein.
    A. *WHO type I (25% of total NPC cases in USA).* Keratinizing squamous cell carcinoma. These tumors show abundant intercellular bridges and keratin production. The histology of this tumor is similar to other upper aerodigestive tract squamous cancers and is not solely characteristic of nasopharyngeal carcinoma.

B. *WHO type II (12%):* Nonkeratinizing squamous cell carcinoma, also known as transitional cell carcinoma because it resembles this form of bladder malignancy.

C. *WHO type III (63%):* Undifferentiated carcinomas forming a diverse group of tumors including lymphoepithelioma, anaplastic, clear cell, and spindle cell variants. A transnasal biopsy was performed in the patient in question and histopathology revealed a lymphoepithelioma.

4. *Immunodiagnostics.* Epstein–Barr virus (EBV) titers in patients with NPC have consistently shown evidence that this virus is considered an etiology for the development of nasopharyngeal carcinoma in sporadic cases as well as in endemic areas. The closest relationship with elevated EBV titers and NPC is with the WHO type II and III tumors. The early antigen (EA) and the viral capsid antigen (VCA-IgA) are the most specific serologic tests for the diagnosis and are strongly associated with the different histopathologic subtypes. The association with WHO type I is weak and no different from control populations. The implications of this test are in the screening of large populations in areas where nasopharyngeal carcinoma is endemic. In addition, in cases of an unknown primary with metastatic cervical adenopathy, EBV titers may suggest NPC and direct random biopsies in the search for the primary tumor. EBV titers were not drawn on the patient.

5. *Chest x-Ray.* Chest x-ray is obtained to rule out distant metastases. Distant metastases occur infrequently in North American population; however, they are more common in endemic areas. A bone scan may also be obtained if patients have symptoms of bone pain in specific areas. The chest x-ray obtained on the patient was negative for metastatic disease.

Staging of nasopharyngeal carcinoma: see Table 19–1.

DIAGNOSIS

1. Lymphoepithelioma WHO type III, stage T4 N2c M0
2. Right serous otitis media

MEDICAL MANAGEMENT

After appropriate histopathologic diagnosis and staging, management consists of external beam radiotherapy. Chemotherapy has been added concurrently with external beam radiotherapy in some studies of advanced stage NPC and these regimens show favorable results when compared with external beam radiotherapy alone. The nasopharynx, skull base, and cervical lymph nodes are included in the ports. Patients are given 6,500 to 7,000 cGy to eradicate the disease.

TABLE 19–1 Staging of Nasopharyngeal Carcinoma

T1: Tumor limited to one subsite of the nasopharynx.
T2: Tumor invades more than one subsite of the nasopharynx.
T3: Tumor invades the nasal cavity and/or oropharynx.
T4: Tumor invades skull and/or cranial nerve(s).

NX: Regional lymph nodes cannot be assessed.
N0: No regional lymph node metastasis.
N1: Metastasis in a single ipsilateral node, 3 cm or less in greatest dimension.
N2a: Metastasis to a single ipsilateral lymph node 3–6 cm in greatest dimension.
N2b: Metastasis in multiple ipsilateral lymph nodes, all less than 6 cm in greatest dimension.
N2c: Metastasis in bilateral or contralateral lymph nodes, all less than 6 cm in greatest dimension.
N3: Metastasis in lymph node more than 6 cm in greatest dimension.

MX: Presence of distant metastasis cannot be assessed.
M0: No distant metastasis.
M1: Distant metastasis.

SURGICAL MANAGEMENT

Surgical management is infrequent. Neck dissection may be required in patients whose primary tumor has been controlled, and residual cervical metastases are palpable. Some authors advocate extensive wide skull base resections for recurrent disease on rare occasions (i.e., Fisch infratemporal fossa approach to the skull base and nasopharynx or transpalatal approach reported by Fee) to relieve pain and pressure symptoms for palliation alone.

A myringotomy with tube insertion should be performed on the patient with serous otitis. This will immediately relieve the symptoms of fullness and decreased hearing. Clinicians wishing to do so should obtain an audiogram prior to surgery on the ear, although Weber and Rinne tests with 512- and 1024-Hz tuning forks should suffice.

REHABILITATION AND FOLLOW-UP

Patients with NPC are followed with monthly examinations for 1 year after the completion of treatment. Bimonthly examinations occur during the second year of follow-up and trimonthly exams during the third year. Yearly examinations are performed after this time for the duration of the patient's life. Long-term sequelae of radiotherapy may develop including multiple cranial neuropathies. If these occur, aggressive workup with CT and MRI should be undertaken to rule out recurrence. Chest x-ray is obtained yearly, as well as a complete physical exam.

SUGGESTED READINGS

Anonymous. Preliminary results of a randomized trial comparing neoadjuvant chemotherapy (cisplatin, epirubicin, bleomycin) plus radiotherapy vs. radiotherapy alone in stage IV (> or = N2, M0) undifferentiated nasopharyngeal carcinoma: a positive effect on progression-free survival. International Nasopharynx Cancer Study Group. VUMCA I trial. *Int J Radiat Oncol Biol Phys.* 1996;35(3):463–469.

Chan AT, Teo PM, Leung TW, et al. A prospective randomized study of chemotherapy adjunctive to definitive radiotherapy in advanced nasopharyngeal carcinoma. *Int J Radiat Oncol Biol Phys.* 1995;33(3): 569–577.

Fee WE Jr, Gilmer PA, Goffinet DR. Surgical management of recurrent nasopharyngeal carcinoma after radiation failure at the primary site. *Laryngoscope.* 1988;98(11):1220–1226.

Lin JC, Jan JS, Hsu CY. Neoadjuvant chemotherapy for advanced nasopharyngeal carcinoma. *Am J Clin Oncol.* 1995;18(2):139–143.

Neel HB III. Benign and malignant neoplasms of the nasopharynx. In: Cummings CW, Frederickson JM, et al., eds. *Otolaryngology—Head and Neck Surgery.* 2nd ed. St. Louis, MO: Mosby-Year Book; 1993.

Santos JA, Gonzalez C, Cuesta P, et al. Impact of changes in the treatment of nasopharyngeal carcinoma: an experience of 30 years. *Radiother Oncol.* 1995;36(2):121–127.

CAROTID ARTERY RUPTURE

Judith M. Czaja, M.D.
Jack L. Gluckman, M.D.

HISTORY

A 55-year-old white male, who underwent a salvage total laryngectomy, partial pharyngectomy, and right modified radical neck dissection with preservation of the spinal accessory nerve approximately 15 days ago, is bleeding from the neck. Full course radiotherapy had been given in the past as part of a laryngeal preservation protocol. This was completed 6 months ago; however, the tumor recurred and salvage surgery was performed. The patient's postoperative course has been complicated by a right lower lobe pneumonia, a wound infection, and a pharyngocutaneous fistula. The fistula, located at the inferior aspect of the apron flap 4 cm to the right of the stoma, has been treated conservatively with opening, drainage, and packing four times daily during the past week. In addition, the skin edges around the fistula have necrosed. A wound infection extends superiorly for 3 to 4 cm. This has also been treated with packing four times daily. The packing was changed the night before, at which time the carotid artery was noted to be visible in the open wound (Fig. 20–1).

On arrival to the patient's room, there is a large amount of bright red blood and blood-soaked sponges covering the patient's pillow. The patient's blood pressure is 90/50 with a pulse of 120. There is active hemorrhage coming from the patient's neck wound.

DIFFERENTIAL DIAGNOSIS— KEY POINTS

1. Risk factors for the development of carotid artery rupture ("blowout") include pharyngocutaneous salivary fistula, previous radiation therapy to the head and neck, early carotid exposure with artery dessication, wound infection, and skin flap necrosis.

2. The prevention of carotid artery rupture begins in the preoperative period. Often, the artery rupture is secondary to technical errors that occur during surgery on high-risk patients. Recognizing those who are at risk for carotid artery rupture will allow the surgeon to tailor the surgical procedure to decrease the incidence of this life-threatening complication. Patients should maintain adequate nutritional status (often hard in this patient population) to help with wound healing. Previous radiotherapy should be noted because its effects on postoperative wound healing can be devastating. Flap viability is also compromised in heavy smokers. Smoking cessation preoperatively (again, often hard in this patient population) may decrease the risk to skin flaps. Careful consideration should be given to the placement of surgical incisions. Incisions directly over the carotid artery should be avoided. If this is not possible, incisions should only cross the carotid once. Trifurcations over the carotid are to be avoided. The surgeon should be familiar and comfortable with many options for skin incisions including the Latyschevsky and Freund, Freund, Crile, modified Shobinger, Conley, and MacFee options.

3. Intraoperatively, closure of mucosal defects resulting in a watertight seal is required to decrease the risk of postoperative fistula. When neck dissection is performed, the surgeon should avoid disrupting the adventitia of the carotid fascia. This layer provides blood supply to the carotid wall and disturbance may lead to vessel wall ischemia. Coverage of the carotid artery with dermal grafts, local muscle flaps (transposed levator scapulae), or regional myofascial or myocutaneous flaps (pectoralis major) should be performed routinely in cases where the carotid is ex-

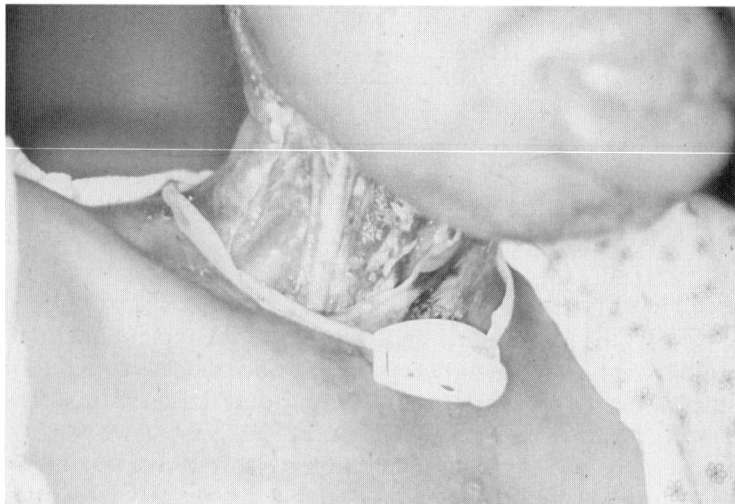

FIGURE 20-1 Carotid artery visible in the open wound.

posed in continuity with an oral cavity or oropharyngeal defect.

4. A carotid artery may undergo sentinel bleeding prior to complete rupture. Intermittent bleeding from a neck wound occurs and stops without massive hemorrhage. This warning sign may give the physician time to assess the situation and plan the therapeutic intervention with the patient. The scenario in which elective carotid artery ligation may be considered is far more ideal than the emergent situation.

5. In addition to the risk factors for carotid artery rupture previously listed, recurrent carcinoma with gross invasion into the artery should be considered as well. **However, bear in mind that the exact etiology of the carotid artery rupture (carcinoma, dessication, necrosis, etc.) is the least important factor in the acute management of the life-threatening emergency.**

TEST INTERPRETION

Some authors advocate the use of angiography with embolization in situations of impending carotid artery rupture, that is, in the face of a sentinel bleed that has ceased. The examination may give the physician an opportunity to test the contralateral blood flow and adequacy of the circle of Willis by temporary balloon occlusion under EEG control. The role of angiography for sentinel bleeding is controversial. There is **no role** for angiography in the case of complete carotid artery rupture.

DIAGNOSIS

Carotid artery rupture.

MEDICAL MANAGEMENT

Immediate response to a call about bleeding from the neck in any patient who has undergone head and neck surgery is absolutely necessary. The situation is treated as a life-threatening emergency. Insist on help from the nursing staff at the patient's bedside and summon further help from any head and neck surgery house staff available in the hospital. Although the steps to care for this emergent situation are listed separately below, a person who has managed a carotid blowout knows that all of the steps below are being carried out simultaneously by many individuals. In other words, the neck vessels are compressed as the airway is secured and the pulse oximeter is attached and the blood is drawn, etc. Of paramount importance is that there is a single person in charge of the situation, not only to keep the resuscitation focused, but to instill a sense of reassurance to the patient that the situation is under control. Commonly, the patient maintains consciousness throughout the ordeal.

1. *Airway:* Patients with acute carotid artery rupture will either have an internal or external "blowout." The vast majority of these will be external, making management of the airway less difficult. Secure the airway immediately. Fortunately, many patients will have a permanent stoma or may have been recently decannulated and a cuffed endotracheal tube or tracheotomy tube should be placed into the tracheostome or through the previous trach site if possible. Do not neglect to inflate the cuff to protect the airway.

2. *Breathing.* Provide supplemental oxygen and place a pulse oximeter on the patient. In the event of a respiratory arrest, patients should be ventilated with an ambubag. Suction catheters that fit the diameter of the tracheotomy tube should be available.

3. *Circulation.* Apply direct external pressure over the site of bleeding. This usually ceases the profuse exsanguination; however, remember that the patient's cerebral perfusion is now compromised. Attempting blindly to clamp the carotid artery at the bedside is mentioned only to be condemned. Often, further damage occurs making eventual ligation difficult. Instruct an assistant to start two or three large-bore intravenous lines (14 to 16 gauge) and replace fluids with lactated Ringer's solution as quickly as possible.

4. *Blood products.* In the sentinel situation, two to four units of packed red cells should be held in the blood bank at all times. Without the "luxury" of a sentinel bleed, an immediate CBC and type and crossmatch for four units of packed red cells should be drawn.

SURGICAL MANAGEMENT

The patient with an acute carotid artery rupture should be transported immediately to the operating room with a physician in attendance. Communication with the operating room staff and anesthesiology team is often done at the point when the patient is brought into the operating suite. An attempt to inform them of the impending case can be made by instructing an assistant to phone ahead as you are securing the airway, breathing, and circulation. The patient is placed under general anesthesia and the blood pressure is kept high in order to increase cerebral perfusion. This unfortunately provides the surgeon with a strong pressure head against which to ligate the vessels. Ligation of both the common and internal and external carotid arteries is necessary to gain vascular control. The most common site of injury is at the carotid bulb. No attempt is made to reconstruct the acutely ruptured vessel. The ends of the ruptured artery are clamped with vascular instruments and hemorrhage is stopped. Hypertension is maintained. The ends of the arteries are ligated with silk suture and should be oversewn as well. Once the ligation is completed, the arterial ends must be covered by a regional flap. A pectoralis major myofascial flap with a skin graft or myocutaneous flap may be used, and attempts to redirect a pharyngocutaneous fistula should be made. Primary closure of a fistula is probably best avoided in the acute setting.

Further considerations include these:

1. Carotid artery exposure should be recognized early in the case of wound breakdown. An artery previously covered by a dermal graft, once exposed, will often readily granulate and reepithelialize with careful wound care. If reepithelialization does not begin within 3 days of vigorous wound care, coverage with regional flaps is indicated. Arteries not previously covered by a dermal graft are at high risk for rupture once exposed and coverage should be provided as soon as possible.

2. The incidence of neurologic sequelae after emergent carotid artery ligation is high. Acute neurologic sequelae may occur in up to 60% of cases with an approximate mortality of 45 to 60%. The incidences of neurologic sequelae and mortality rate are significantly lower when the procedure is done electively.

3. An intraoral carotid blowout is a difficult situation; however, it can be handled adequately. The patient may be bleeding from one of the branches of the external carotid or the internal carotid that is surrounded by tumor. The same protocol—securing the air-

way, external neck compression, and maintaining adequate circulation—must be followed. Intraoral compression of the region in question may be performed as well, with tonsil sponges on a tonsillar tenaculum. Securing the airway is more tenuous in these situations.

REHABILITATION AND FOLLOW-UP

Even after successful management of an acute carotid artery rupture, the patient may require long-term care either for the neurologic sequelae of the injury or wound care for the neck process. In patients who have recurrent nonresectable and rapidly progressing disease, palliative psychosocial therapy and analgesic therapy are important parts of the overall treatment regimen. On the other hand, if there is no evidence of recurrent carcinoma, aggressive local wound care, as well as neurologic rehabilitation, should be instituted so that the quality of life can be optimized in these patients.

SUGGESTED READINGS

COLEMAN JJ III. Treatment of ruptured or exposed carotid artery: a rational approach. *South Med J.* 1985;78(3):262–267.

HELLER KS, STRONG EW. Carotid arterial hemorrhage after radical head and neck surgery. *Am J Surg.* 1979;138:607–610.

HILLERMAN BL, KENNEDY TL. Carotid rupture and tissue coverage. *Laryngoscope.* 1982;92:985–988.

LEIKENSOHN J, MILKO D, COTTON R. Carotid artery rupture. *Arch Otol.* 1978;104:307–310.

MAVES MD, BRUNS MD, KEENAN MJ. Carotid artery resection for head and neck cancer. *Ann Otol Rhinol Laryngol.* 1992;101:778–781.

SHUMRICK DA. Carotid artery rupture. *Laryngoscope.* 1973;83:1051–1061.

Case 21

ODONTOGENIC TUMORS

Judith M. Czaja, M.D.
Jack L. Gluckman, M.D.

HISTORY

A 35-year-old white female is referred by her dentist for evaluation of a swelling in the right mandible. The patient noted a fullness in the right side of her face approximately 6 weeks ago. She went to the dentist for a presumed tooth infection and fullness of the right mandible was noted intraorally and externally at that time and was referred to otolaryngology. On further history, she denies any malocclusion, pain, or numbness of her teeth or lips. She has no history of previous exposure to radiotherapy.

On physical exam, a firm 3- × 3-cm nontender mass is noted intraorally in the mandibular body on both lingual and buccal surfaces. Teeth 27 through 29 are loose. Sensation over the gingiva is normal. Externally, the mass deforms the lower face, causing asymmetry of the mandible. Sensation of the lower lip is normal. Auscultation of the mass reveals no bruit. The remainder of the exam is normal.

DIFFERENTIAL DIAGNOSIS— KEY POINTS

1. Painless swelling of the jaw, either upper or lower, is a common presentation of jaw cysts and tumors. Dysesthesias, pain, and loose dentition suggest malignancy. Another common finding in the history suggesting malignancy is a nonhealing tooth socket after extraction. Osteogenic sarcoma may occur in the mandible or maxilla and may mimic an odontogenic tumor. Vascular malformations, more common in children, may also present as slow-growing mandibular masses. A bruit heard on auscultation requires further evaluation with magnetic resonance imaging (MRI), magnetic resonance angiography

(MRA), or angiography. If embolization is chosen as definitive treatment or preoperatively, angiography is the best study.

2. Panorex evaluation of the maxilla and mandible can assist with differential diagnosis of jaw cysts and tumors; however, definitive diagnosis is made on biopsy and histopathologic examination. Slowly growing lesions will have thin sclerotic bony walls that are well demarcated. Aggressive cysts and tumors will show lysis of surrounding bone, tooth root displacement, and bone expansion.

3. Inflammatory and developmental cysts include periapical, dentigerous, globulomaxillary, and nasopalatine cysts. The most common is the periapical cyst, while the dentigerous cyst, often associated with the crown of an unerupted molar, may rarely give rise to ameloblastoma or squamous cell carcinoma. Odontogenic keratocyst (OKC) is considered a multicystic benign neoplasm with an increased propensity for recurrence after inadequate currettage. Multiple keratocysts with recurrence may occur with basal cell nevus syndrome (BCNS). The diagnosis of BCNS must be entertained in patients with findings of bifid ribs, hypertelorism, widened nasal dorsum, mandibular cysts, and early development of basal cell carcinomas of the face and trunk.

4. True odontogenic tumors arise from cells of the enamel organ and include ameloblastoma, calcifying epithelial odontogenic tumor (Pindborg tumor), squamous odontogenic tumor, calcified odontogenic tumor (Gorlin's cyst), odontogenic myxoma, cementoblastoma, ameloblastic fibroma, and odontoma. Ameloblastoma is considered the most primitive of the odontogenic tumors, while the odontoma is the most differentiated, showing histologic evidence of tooth

formation. Other more rare tumors occur and are not mentioned here.

5. Tumors typically involving the mandible include ameloblastoma, OKC, calcifying epithelial odontogenic tumor, squamous odontogenic tumor, cementoblastoma, ameloblastic fibroma. Tumors typically involving the maxilla include Gorlin's cyst (also affects mandible) and odontoma.

6. Metastatic tumor from breast carcinoma, renal cell carcinoma, and other primaries, as well as contiguous involvement of oral cavity and oropharyngeal squamous cell carcinoma, may occur in the jaws. A history of previous or concurrent malignancy may suggest this in the differential diagnosis.

TEST INTERPRETATION

Workup of a patient with a jaw mass includes a full head and neck exam, panorex, computed tomography (CT) scan, and preoperative laboratory studies.

1. *Panorex.* A multiloculated soap-bubble radiolucency in the right body of the mandible extending to the angle.

2. *CT scan.* Extensive inner cortical destruction with multiple areas of thinning external cortical bone by a multiloculated cystic mass.

3. Chest x-ray, complete blood count, and electrolytes are normal.

4. *Biopsy.* Fine-needle aspiration biopsy of a solid jaw mass is difficult, if not impossible, to perform adequately. Therefore, an open biopsy should be performed. Biopsy is either complete enucleation in the case of small lesions or incisional in cases of suspected malignancy or larger tumors where preoperative counseling regarding treatment is necessary. Histopathologic exam of the biopsy is needed for diagnosis.

Biopsy of the tumor in the case presented shows a lesion composed of epithelial follicles surrounded by a fibrous stroma. The epithelium resembles the enamel organ, with peripheral tall columnar ameloblastic cells with palisading nuclei (similar in appearance to basal cell carcinoma) surrounding a stellate reticular formation (Fig. 21–1). On high-powered microscopy, the columnar cell nuclei appear polarized away from the basement membrane (Fig. 21–2).

DIAGNOSIS

Ameloblastoma right mandibular body.

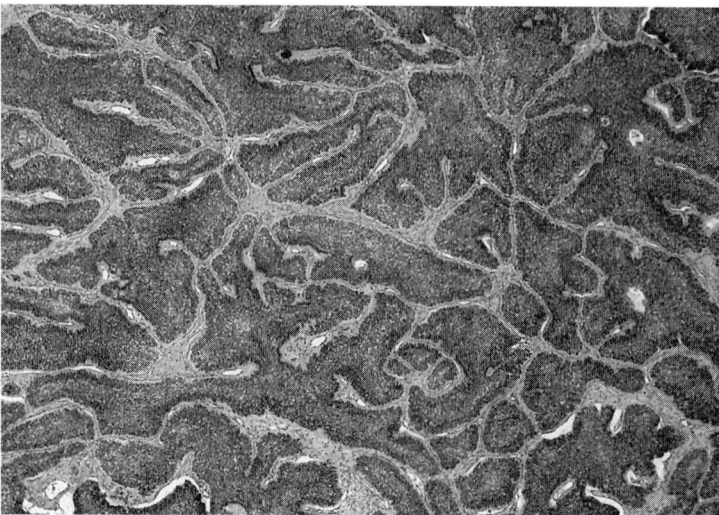

FIGURE 21–1 Epithelium resembles the enamel organ, with peripheral tall columnar ameloblastic cells with palisading nuclei surrounding a stellate reticular formation.

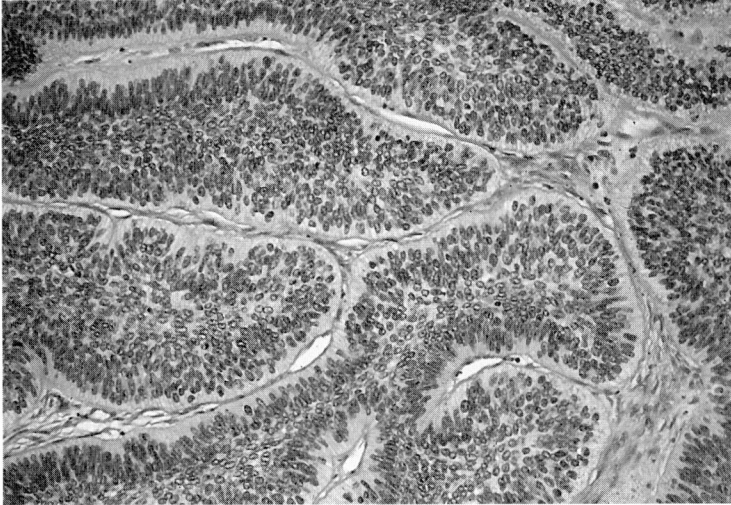

FIGURE 21–2 On high-powered microscopy, the columnar cell nuclei appear polarized away from the basement membrane.

MEDICAL MANAGEMENT

There is no role for medical management of this problem.

SURGICAL MANAGEMENT

The various forms of odontogenic tumors are usually adequately treated with enucleation. In cases of OKC, there is a tendency for recurrence if simple enucleation is performed. A more aggressive approach, with extensive curettage and drilling of all bony loculations should be performed. The surgeon should not be reluctant to perform a marginal mandibulectomy if there is extensive disease that cannot be adequately accessed with curettage and drilling. Recurrent OKC typically requires segmental mandibulectomy for adequate gross removal.

Opinions in the literature vary regarding the appropriate treatment of ameloblastoma. Although it is a benign disease histologically with rare metastases, ameloblastoma has a propensity for aggressive behavior with significant destruction of local structures. When inadequately treated with simple enucleation or curettage, ameloblastoma recurs readily. In the case of small and moderately sized tumors, a marginal mandibulectomy is performed, leaving a rim of inferior mandible intact. Large destructive lesions with multiple loculations and obvious bony destruction of the cortices require segmental mandibulectomy for complete removal. Reconstruction is best performed with a free tissue transfer. There is no role for radiotherapy in the management of odontogenic tumors.

REHABILITATION AND FOLLOW-UP

Close follow-up is required, particularly in cases where enucleation was performed for OKC or ameloblastoma. Recurrence is the most common complication of these tumors, especially when the enamel organ is not entirely removed. Malignant transformation may develop in the recurrence and, although rare, requires extensive revision surgery for treatment.

SUGGESTED READINGS

Anand VK, Arrowood JP Jr, Krolls SO. Odontogenic keratocysts: a study of 50 patients. *Laryngoscope.* 1995;105(1):14–16.

Chehade A, Daley TD, Wysocki GP, Miller AS. Peripheral odontogenic keratocyst. *Oral Surg Med Pathol.* 1994;77(5):494–497.

Dierks EJ, Bernstein ML. Odontogenic cysts, tumors,

and related jaw lesions. In: Bailey BJ, Johnson JT, Kohut RI, et al, eds. *Head and Neck Surgery—Otolaryngology*. Philadelphia, PA: JB Lippincott; 1993.

FEINBERG SE, STEINBERG B. Surgical management of ameloblastoma. Current status of the literature. *Oral Surg Med Pathol Radiol*. 1996;81(4):383–388.

HARING, JI, VAN DIS ML. Odontogenic keratocysts: a clinical, radiographic, and histopathologic study. *Oral Surg Med Pathol*. 1988;66(1):145–153.

PINSOLLE J, MICHELET V, COUSTAL B, et al. Treatment of ameloblastoma of the jaws. *Arch Otol Head Neck Surg*. 1995;121(9):994–996.

SHEAR M. Developmental odontogenic cysts. An update. *J Oral Pathol Med*. 1994;23(1):1–11.

TONSILLAR CARCINOMA

Judith M. Czaja, M.D.
Jack L. Gluckman, M.D.

HISTORY

A 52-year-old white male is referred for evaluation of persistent sore throat and some odynophagia of approximately 3 months duration. He has lost 10 pounds during this time as a result of decreased dietary intake. He admits to occasional right-sided otalgia. His medical history is significant for hypertension that is well controlled with oral medications. He smokes 1½ packs of cigarettes and drinks 6 to 12 beers per day. He is currently employed as a punch press operator, is married, and has three children.

On physical examination, there is a large exophytic friable mass in the right tonsillar area that extends superiorly onto the soft palate and inferiorly to the base of the tongue along the glossotonsillar fold (Fig. 22–1). The tumor measures 4.5 cm in greatest dimension. Palpation of the neck reveals a solitary 3-cm firm mass in the midjugular region. By palpation, the tumor mass does not appear to involve the mandible. The remainder of the head and neck exam is normal.

DIFFERENTIAL DIAGNOSIS— KEY POINTS

1. There is little doubt that in the patient presented, persistent sore throat, a large friable mass in the oropharynx, and a firm mass in the neck indicate malignancy. The differential diagnosis therefore becomes the variety of histopathologic tumor types found in this area including squamous cell carcinoma and variants (spindle cell carcinoma, verrucous carcinoma, lymphoepithelioma), lymphoma, sarcoma, and occasionally minor salivary gland malignancies. Biopsy and histopathologic exam will reveal the definitive diagnosis.

2. Important factors in the management of the patient presented include both patient and tumor considerations. The essential patient factors include adequate assessment of the patient's nutritional status, underlying baseline health status, social support, and patient expectations and motivations.

A. *Nutritional status.* Patients with advanced head and neck malignancies usually have poor nutritional status secondary to poor diet and alcoholism. Baseline weight is measured at the initial visit. Serum albumin, liver function tests, complete blood count (CBC), blood chemistries, glucose, and often thyroid function tests should be drawn preoperatively as an indicator of general nutritional status. Some physicians prefer to defer surgery until the nutritional status of the patient is improved either with dietary supplements or gastrostomy tube placement; however, this is not a universal opinion.

B. *General health.* Patients with advanced head and neck malignancy often admit to much less alcohol and tobacco than they actually abuse. The more critical of these is the alcohol abuse because alcohol withdrawal can be severe enough to cause death postoperatively. A carefully directed history, with open and honest communication between patient and physician about this sensitive topic, will often reveal the exact amount of alcohol used without the patient becoming overly defensive. Careful perioperative monitoring for delirium tremens and the judicious use of short- or long-acting benzodiazapines or alcohol infusion at the first sign of symptoms are necessary. The symptoms of delirium tremens include tachycardia, hyperventilation, profuse diaphoresis, agitation, confusion, hallucinations, and seizures.

C. *Social support.* Inquiry about the patient's

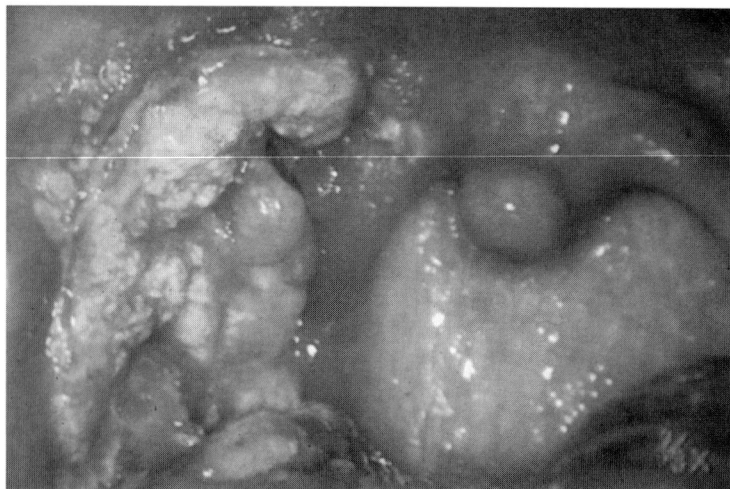

FIGURE 22–1 Mass in the right tonsillar area extends superiorly on to the soft palate and inferiorly to the base of the tongue along the glossotonsillar fold.

living situation and social support is critical. The patient who has supportive family and friends may have an easier recovery than those patients who lack such support. The physician must also assess the patient's home situation and the need for social workers and home care nurses in the postoperative period. The physician's concern for the patient's personal life, in addition to his or her physical condition, allows a strong, trustful physician–patient relationship to develop.

D. *Patient expectations and motivation.* The patient must be fully aware of the anticipated surgery and potential outcomes as well as alternatives to surgery before informed consent is obtained. Frank discussions with patient and family regarding potentially disfiguring surgery, permanent tracheotomy and gastrostomy, and loss of voice or swallowing should be discussed openly with all questions asked and answered prior to proceeding with surgery.

3. Tonsillar carcinoma may involve the mandible or may be contiguous into the neck by direct extension, surrounding the carotid artery. Accurate assessment of the primary tumor is necessary to determine what surgical procedure and approach is appropriate. To-

gether with physical exam, a computed tomography (CT) scan or magnetic resonance image will give accurate information about the mandible and neck vessels.

4. Panendoscopy to evaluate the remainder of the upper aerodigestive tract should be performed to rule out a second primary.

TEST INTERPRETATION

1. Chest x-ray *(CXR).* This is performed routinely to screen for metastatic disease. In the case presented, the CXR is normal.

2. *Laboratory.* CBC, electrolytes, and urinalysis are normal.

3. *CT scan.* This shows a large mass filling the right tonsillar fossa extending laterally; however, the mandible appears uninvolved. Neck examination shows an isolated mass in the right midjugular region, with no other masses noted. Occasionally the involved lymph nodes seen on CT scan will be cystic. This finding is more commonly associated with carcinomas originating from Waldeyer's ring and may provide guidance for directed biopsies in the case of an upper aerodigestive tract unknown primary malignancy.

4. *Biopsy.* The biopsy specimen is consistent

TABLE 22–1 Staging Systems for Oropharyngeal Carcinoma

T1: Primary tumor less than 2 cm in greatest dimension.
T2: Primary tumor between 2 and 4 cm in greatest dimension.
T3: Primary tumor greater than 4 cm in greatest dimension.
T4: Primary tumor involving surrounding structures: bone, soft tissue of neck, tongue.

NX: Nodal status cannot be determined.
N0: No evidence of metastatic nodes.
N1: Metastasis to a single ipsilateral node less than or equal to 3 cm.
N2a: Metastasis to a single ipsilateral node between 3 and 6 cm in greatest dimension.
N2b: Metastasis to multiple ipsilateral nodes none greater than 6 cm.
N2c: Metastasis to bilateral or contralateral nodes none greater than 6 cm.
N3: Metastasis to a lymph node greater than 6 cm.

MX: Distant metastasis cannot be determined.
M0: No distant metastasis.
M1: Distant metastasis.

with keratinizing squamous cell carcinoma (Table 22–1).

DIAGNOSIS

T3N1M0 squamous cell carcinoma of the right tonsillar fossa.

MEDICAL MANAGEMENT

Advanced stage tonsillar carcinomas require combined modality therapy to attempt a cure. In cases where the patient is unable or unwilling to undergo an extensive tumor resection, palliative radiotherapy with or without chemotherapy may be given. Stage I tonsillar carcinoma (T1) may be treated effectively for cure with radiotherapy. The results appear to be equal to surgery alone in patients unable or unwilling to undergo resection. Likewise, lymphoepithelioma of the tonsillar fossa with cystic neck metastases responds extremely well to radiotherapy and should be treated with this modality.

SURGICAL MANAGEMENT

In a patient who is able to undergo surgery, the best treatment option for advanced stage tonsillar carcinoma is combined modalities including surgery followed by full-course postoperative radiotherapy. Tonsillar carcinoma can be an aggressive malignancy with a high rate of regional metastases and extensive surgical excision is usually required.

The assessment of the primary tumor determines the surgical approach that is appropriate. Most T1 and some smaller T2 carcinomas can be adequately excised transorally with good margins. The surgical defects are closed either primarily or with a split-thickness skin graft. In addition, a complete modified neck dissection (sparing spinal accessory nerve if possible) should be performed.

T3 and T4 carcinomas require wide exposure for accurate excision. Parasymphyseal mandibulotomy is the favored approach of the author. The mandibulotomy is easy to perform and provides excellent exposure to large tonsillar carcinomas that extend onto the lateral tongue base and soft palate. This approach also provides excellent exposure of the parapharyngeal space. In cases where the mandible is to be preserved, the mandible is readily reapproximated with two miniplates secured over the stairstep osteotomy after resection and reconstruction. Lateral mandibulotomy may also be performed; however, this divides the inferior alveolar nerve, leaving the lower teeth and lip anesthetized. The site of the lateral osteotomy is in the region of the radiation field, which may lead to poor union, devitalized bone, and osteomyelitis with bone exposure. These complications are very difficult to manage and are best avoided by careful placement of osteotomies.

Mandibulectomy is required for obvious

gross tumor invasion into the bone or in cases where the tumor is firmly adherent to or invading into the mandibular periosteum. Hemimandibulectomy is performed, leaving a remnant of ascending ramus and condyle, with removal of the coronoid in most cases. The distal osteotomy is in the parasymphyseal region.

Reconstruction of mandibular defects may be performed with a plate and myocutaneous flap, a myocutaneous flap alone, or a free tissue transfer. Most commonly, the pectoralis major myocutaneous flap or the fibular free graft is used.

Postoperative adjuvant radiation therapy is added to the treatment protocol in all patients with advanced (T2–T4) tonsillar carcinoma and many T1 tonsillar carcinomas to decrease the incidence of local recurrence and recurrence in the retropharyngeal lymph nodes.

REHABILITATION AND FOLLOW-UP

Patients with advanced squamous cell carcinoma of the head and neck should be followed regularly for the patient's lifetime. Continuous surveillance will diagnose not only recurrence at the primary site, but second primary tumors that tend to develop regularly in head and neck tumor patients. Yearly CXR and physical exam are performed. Alcohol and tobacco dependence should be addressed and managed appropriately. Modifications of the patient's lifestyle must be undertaken with the help of other professionals.

SUGGESTED READINGS

FOOTE RL, SCHILD SE, THOMPSON WM, et al. Tonsil cancer. Patterns of failure after surgery alone and surgery combined with postoperative radiation therapy. *Cancer.* 1994;73(10):2638–2647.

GUAY ME, LAVERTU P. Tonsillar carcinoma. *Eur Arch Otol Rhinol Laryngol.* 1995;252(5):259–264.

HASEGAWA M. Primary and salvage surgery for cancer of the tonsillar region: a retrospective study of 120 patients. *Head Neck.* 1994;16(5):463–466.

THOMPSON WM, FOOTE RL, OLSEN KD, et al. Postoperative irradiation for tonsillar carcinoma. *Mayo Clin Proc.* 1993;68(7):665–669.

Case 23

GLOTTIC CARCINOMA

Lyon L. Gleich, M.D.

HISTORY

A 63-year-old male presents with a 2-month history of progressive hoarseness. This is accompanied by mild dysphagia. He has lost no weight. He is otherwise in good health and uses no medication. He has smoked two packs of cigarettes/day for 50 years. He drinks beer regularly. He can walk two flights of steps without difficulty. He has had no prior surgery or major illnesses.

The physical examination is significant for a lesion involving the right laryngeal surface of the epiglottis. The tumor extends inferiorly to involve the false and true vocal folds. The lesion crosses the midline. The right true vocal fold is fixed. The larynx is freely mobile. There are palpable nodes in the right middle and upper jugular chain, the largest of which is 3 cm. There is no palpable adenopathy on the left.

DIFFERENTIAL DIAGNOSIS— KEY POINTS

1. This patient appears to have an advanced laryngeal tumor. Given the history of smoking and alcohol use, this can be presumed to be a squamous cell carcinoma until proven otherwise. However, biopsy confirmation is needed before actually proceeding with treatment.

2. The differential diagnosis must include other

neoplastic processes. Tuberculosis and invasive fungal infection, must be considered even if low on the list of differential diagnoses.

3. The lesion can be tentatively staged as a T3 tumor due to cord fixation and N2b due to multiple lymph nodes. Other lesions that occur in the larynx and can mimic squamous cell carcinoma include lymphoma, tuberculosis, and chondrosarcoma.

DIAGNOSTIC TESTS

A metastatic evaluation is necessary. At a minimum a chest x-ray and routine hematologic and chemistry evaluation should be performed. Given the advanced neck disease additional testing for metastases, such as a bone scan or chest or abdominal computed tomography (CT) may be considered, but are generally not cost effective. In an advanced tumor such as this a CT scan of the larynx and neck is often helpful because it will aid in determining the extent of disease, location of involved nodes, and cartilage involvement.

It is then necessary to confirm the diagnosis. A fine-needle aspiration biopsy can be performed on the lymph nodes to rapidly confirm the diagnosis. The patient should then undergo a complete endoscopic examination. The purpose of this examination would be to determine the extent of the tumor and to obtain biopsies. An esophagoscopy and bronchoscopy can also be performed to search for second primary tumors, though the cost effectiveness of these added procedures is poor.

For this patient the following tests were done: chest x-ray, hematologic, renal, hepatic, and bone blood profiles, CT scan of the larynx and necks with contrast, and panendoscopy with biopsy.

TEST INTERPRETATION

The chest x-ray and blood profiles are all within normal limits except for mild elevations of liver enzymes. The CT scan is shown in Figure 23–1. The scan revealed that the tumor extended from the supraglottis to involve the preepiglottic space. Additionally, the tumor extended inferiorly to the level of the inferior border of the thyroid cartilage. There was no definite evidence of cartilage involvement. The right neck nodes extended along the jugular chain, and in areas approached, but did not surround, the carotid artery. Many of the nodes had necrotic centers. There were two nodes, each <1 cm and without any evidence of necrosis, in the left jugulodigastric region.

At panendoscopy the tumor was noted to involve both the lingual and laryngeal surfaces of the epiglottis and to cross the midline. The tumor extended inferiorly to the inferior

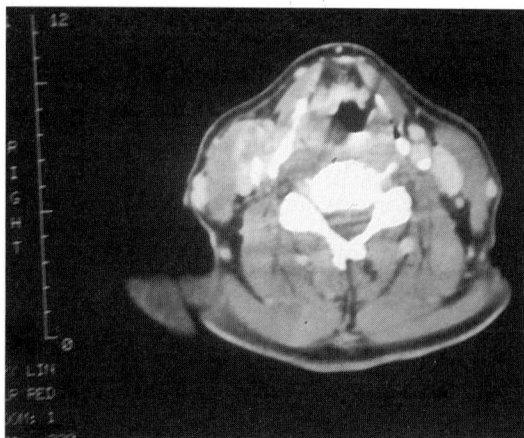

FIGURE 23–1 CT scan demonstrates a tumor extending from the supraglottis to the preepiglottic space. Note that it also extends inferiorly to the level of the inferior border of the thyroid cartilage but does not appear to involve the cartilage.

surface of the true vocal fold. Bimanual palpation of the preepiglottic region revealed fullness. The tongue base was soft. No other lesions were seen. Biopsies were sent and revealed moderately differentiated squamous cell carcinoma.

DIAGNOSIS

T3N2b (stage IV) squamous cell carcinoma of the supraglottic larynx.

MEDICAL MANAGEMENT

This patient has a confirmed stage IV squamous cell carcinoma of the supraglottic larynx without evidence of distant metastases. The options for treatment must now be discussed with the patient and are as follows.

The VA study demonstrated that an organ preservation treatment consisting of induction chemotherapy followed by radiation therapy in those patients responding to chemotherapy yields comparable survival to traditional surgery followed by radiation therapy in advanced laryngeal study. The European Organization for Research and Treatment of Cancer (EORTC) recently reported a similar randomized study of hypopharyngeal cancers. Radiotherapy alone with surgical salvage can also yield comparable cure rates for T3 laryngeal cancers. Radiation alone can yield particularly good results if the tumor volume is small (<6 cm^3 for supraglottic tumors). Given this evidence regarding organ preservation, this information should be relayed to the patient.

The patient should be informed what treatment with radiation alone would entail. While the obvious advantage of possibly preserving a functioning larynx is important to discuss, the patient must be informed of the risks. Most specifically, the risk of persistent disease and the difficulty detecting this in an irradiated patient should be discussed. Additionally, the patient must realize that their larynx may be successfully preserved, but be edematous, necessitating a permanent tracheostomy and even a gastrostomy tube.

The patient should be informed of the role chemotherapy may play. Although chemotherapy has not demonstrated a definitive survival advantage in larynx cancer, the use of neoadjuvant chemotherapy in both the VA and EORTC trials permitted patients that failed to respond to chemotherapy, and were therefore less likely to respond to radiotherapy, to undergo salvage laryngectomy prior to radiation therapy, and thus have a potentially lower complication rate. Additionally, chemotherapy may increase the rate of laryngeal preservation, though this is not proven.

If this patient elects an organ preservation treatment he should also be informed that he has extensive lymph node disease which is not likely to respond completely to nonsurgical therapy. A neck dissection should be performed if the disease fails to respond completely to the chemotherapy. I perform a neck dissection in all N2 or N3 necks that undergo organ-preserving therapy 4 to 6 weeks after the radiation, because at this time the inflammation is decreasing and the fibrosis is only mild.

SURGICAL MANAGEMENT

If this patient is treated surgically the lesion is too extensive for a supraglottic laryngectomy. Both cord fixation and extension inferiorly to the ventricle and true cord are contraindications to a supraglottic laryngectomy. Supracricoid laryngectomy, such as a cricohyoidoepiglotto-pexy, can be considered, but given the extensive preepiglottic involvement and cord fixation, is contraindicated. The only surgical options therefore are extensive laryngeal procedures. The standard treatment of this laryngeal tumor would be a total laryngectomy. At centers where near-total laryngectomies are performed routinely this can also be considered. A total laryngectomy would offer the advantages of permitting complete oncologic resection of the primary tumor. The pharynx is not involved and closure would be possible primarily. It is necessary to inform the patient of the changes wrought by a total laryngectomy related to breathing and coughing through the stoma, the loss of speech, and possible dysphagia.

This patient has a supraglottic cancer and ipsilateral neck disease. There is a high risk of contralateral neck disease. The ipsilateral neck disease is in the region of the jugular chain, and treatment will therefore require a complete neck dissection. Cranial nerve XI can be preserved if uninvolved by tumor. The contralateral neck requires treatment. There is no evidence of extensive cancer in this neck, but the primary tumor is in the supraglottis and crosses the midline, and the left neck is therefore at risk. This neck can be treated surgically by a complete neck dissection, preserving cranial nerve XI, the sternocleidomastoid muscle, and the internal jugular vein, or by a selective neck dissection of levels II, III, and IV. Additionally, because there is no gross neck disease, radiation alone for the contralateral neck is probably sufficient.

REHABILITATION AND FOLLOW-UP

This patient spoke with a radiotherapist about organ preservation treatments. Given the large size of his tumor it was recommended he undergo surgical therapy. The surgery consisted of a total laryngectomy with a right radical neck dissection and a left selective dissection of levels II–IV. A tracheoesophageal puncture was also performed. The margins were clear and the laryngeal cartilage was uninvolved. The lymph nodes in the right neck had extracapsular spread. The nodes in the left neck were negative.

Due to the extensive neck disease with extracapsular spread the patient underwent radiation therapy starting at 5 weeks after surgery. The patient has received smoking cessation treatments. He has been followed with regular examinations to assess for disease recurrence or second primaries. An annual chest x-ray is done. Thyroid function tests were done 3 months after radiotherapy and revealed hypothyroidism, for which he is receiving levothyroxine sodium.

SUGGESTED READINGS

LEE WR, MANCUSO AA, SALEH EM, et al. Can pretreatment computed tomography findings predict local control in T3 squamous cell carcinoma of the glottic larynx treated with radiotherapy alone? *Int J Rad Oncol Biol Phys*. 1993;25:683–687.

Lefebvre JL, Chevalier D, Luboinski B, et al. Larynx preservation in pyriform sinus cancer: preliminary results of a European Organization for Research and Treatment of Cancer Phase III trial. *J Nat Cancer Inst.* 1996;88:890–899.

Wolf GT, Hong WK, Fisher SG, et al. Induction chemotherapy plus radiation compared with surgery plus radiation in patients with advanced laryngeal cancer. *N Engl J Med.* 1991;324:1685–1690.

Case 24

POSTRADIATION LARYNGEAL FRAMEWORK CHONDRITIS

Lyon L. Gleich, M.D.

HISTORY

A 60-year-old male returns 1 year after having received 7,000 cGy of radiation for a T3N0M0 glottic squamous cell carcinoma. During therapy he had significant edema and required a tracheostomy, which was removed 1 month later. He failed to return thereafter, but now presents complaining of progressive throat pain, hoarseness, and difficulty breathing, which has been progressing over a 3-week period. His speech has been muffled for 1 week. He has decreased his oral intake due to pain on swallowing and has lost 5 pounds. He decreased his cigarette intake to one-half pack per day.

On physical examination the vital signs are normal except for a respiratory rate of 25. The neck is visibly erythematous over the larynx. The larynx is tender to palpation. Flexible laryngoscopy reveals severe bilateral arytenoid edema with ulcerative regions on the laryngeal surface of epiglottis. The motion of the left vocal cord is impaired. The airway is judged to be significantly compromised.

DIFFERENTIAL DIAGNOSIS— KEY POINTS

1. This patient is difficult to evaluate since the larynx underwent significant radiotherapy and the patient has not had regular follow-up visits. These findings may well represent recurrent carcinoma, but could also be due to chondronecrosis.

2. Chondronecrosis of the larynx following radiotherapy is relatively rare, occurring in approximately 1% of patients who receive full-course radiation. The risk of chondronecrosis increases with larger daily fractions, larger treatment volumes, prior laryngeal surgery, surgical manipulations for biopsy, and continued smoking.

3. A computed tomography (CT) scan may aid in directing biopsies toward a deep recurrence that is minimally visible at the surface. It can, however, be very difficult to distinguish recurrent cancer from radiation necrosis if there is not a discrete focus of disease. Additionally, in this patient, the airway is at risk and must be managed before there is further decompensation.

TEST INTERPRETATION

A metastatic workup should be started, consisting of at a minimum a chest x-ray and screening blood chemistry to include liver enzymes and thyroid function tests.

The chest x-ray and laboratory values were obtained and were within normal limits. A CT scan was not obtained in this case due to the patient's limited airway. However, in cases where the airway is stable, a CT scan can add valuable information. Figure 24–1, while not a scan of this particular case, reveals findings typical of laryngeal chondronecrosis with loss of laryngeal cartilage and subperichondrial edema and fluid accumulations. Potentially critical patients should not be sent for testing that is not absolutely required.

At the time of direct laryngoscopy, a biopsy was performed that revealed no evidence of residual carcinoma.

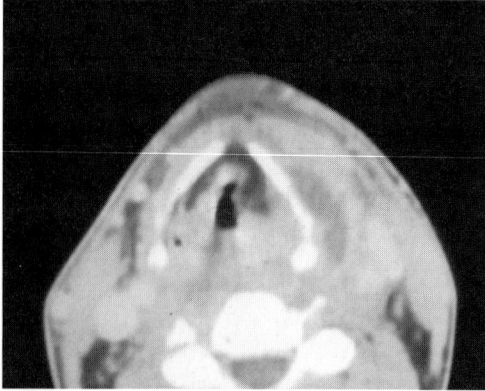

FIGURE 24–1 CT scan reveals findings typical of laryngeal chondronecrosis, with loss of laryngeal cartilage and subperichondrial edema and fluid accumulations.

DIAGNOSIS

Postradiation laryngeal chondronecrosis.

MEDICAL MANAGEMENT

Following radiation therapy for laryngeal carcinoma an ulcerated lesion most frequently represents recurrent disease, and this possibility must be considered. Radiation changes may complicate the interpretation of biopsies, but biopsies and a metastatic evaluation must be done. If there is recurrent cancer at the primary site, without distant metastases, a salvage laryngectomy can be considered, but the complication rate would be higher than that for a standard nonradiated laryngectomy. If there is no recurrent cancer, then his laryngeal disorder is due to radiation injury or the biopsy was insufficient.

Early changes suggestive of laryngeal chondronecrosis can, in select cases, be managed conservatively with a tracheostomy, humidification, and antibiotics. In these less advanced cases hyperbaric oxygen therapy may also aid in recovery. Significant radiation-induced laryngeal chondronecrosis is uncommon. The best treatment is total laryngectomy because this will remove the infected and dead tissue, and will aid in further treating potential tumor recurrence. Most significantly, with significant laryngeal chondronecrosis, laryngeal function is poor and the surgery may even improve function.

After extensive explanation, consent was obtained in this case for a tracheostomy under local anesthesia. The patient then underwent a complete medical evaluation, which in this case revealed no other significant findings. Narcotics were given to alleviate the laryngeal pain. The edema of the larynx persisted, and given his risk of recurrent disease and poor laryngeal function surgical management was recommended.

SURGICAL MANAGEMENT

After obtaining informed consent, the patient should be brought to the operating room for panendoscopy, biopsy, and possible total laryngectomy. Laryngoscopy should be performed and the laryngeal tissues palpated. Biopsies can be obtained and reviewed at frozen section. If a total laryngectomy is performed (the surgical specimen shown in Fig. 24–2 shows typical chondroradionecrotic changes in the anterior laryngeal region), the pharynx can be closed primarily and a cricopharyngeal myotomy per-

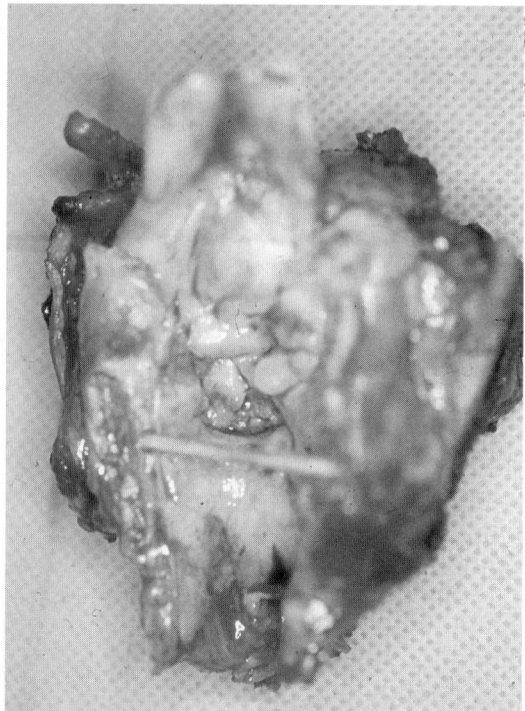

FIGURE 24–2 Surgical specimen demonstrates typical chondroradionecrotic changes in the anterior laryngeal region.

formed. The final pathology in this case revealed chondronecrosis and no residual tumor.

In cases such as this, where laryngeal function is severely compromised, total laryngectomy is the safest treatment. Total laryngectomy is, unfortunately, also the best method of evaluating for persistent disease. Additionally the patient can be rehabilitated, resume an adequate diet, and decrease the need for narcotics. Although a total laryngectomy should not be immediately performed in patients presenting with an impaired larynx after radiation, if recurrent disease is still a significant risk, or if the patient remains in severe pain from the necrosis despite medical treatment, it must be considered.

REHABILITATION AND FOLLOW-UP

Because postradiation surgery carries the potential for increased local complications, the wound should be cautiously observed prior to oral feeding. Oral alimentation can usually be resumed on the 10th postoperative day. Speech can be initially rehabilitated with an electrolarynx, and later with esophageal or T-E fistula speech. Patients should be monitored for disease recurrence.

SUGGESTED READINGS

FERGUSON BJ, HUDSON WR, FARMER JC JR. Hyperbaric oxygen therapy for laryngeal chondronecrosis. *Ann Otol Rhinol Laryngol.* 1987;96:1–6.

PARSONS JT, MENDENHALL WM, MILLION RR. Complications of radiotherapy for head and neck neoplasms. In: Weissler MC, Pillsbury HC III, eds. *Complications of Head and Neck Surgery.* New York: Thieme, 1995: Chapter 15.

STELL PM, MORRISON MD. Radiation necrosis of the larynx: etiology and management. *Arch Otol.* 1973; 98:111–113.

Case 25

POST-THYROIDECTOMY HYPOPARATHYROIDISM

Lyon L. Gleich, M.D.

HISTORY

A 68-year-old male underwent a total thyroid-ectomy for a rapidly enlarging 9-cm thyroid mass the previous day. Frozen section was consistent with papillary carcinoma. The surgery was difficult due to extensive inflammatory and fibrotic reaction surrounding the thyroid gland. The surgeon was able to identify the recurrent laryngeal nerves bilaterally, but the parathyroid glands were difficult to distinguish. There was no palpable adenopathy and the necks were not treated. A calcium level was obtained in the recovery room and was 8.4 mg/dL. The albumin level measured at that time was 3.0 g/dL. The patient is now anxious and having paresthesias of the extremities. He is also having muscle cramping in his upper extremities. He is breathing well and tolerating a soft diet.

On physical examination the surgical site is neither swollen nor erythematous. A Jackson–Pratt drain is in place and is having minimal output. The patient can extend his arms, but has slight spasms at the wrist. The patient has difficulty sensing a pin prick on his toes bilaterally. When the face is tapped by the facial nerve trunk twitching is seen.

DIFFERENTIAL DIAGNOSIS/ KEY POINTS

1. This patient has signs and symptoms strongly suggesting hypoparathyroidism. After total thyroidectomy temporary hypocalcemia is a common finding. Many factors can contribute to the occurrence of significant hypoparathyroidism such as the extent of the thyroid disease, the extent of the surgery, the presence of intrathyroidal parathyroid glands, the reaction of the surrounding tissue to the thyroid disease, and the care, diligence, and experience of the surgeon. In this situation a total thyroidectomy was performed for a large mass and the parathyroid glands were not successfully identified. This patient was therefore at high risk of hypoparathyroidism.

2. Serum calcium levels should be checked in patients after total thyroidectomy twice daily until stable. In this patient the initial postoperative level is below normal, but the albumin is also decreased. Since each gram of albumin binds 0.7 mg of calcium, at that time the patient was not significantly hypocalcemic. This drop in albumin levels is typically seen during surgery and is related to an Antidiuretic hormone release. However, a calcium level should have been checked the next morning. Ionized calcium levels are now widely available and eliminate the need to account for protein binding. Familiarity with serum levels though is important, because in an emergency situation ionized levels cannot always be obtained.

3. Hypocalcemia can cause anxiety, paresthesias, tetany, carpopedal spasm, neuromuscular excitability, laryngospasm, and convulsions. Increased neuroexcitability is often present and can be demonstrated by tapping the facial nerve trunk and seeing twitching

(Chovstek's sign), or by occluding the brachial artery to cause carpal spasm (Trousseau's sign).

DIAGNOSTIC TESTS

This history is highly suggestive of hypocalcemia that needs urgent treatment. Complex diagnostic tests should be avoided for expediency. Chovstek's sign should be checked as described above. A calcium level should be sent stat. If this will require >30 minutes to perform at your hospital, treatment with calcium replacement should begin. In addition, an albumin level should be sent, because this will aid in interpretation of the serum calcium level. Magnesium affects parathyroid hormone function and calcium metabolism, and hypomagnesemia can stress the situation. A magnesium level should therefore be checked.

TEST INTERPRETATION

Serum calcium	5.9 mg/dL
Albumin	2.7 mg/dL
Magnesium	pending at this time

DIAGNOSIS

Even correcting for this patient's hypoalbuminemea, this patient has severe hypocalcemia requiring urgent therapy.

MEDICAL MANAGEMENT

This patient has signs suggesting approaching tetany and could have been treated with intravenous calcium even before the blood levels were confirmed. At this time calcium gluconate 10%, 2 ampules in 100 mL of D5W should be given. Each ampule can be administered during a 15-minute period. In less severe instances of hypocalcemia calcium gluconate can be given one ampule at a time. Each ampule of calcium gluconate delivers 90 mg of elemental calcium.

This patient should be monitored after the initial dose for any further clinical signs of hypocalcemia. The serum calcium or ionized calcium level should be repeated after the calcium injection. If the calcium level remains very low (<7 mg/dL) ampules of calcium gluconate can be given, with levels rechecked after each injection until the calcium level begins to equilibrate. The calcium gluconate can then be given as 1 mg/kg/hr for 6 hours to stabilize the patient at a level >8 mg/dL. Magnesium replacement should also be given to reach a normal level.

After the calcium level is initially stabilized and magnesium replacement initiated, oral calcium replacement can start. If a patient has only a mild or moderate hypocalcemia after total thyroidectomy, oral replacement may not be needed, because this may be only a transient problem. When the hypocalcemia is severe, the injury to the parathyroids is more extensive and long-term calcium replacement may be required. If the parathyroids were inadvertently removed, long-term therapy will always be required. The surgical pathology should therefore be reviewed for the presence of parathyroid tissue. More frequently though, the hypoparathyroidism is the result of devascularization of the parathyroid glands. Calcium carbonate should be used for oral replacement. Replacement of vitamin D enhances the calcium absorption, and ergocalciferol, 50,000 U/day, is frequently used. During the hospitalization the oral calcium should be adjusted until a stable serum level is achieved without the need for intravenous replacement.

REHABILITATION AND FOLLOW-UP

The serum calcium level will need frequent long-term monitoring while the patient is using calcium replacement. The vitamin D dosage may also require adjustments, because the therapeutic and toxic doses are similar. If parathyroid glands are not present in the pathology specimen, and the hypoparathyroidism is therefore from disturbing the vascular supply of the glands and the calcium level is stable or rising, attempts can be made to cautiously wean the patient from calcium replacement. Thyroid function tests should also be monitored more frequently in this patient. This patient had a total thyroidectomy and will therefore need levothyroxine sodium. Hypothyroidism can affect calcium metabolism, and a euthyroid state is therefore optimal.

SUGGESTED REFERENCES

FALK SA. Complications of thyroid surgery. In: Falk SA, ed. *Thyroid Disease: Endocrinology, Surgery, Nuclear Medicine, and Radiotherapy*. New York: Raven Press; 1990:Chapter 38.

FALK SA, BIRKEN EA, BARAN DT. Temporary postthyroidectomy hypocalcemia. *Arch Otol Head Neck Surg.* 1988;114:168–174.

NETTERVILLE JL, ALY A, OSSOFF RH. Evaluation and treatment of complications of thyroid and parathyroid surgery. *Otol Clin North Am.* 1990;23: 529–552.

PAPILLARY CARCINOMA

Lyon L. Gleich, M.D.

HISTORY

A 40-year-old female is referred by her internist. On a routine annual physical her internist detected a right-sided thyroid mass. The patient was unaware of this mass prior to her annual physical, but is now concerned. She is in good health and on no medication. She does not smoke and drinks rarely. She has no change in weight, tremors, palpitations, changes in hair or skin. She has no dysphagia, dyspnea, or changes in her voice. She has not had any radiation exposure. Two of her aunts have had thyroid disease that has been treated with just levothyroxine sodium.

The physical examination is significant for a 3- × 3-cm right-sided thyroid nodule. The lesion moves with deglutition. The remainder of the gland is soft, and the left side is barely palpable. There is no palpable cervical adenopathy. The laryngeal exam reveals normal appearing vocal folds with normal mobility.

DIFFERENTIAL DIAGNOSIS— KEY POINTS

1. This patient has an asymptomatic solitary thyroid nodule. The aim in evaluating her will be to determine if this lesion has a significant malignant potential and thereby requires surgery. Females are more likely than males to develop thyroid masses. However, even though thyroid cancer has a greater predilection for females, a thyroid mass in a male is more worrisome because benign lesions are less common in males. This woman is 40, an age at which both benign and malignant lesions have a high rate of onset. There is a family history of benign thyroid disease in her aunts. While benign thyroid disease does have a genetic predisposition, there is not a

significant genetic predisposition with thyroid cancer except for familial medullary cancer and the multiple endocrine neoplasia syndromes.

2. She has no symptoms to suggest hypothyroidism or hyperthyroidism, but thyroid function tests are still indicated prior to therapy. She also has no signs or symptoms that strongly suggest cancer, such as adenopathy, vocal fold impairment, or a history of irradiation. She does, however, have a solitary nodule, which has a 10 to 15% risk of carcinoma and this will require further evaluation.

DIAGNOSTIC TESTS

The available tests for evaluating thyroid masses are extensive, but it is necessary to be selective to be sensitive, specific, and effective.

1. *Fine-needle aspiration biopsy (FNAB).* Although FNAB is a highly sensitive and specific technique for evaluating thyroid masses, it has limitations, and familiarity with the other studies is important. FNAB is easily performed in the office, but requires a skilled cytopathologist for accurate interpretation. Underlying benign disease can confuse the cytopathologist's ability to render an accurate diagnosis. For example, let us presume a patient has Hashimoto's thyroiditis with a thyroid mass and Hurthle cells are seen on the FNAB. No cytopathologist can determine if the Hurthle cells were from the nodule, which would then be either a Hurthle cell adenoma or carcinoma, or if the Hurthle cells were obtained from the surrounding thyroid gland, which had Hurthle cells due to the thyroiditis.

The most frequent diagnosis that limits the cytopathologist is when the aspirate is consistent with a follicular tumor. The diagnosis of follicular carcinoma is not based on cellular changes, but on pathologic evidence of vascular invasion or capsular invasion. A cytopathologist can only see cellular changes, and therefore cannot render this diagnosis. Therefore, when a cytopathologist sees evidence of a follicular neoplasm, the FNAB will generally be reported as "follicular neoplasm, cannot specify." With other pathologic entities though, such as papillary carcinoma, distinct cellular changes can be diagnostic, and FNAB is therefore often of great value in planning treatment.

The FNAB can also be valuable in determining the characteristic of the mass. A FNAB can obtain cystic fluid, which can then be sent for cytopathology. A cystic thyroid mass has a lower incidence of carcinoma, and if there are no other signs of cancer these patients can be treated with thyroid suppression.

2. *Ultrasonography.* Ultrasound is of value in assessing thyroid masses because it can objectively measure the size and extent of the lesion. It will also determine if a clinically solitary thyroid mass is the only thyroid lesion. If other masses are present, the lone palpable mass is a dominant nodule, and while still at risk for cancer, the risk is lower. Ultrasound will also determine if the mass is solid or cystic, but FNAB gives this same information. Ultrasound involves no ionizing radiation, and therefore is a low-risk examination for patients and is of particular value to document a lesion's size if the plan is initially nonsurgical. Ultrasound can be of limited value if the tumor extends significantly below the clavicles, because ultrasound cannot penetrate bone.

3. *Thyroid scan.* Thyroid scanning was popular in the past, prior to the popularity of ultrasonography and FNAB. On thyroid scans, lesions with minimal hormonal production appear cold, and have a higher incidence of carcinoma. Due to cost, radiation exposure, and the minimal amount of information obtained, this test is employed less commonly.

4. *Computed tomography (CT) scans or magnetic resonance imaging.* These tests are not necessary for small lesions, as in this patient where the dimensions can be determined by exami-

nation or ultrasound. In cases where the mass extends into the superior mediastinum, these studies are of great value to determine the relationship of the mass with the great vessels and trachea. Additionally, in large masses, CT is valuable to assess tracheal compression. If there are palpable nodes, scanning may aid in planning the type of neck dissection, though if a complete neck dissection is planned this may be superfluous.

5. *Chest x-ray.* This is needed in all cases prior to treatment to assess for any metastatic disease and to evaluate the position of the trachea.

6. *Thyroid function tests (TFTs).* A TSH determination is the most sensitive marker of abnormal thyroid function. Prior to any thyroid surgery or medical therapy the TFTs should be checked.

7. *Special blood tests.* Calcitonin levels are elevated with medullary thyroid cancer. This should be checked in patients with a family history of medullary cancer or with a history suggesting an aggressive thyroid cancer. Thyroglobulin can be valuable in following patients after treatment of well-differentiated thyroid neoplasms. In these lesions thyroglobulin decreases after resection and elevates if there is recurrence. The presenting thyroglobulin level though is minimally predictive of either tumor type or disease.

For this patient TFTs are obtained followed by an FNAB and chest x-ray.

TEST INTERPRETATION

The chest x-ray is normal. The patient is euthyroid. Her annual examination included a normal EKG, hematologic, and chemistry profile. The FNAB is shown in Figure 26–1. The FNAB demonstrates a papillary growth pattern along with a nuclear pseudoinclusion in the cell in the upper right portion of the field. These findings together are pathognomonic for papillary carcinoma. This information is discussed with the patient and surgery is recommended.

MEDICAL MANAGEMENT

No medical management is available for papillary carcinoma.

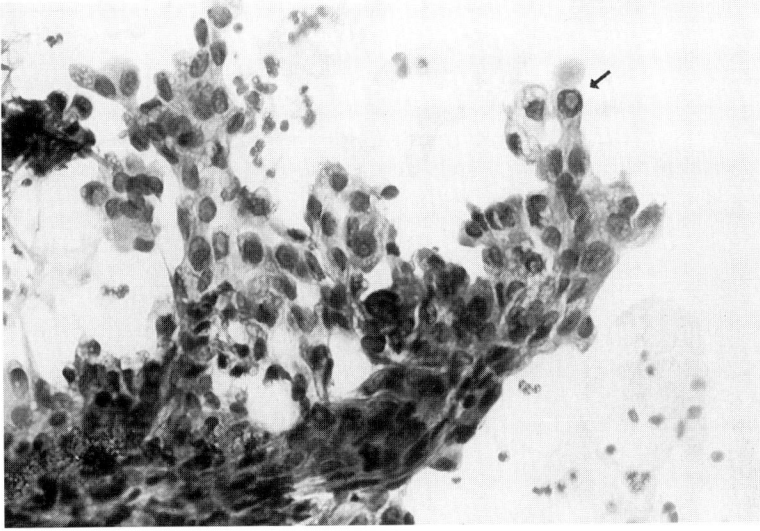

FIGURE 26-1 FNAB reveals a papillary growth pattern and pseudoinclusion in the cell in the upper right portion of the field, pathognomonic for papillary carcinoma.

SURGICAL MANAGEMENT

Papillary thyroid cancer is a well-differentiated thyroid cancer. The informed consent needs to include a right hemithyroidectomy and possible total thyroidectomy. The patient must also understand the risk of cervical metastases, and that a neck dissection will be performed if nodes are found. Major risks include recurrent nerve injury with resulting changes in voice and aspiration; superior laryngeal nerve injury, which can affect vocal range and strength; hypoparathyroidism with resultant need for calcium replacement therapy; hematoma; and general surgical risks such as infection or anesthetic reaction. Once the patient understands the risks of surgery one can proceed.

The initial procedure was a right hemithyroidectomy. Frozen section revealed a 3- × 3- × 3-cm papillary carcinoma contained in the right thyroid gland. There are no palpable nodes and the left gland feels normal. This is consistent with a T2N0 stage I papillary carcinoma. In this patient a completion thyroidectomy was performed due to the high frequency of multicentric papillary thyroid cancer. In small lesions in younger females there are surgeons who do not believe the risk of developing a significant cancer in the contralateral lobe is high enough to warrant a completion thyroidectomy, with its increased risk to the parathyroid gland. Either option is therefore acceptable at this time.

After the completion thyroidectomy calcium levels were checked twice daily during her 2-day hospitalization and were stable. The patient was then discharged.

REHABILITATION AND FOLLOW-UP

A thyroid scan was performed 1 month after her surgery and revealed sparse uptake in the thyroid bed only. The patient was treated with radioactive iodine. This combination of total thyroidectomy followed by radioactive iodine has been demonstrated to yield the best long-term survival in patients with tumors > 1.5 cm. After radioactive iodine therapy she began levothyroxine sodium daily for life.

With this low-stage disease and appropriate therapy, her prognosis is excellent. Follow-up is necessary to monitor her levothyroxine sodium and assess for any disease recurrence. Disease recurrence can be monitored by thyroglobulin assays and/or total body iodine scanning. Either method is acceptable as a monitoring modality. Combining the two monitoring methods though does increase sensitivity, but is less cost effective.

SUGGESTED REFERENCES

Harvey HK. Diagnosis and management of the thyroid nodule: an overview. *Otol Clin North Am.* 1990;23:303–338.

Shah JP, Loree TR, Dharker D, Strong EW. Lobectomy versus total thyroidectomy for differentiated carcinoma of the thyroid: a matched pair analysis. *Am J Surg.* 1993;166:331–335.

Strong EW. Evaluation and surgical treatment of papillary and follicular carcinoma. In: Falk SA eds. *Thyroid Disease: Endocrinology, Surgery, Nuclear Medicine, and Radiotherapy.* New York: Raven Press; 1990:Chapter 27.

Case 27

ESTHESIONEURO-BLASTOMA

Keith M. Wilson, M.D.

HISTORY

A 33-year-old man presents with a 3-month history of left nasal obstruction, midfacial pressure, and occasional epistaxis. He denies purulent nasal discharge and postnasal drainage. He reports that during the last 2 months he has been on three courses of antibiotics, each course being 7 days in duration. He has also been on multiple antihistamine/decongestion/mucolytic medications without any relief.

His medical history is unremarkable. He admits to smoking 1½ packs of cigarettes per day but denies alcohol use. He is a carpenter by trade.

On physical examination he is found to have a red polypoid mass originating high in the left nasal chamber that is causing near complete nasal obstruction. Evidence of prior bleeding can be found. The right nasal chamber is narrowed but does not have an obvious mass lesion. The eyes have normal mobility without evidence of proptosis. Vision is grossly normal. Examination of the neck reveals no palpable masses. Neurologic examination is grossly within normal limits.

DIFFERENTIAL DIAGNOSIS— KEY POINTS

1. The presentation of a unilateral nasal mass causing obstruction and bleeding raises concern for a malignancy. Although the most common primary malignancy of the sinonasal tract is squamous cell carcinoma, adenocarcinoma, esthesioneuroblastoma, and minor salivary gland tumors must be considered (see Table 27–1). Sinonasal tract malignancies tend to present late and lack known risk factors. Certain occupations, such as nickel workers, woodworkers, and leather workers have been determined to be high risk for the development of cancers of the sinonasal area. Unfortunately, most tumors in this area tend to have a similar presentation. Radiographic imaging provides information about the extent of disease and potentially destructive nature of the tumor. Definitive diagnosis is made by biopsy and, if needed, immunohistochemical staining.

2. There are many benign tumors that may have this same presentation; papillomas, juvenile angiofibromas and neurogenous tumors to name a few (see Table 27–2). Age, gender, and medical history can help in the diagnosis. Biopsy is ultimately needed for diagnosis. Radiographic imaging helps define the disease process.

3. Nasal polyposis is part of the differential diagnosis for this patient. However, bleeding would not be expected as a major presenting complaint and most patients tend to present with bilateral nasal symptoms.

TABLE 27-1 Benign Sinonasal Tumors

Epithelial
  Papilloma
    fungiform
    inverting
  Adenoma
  Nevus
  Mixed tumor
  Oncocytoma

Mesenchymal
  Angiofibroma
  Hemangioma
  Lymphangioma
  Neurogenous
    neurilemoma
    neurofibroma
  Fibroma
  Lipoma
  Chondroma
  Hamartoma
  Meningioma

Osseous
  Osteoma
  Exostosis (torus palatinus)
  Osteoid osteoma
  Giant cell tumors
    reparative granuloma
    giant cell tumor
    osteitis fibrosa cystica
    cherubism
  Ossifying fibroma
  Fibrous dysplasia
  Desmoplastic fibroma
  Chondromyxoid fibroma

Odontogenic
  Ameloblastoma
  Pindborg tumor
  Adenoblastoma
  Myxoma
  Odontogenic fibroma
  Odontogenic fibromyxoma
  Cementoma
  Mixed odontogenic tumors

TABLE 27-2 Malignant Sinonasal Tumors

Epithelial
  Squamous cell carcinoma
  Minor salivary gland cancers
  Adenocarcinoma
  Undifferentiated carcinoma
  Malignant melanoma
  Esthesioneuroblastoma

Mesenchymal
  Sarcoma
    chondrosarcoma
    rhabdomyosarcoma
    fibrosarcoma
    angiosarcoma
    neurofibrosarcoma
  Hemangiopericytoma
  Fibrous histiocytoma
  Lymphoreticular tumors
    lymphoma
    plasmacytoma

Osseous
  Osteogenic sarcoma
  Ewing's sarcoma

Odontogenic

Metastasis

lobe. There is no involvement of the soft tissues of the orbit. The sphenoid sinuses are clear (Fig. 27–1).

3. *Biopsy.* Small, round cells arranged in a rosette pattern with surrounding stroma composed of undifferentiated nuclei and fibrillary cords, marked microvascularity and palisading cells around blood vessels (Fig. 27–2). Immunohistochemical analysis reveals positive staining for S-100, neuron-specific enolase, synaptophysin, and chromagranin. Negative stains were found for epithelial membrane antigen and cytokeratin.

DIAGNOSIS

Esthesioneuroblastoma, group B (see Table 27–3).

MEDICAL MANAGEMENT

The treatment of esthesioneuroblastoma is usually surgical. However, medical management of esthesioneuroblastoma is the treatment of choice if the patient is a poor surgical candidate, has extensive local disease, has distant metasta-

TEST INTERPRETATION

1. *Computed tomography scan.* Destructive lesion in the superior aspect of the left nasal chamber showing signs of destruction. The tumor involves the medial wall of the orbit. The sphenoid sinuses are clear.

2. *Magnetic resonance imaging (MRI) scan.* There is a soft tissue density present in the left ethmoid sinus. The mass extends to the dura with questionable involvement of the frontal

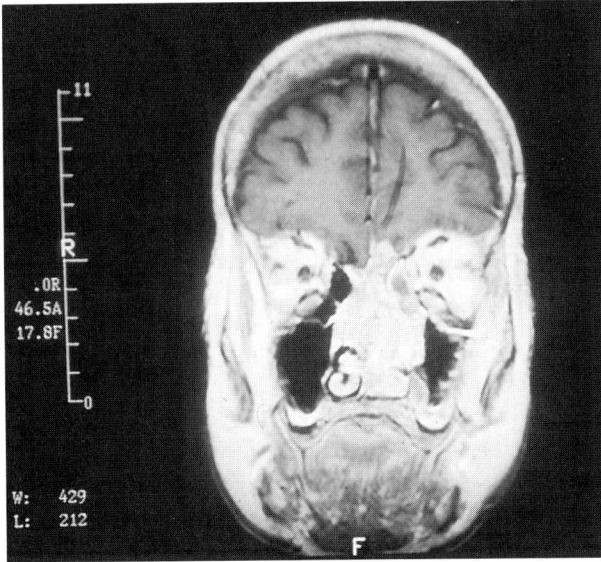

FIGURE 27–1 MRI demonstrates a soft tissue density in the left ethmoid sinus, extending to the dura and possibly the frontal lobe.

ses, or refuses surgery. Medical management would consist of chemotherapy and radiation therapy. Chemotherapeutic agents that have shown efficacy in the treatment of esthesioneuroblastoma include cisplatin, etoposide, fluorouracil, cyclophosphamide, and vincristine.

While radiation therapy tends to be used either preoperatively or postoperatively, curative doses, ranging from 50 to 65 Gy, have been reported. There is some evidence to support using stereotaxic proton irradiation for esthesioneuroblastoma. This technique allows higher doses of radiation to be delivered to a tumor while minimizing the radiation to adjacent vital structures.

Surgical salvage for local recurrences after chemotherapy/radiation is reported to provide 80% 5-year survival rates.

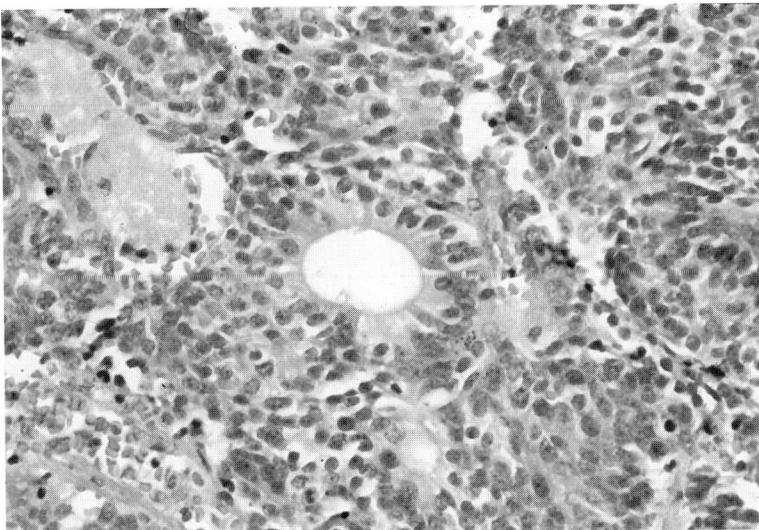

FIGURE 27–2 Biopsy reveals small round cells arranged in a rosette pattern.

TABLE 27–3 Staging for Esthesioneuroblastoma

Group A	Tumor confined to the nasal cavity
Group B	Tumor extending beyond nasal cavity into paranasal sinuses
Group C	Tumor spread beyond nasal cavities and paranasal sinuses

SURGICAL MANAGEMENT

Craniofacial resection combined with radiation therapy has become the accepted treatment for esthesioneuroblastoma. This includes the midline anterior cranial base, involved paranasal sinuses, dura, and frontal lobe if necessary. Cervical lymph nodes are the most common site of metastatic disease with rates varying from 17 to 48%. Although neck dissection is usually performed in the face of overt cervical metastases, an argument can be made for elective cervical lymphadenectomy in patients with esthesioneuroblastoma. Radiation therapy is usually administered postoperatively but in certain instances is delivered preoperatively. Survival rates are reported in the range of 75 to 92% with follow-up ranging from 2 to 5 years.

Craniofacial resection does have significant risks associated with the procedure. Potential complications include those associated with neurosurgery, like cerebrospinal fluid leaks, symptomatic pneumocephalus, and those seen in sinus surgery, like enophthalmos or injury to orbital structures. All patients have anosmia as a result of the loss of the olfactory cleft.

REHABILITATION AND FOLLOW-UP

In the immediate postoperative period, patients should be closely monitored for the potential neurologic sequelae of cerebrospinal fluid leak or pneumocephalus. Any evidence of meningitis should be identified rapidly and corrected as appropriate.

From a long-term prospective, these patients require vigilant monitoring for evidence of local or distant recurrence. MRI scan is an ideal tool for monitoring these patients for local recurrence.

SUGGESTED READINGS

BHATTACHARYYA N, THORNTON AF, JOSEPH MP, et al. Successful treatment of esthesioneuroblastoma and neuroendocrine carcinoma with combined chemotherapy and proton radiation. *Arch Otolaryngol Head Neck Surg.* 1997;123:34–40.

GLUCKMAN JL. Tumors of the nose and paranasal sinuses. In: Donald PJ, Gluckman JL, Rice DH, eds. *The Sinuses.* New York: Raven Press; 1995:423–444.

LEVINE PA, STEWART FM, CANTRELL RW, et al. Esthesioneuroblastoma: long-term outcome and patterns of failure—the University of Virginia experience. *Cancer.* 1994;73:2556–2562.

MAXILLARY SINUS CARCINOMA

Douglas B. Villaret, M.D.
Keith M. Wilson, M.D.

HISTORY

A 52-year-old male presented with a 6-month history of nasal congestion and headaches, predominately right sided. He had been treated with multiple courses of antibiotics with partial resolution of his symptoms. Recently, short episodes of epistaxis began troubling him.

His medical history was noncontributory for seasonal allergies or industrial exposure, although he did work with wood as a hobby. Additionally, he was being treated with an aspirin a day for cardiovascular disease.

On physical examination there was mild tenderness over the right maxillary sinus, but no orbital proptosis, ulcerations, or purulence in the nasal cavity. A soft tissue mass could be visualized superiorly in the right nares. The neck examination was negative for adenopathy.

A thin-cut computed tomography (CT) scan of the sinuses was ordered.

DIFFERENTIAL DIAGNOSIS— KEY POINTS

1. The triad of unilateral facial pain, nasal obstruction, and epistaxis requires that malignant tumor be ruled out. Squamous cell CA would most commonly be found in the maxillary sinus followed by minor salivary gland tumors and adenocarcinoma of mucosal origin (associated with woodworkers).

2. Antral and ethmoid polyps usually are apparent on nasal endoscopy, have a characteristic fleshly appearance, and show bony remodeling.

3. Papillomas, especially inverting papilloma based on the lateral nasal wall, are a real possibility.

4. Other benign tumors such as neurilemmoma, neurofibroma, and giant cell tumors have been reported in this area.

5. The presenting symptoms are consistent with bacterial or fungal sinusitis with polypoid changes. The antibiotics provided partial relief and pyogenic or fungal sinusitis can erode bone, although the nasal cavity should have shown more inflammation.

6. Lymphomas, osteogenic and odontogenic tumors, as well as metastases (primarily renal) also occur in the maxillary sinus.

TEST INTERPRETATION

The CT scan revealed a soft tissue mass filling the right superior nasal cavity and maxillary sinus. The septum was bowed to the contralateral side. There was evidence of bony erosion and extension into the ethmoid sinuses. No calcifications were seen within the soft tissues nor was there any sclerosis of the adjacent bony walls. The posterior ethmoids were surprisingly not involved (Fig. 28–1).

Maxillary sinus malignancies are usually of soft tissue density on CT, which separates them from acute inflammatory mucosa as well as markedly desiccated secretions. Bony remodeling, sclerosis, and calcifications within the soft tissue mass are most consistent with a benign process. A CT scan is necessary for suspected tumors to evaluate the extent of the mass and any bony erosion.

Magnetic resonance imaging is a better modality for distinguishing inflammation from tumor, should clinical signs be nonspecific. Tumors will be of intermediate intensity on T2-weighted images, while the inflammatory component will be of high signal intensity. Additionally, the tumors will have intermedi-

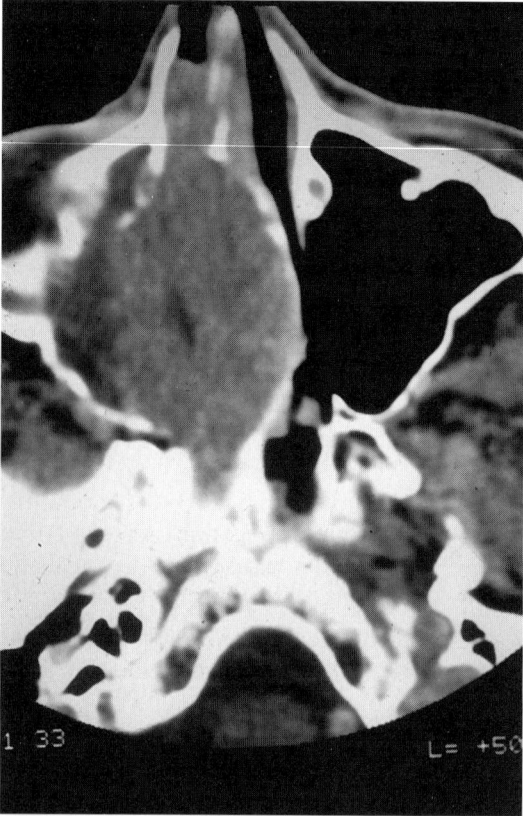

FIGURE 28–1 CT scan demonstrates soft tissue mass filling the right superior nasal cavity and maxillary sinus.

ate intensity on T1 images with intravenous gadolinium enhancement: Secretions will not enhance but will be rimmed by a bright signal from the inflamed mucosa. Also, this will help answer questions as to the extent of orbital or dural involvement.

Open biopsy through the nose showed a firm, tan mass adhering superiorly and laterally. The specimen showed squamous cells with cellular atypia, nuclear pleomorphism, and keratin pearl formation. Prognosis for these tumors is influenced most by the extent of invasion; therefore, increasing numbers of associated symptoms result in decreasing 5-year survival.

DIAGNOSIS

T3N0 Squamous Cell Carcinoma (SCCA) of the maxillary sinus.

MEDICAL MANAGEMENT

Maxillary sinus malignancies tend to grow to a large size before they signal their existence by interfering with the sinus ostia, invading bone, interrupting the infraorbital nerve, or involving the eye. Öhngren separated the tumors into those growing anteroinferiorly versus posterosuperiorly; the latter having a graver prognosis (Öhngren's line joins the angle of the mandible to the medial canthus). This is reflected in the staging system of these tumors (Table 28–1).

Due to the poor 5-year survival rate, multimodality therapy is most often used. T1 tumors have a 60% 5-year survival, decreasing to 10 to 20% for T4 tumors. Overall, there is a 30% 5-year survival rate for squamous cell carcinomas of the paranasal sinuses.

Although chemotherapy definitely has a role in lymphomas and rhabdomyosarcomas of the maxilla, there are no studies showing efficacy of this as single modality treatment in squamous cell carcinomas. However, its use as a palliative agent for inoperative, advanced cancers should be considered.

Occasionally, radiation is used for cure, especially for lymphoma, plasmacytoma, and juvenile angiofibroma. Approximately 50 to 55 Gy are used over a period of 5 to 6 weeks. Most tumors of the maxillary sinus are relatively radioresistant and, therefore, radiotherapy is commonly reserved for adjunct treatment postoperatively or as palliation.

TABLE 28–1 Staging of Maxillary Sinus Cancer

Tis	Carcinoma *in situ*.
T1	Tumor limited to the antral mucosa with no erosion or destruction of bone.
T2	Tumor with erosion or destruction of the infrastructure including the hard palate and/or the middle nasal meatus.
T3	Tumor invades skin of the cheek, posterior wall of the maxillary sinus, floor or medial wall of the orbital, anterior ethmoid sinus.
T4	Tumor invades orbital contents and/or cribiform plate, posterior ethmoid or sphenoid sinuses, nasopharynx, soft palate, pterygia maxillary or temporal fossa or base of skull.

SURGICAL MANAGEMENT

This patient underwent a radical maxillectomy, preserving the orbit, with obturator placement.

The treatment philosophy is dictated by the type and stage of the tumor, the patient's wishes, and the comfort level of the surgeon. Maxillary tumors often present at an advanced stage as there is room for growth with minimal symptoms. The psychological state of the patient must be assessed as to his or her ability to withstand a disfiguring operation and possibly the loss of an eye. Finally, an experienced prosthodontist is essential for the rehabilitation of the patient.

The surgical management is varied and tailored to the extent of the tumor. The basic procedures are:

1. *Medial maxillectomy.* Exposure is achieved via a lateral rhinotomy or midfacial degloving procedure. The bony skeleton is separated from the pyriform aperture to the frontoethmoid suture line; across the medial, inferior aspects of the orbit with the lateral limit being the infraorbital nerve. This dissection is carried inferiorly to the bottom of the maxillary sinus and then medially across the pyriform rim. The lateral nasal wall is then removed while separating the last attachments to the pterygoid plates.

2. *Suprastructure maxillectomy.* Used for ethmoid tumors that encroach upon the orbit. The superior half of the maxillary sinus is removed and possibly the ethmoid air cells, floor of the orbit, and its contents.

3. *Infrastructure maxillectomy.* This can be used for tumors of the alveolar ridge, hard palate, and floor of the maxillary antrum. A maxillary antrostomy is performed and the sinus is checked for tumor extending beyond the floor. The palate is then divided (usually at the midline), and the attachment to the pterygoid plates is divided. An obturator is then attached to the remaining hard palate with screws from a miniplating system.

4. *Radical maxillectomy.* Used for all maxillary or ethmoid tumors that are not localized to a small area. Includes hard palate, part of the body of the zygoma, anteromedial portion of the orbit, lateral nasal wall, and maxillary sinus. It can be extended in any direction to include adjacent structures. Contraindications include involvement of the sphenoid sinus, nasopharynx, middle cranial fossa, infratemporal fossa (extensive), and distant metastases. A relative contraindication is bilateral neck disease (due to very poor 2-year survival rates).

All procedures can be extended to include the orbit, the infratemporal fossa, the contralateral maxilla, and finally a craniofacial resection.

REHABILITATION AND FOLLOW-UP

This is arguably the most important aspect of this disease given the 30% 5-year survival rate for all patients with cancers of the maxillary sinus who have undergone these disfiguring operations. A team approach is essential, including a prosthodontist, speech therapist, social worker, and psychologist with the surgeon as coordinator.

A well-fitting prosthesis is of paramount importance. To help in this regard, it is important to place a skin graft at the time of surgery to prevent contracture, to leave as many teeth and as much anterior maxilla as possible, and to remove all bony projections that would interfere with the placement of the obturator. Preoperative evaluation by the prosthodontist assists not only with the intraoperative obturator, but also sets the stage for long-term rehabilitation.

SUGGESTED READINGS

BEAHRS OH, HENSON DE, KENNEDY BJ, eds. American Joint Committee on Cancer. *Manual for Staging Cancer.* 4th ed. Philadelphia, PA: JB Lippincott, 1992.

DONALD PJ, GLUCKMAN JL, RICE DH. Tumors of the nose and paranasal sinuses. In: *The Sinuses.* New York: Raven Press; 1995:423–444.

GLUCKMAN JL, GULANE P, JOHNSON J. Nasal cavity and paranasal sinus. In: *Practical Approach to Head and Neck Tumors.* New York: Raven Press; 1994:113–130.

Myers E, Suen J, eds. Cancer of the nasal cavity and paranasal sinuses. In: *Cancer of the Head and Neck*. Philadelphia, PA: WB Saunders; 1996:205–233.

Osguthorpe JD, ed. Paranasal sinus tumors. *Otol Clin North Am*. 1995;28(6).

Paparella MM, Shumrick DA, Gluckman JL, Meyerhoff WL, eds. Tumors of the nose and paranasal sinuses. In: *Otolaryngolgy*. Philadelphia, PA: WB Saunders; 1991:1935–1958.

INVERTING PAPILLOMA

Michelle M. Cullen, M.D.
Thomas A. Tami, M.D.

HISTORY

A 55-year-old white male presents with a history of recurrent right-sided epistaxis and right-sided nasal obstruction for several months. The patient denies trauma, sneezing, itchy eyes, nasal pain, diplopia, otalgia, facial numbness, purulent drainage, ill-fitting dentures, trismus, or chronic sinusitis. The patient's medical history is unremarkable. He neither drinks nor smokes; he works as an accountant.

The physical examination reveals a very slight swelling of the right midface and infraorbital skin, with a normal appearance to the external nose. Anterior rhinoscopy reveals a unilateral polypoid, granular, erythematous mass in the right nasal cavity. On nasal endoscopy, a mass is emanating from the lateral nasal wall in the approximate region of the right middle meatus.

DIFFERENTIAL DIAGNOSIS— KEY POINTS

1. Unilateral nasal polyp/mass must immediately raise the possiblity of a diagnoisis other than inflammatory nasal polyposis such as malignancy or aggressive infection (mucormycosis or invasive aspergillosis).

2. Inverting papilloma may present in all age groups, although it has a peak incidence in the fifth and sixth decades of life, with a male to female ratio of 3 to 1. The most common symptom is unilateral nasal obstruction. Pain is uncommon unless associated with a secondary bacterial superinfection or malignancy.

3. Trismus is an ominous sign of malignancy and can indicate invasion of the masseter and pterygoid muscles. Ill-fitting dentures can be indicative of tumor invasion into the floor of the maxillary antrum. Edema and/or hypesthesia in the distribution of the second division of the trigeminal nerve can occur due to skull base or pterygopalatine fossa extension.

4. The location of *nasal papilloma* is an important predictor of histology. **Fungiform papillomas** have little if any propensity for malignant transformation and usually arise anteriorly on the nasal septum. These are caused by the common cutaneous papilloma virus.

   In contrast, *inverting papilloma,* also known as Schneiderian papilloma or soft papilloma, is a true epithelial neoplasm characterized by hyperplastic epithelium that inverts into the underlying stroma. The basement membrane is intact and there is no histologic evidence of malignancy. There are no associated keratin pearls, and a normal number of mitoses are seen. Although the lesion appears benign histologically, it can behave aggressively with destruction of the lateral nasal wall, which is where the lesion is most commonly located.

   The human papilloma virus types 6, 11, 16, and 18 have been implicated in the disease and a majority of these that undergo malignant transformation harbor types 6, 11, or 16 Also, those tumors with HPV DNA are more likely to recur.

5. Biopsy can be deferred until after a computed tomography (CT) scan is obtained. If a biopsy is performed in the office, materials and supplies for treatment of epistaxis should be readily available.

6. Inverting papilloma is a benign lesion; however, its incidence of malignant transformation to squamous cell carcinoma is between 5 and 80%. An acceptable figure by most is that of 13%. Direction of the lymphatic spread, should malignancy arise, is dependent on the site of the tumor. Cancers of the

nasal vestibule and anterior nose drain into the submental, parotid, submandibular, and facial nodes prior to reaching the second echelon upper deep cervical nodes. Tumors of the paranasal sinuses and nose spread initially to plexus of lymphatics in the region of the torus tuberalis, followed by spread to the retropharyngeal and upper deep cervical nodes.

7. Other benign tumors include juvenile angiofibroma (which is a highly vascular tumor with a propensity for local extension and is usually found in young males), minor salivary gland tumors (the most common of which is pleomorphic adenoma, followed by basal cell adenoma and oncocytoma), neurinomas, neurofibromas, meningiomas, osteomas, and giant cell tumors. Malignant neoplasms include squamous cell carcinoma, adenocarcinoma, mucosal melanoma, esthesioneuroblastoma, chondrosarcoma, rhabdomyosarcoma, fibrosarcoma, fibrous histiocytoma, hemangiopericytoma, lymphoma, plasmacytoma, osteogenic sarcoma, as well as metastases and odontogenic tumors. Furthermore, antral choanal polyp and benign rhinolith with retained foreign body and granuloma should be considered.

TEST INTERPRETATION

1. *CT scan.* In evaluating a unilateral nasal mass, a CT scan is a valuable diagnostic test to ascertain the extent of the mass and evidence of bony change. Destruction is associated with a malignancy, whereas bony remodeling is consistent with benign or slow-growing neoplasm. Evaluation of the extent of the disease (skull base, retropharynx, midface, orbit, cribriform plate, and maxillary sinus extension) is important. The CT scan of the sinuses of this patient (Fig. 29–1) demonstrates a unilateral nasal mass with bony destruction of the lateral nasal wall. The maxillary sinus involvement may represent postobstructive inflammatory changes or neoplasm.

2. *Magnetic resonance imaging scan.* It is helpful to perform an MRI as well as a CT when evaluating nasal or nasopharyngeal masses because MRI can more clearly define the dif-

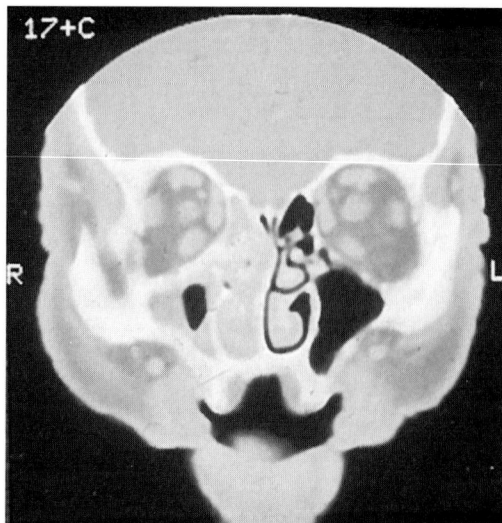

FIGURE 29–1 CT scan demonstrates a unilateral nasal mass with bony destruction of the lateral nasal wall.

ference between mucosal thickening and tumor whereas CT cannot. A combination of T1, T2, and gadolinium enhancement may be used to delineate the tumor extent.

3. Angiography or magnetic resonance angiography. These tests can be used to evaluate the arterial circulation and its proximity or involvement with tumor for adequate assessment of resectability and preoperative planning. These tests are usually not necessary unless a vascular mass is being considered.

4. Biopsy. Biopsy of the nasal mass of this patient shows hyperplastic endothelium with epithelial tissue inverting into the underlying stroma. The basement membrane is intact and there is no evidence of squamous cell carcinoma.

DIAGNOSIS

Inverting papilloma of the right nasal cavity involving the ethmoid sinuses.

MEDICAL MANAGEMENT

Radiation is not recommended as the only treatment for inverting papilloma; however, it can be used for those patients who are poor surgical risks, are unresectable, or have extremely aggressive disease. It is suggested that malignant transformation can occur following radiation therapy.

SURGICAL MANAGEMENT

Complete excision of the lesion with adequate margins is the treatment for this disease. The best chance for cure is at the time of initial resection and, therefore, the surgical resection should be complete. The extent of the lesion in this patient would be treated with a medial maxillectomy via a lateral rhinotomy. Despite careful surgical technique a recurrence rate of 9 to 43% can occur and multiple surgeries may be necessary for cure.

Recently, the nasal endoscopic approach has been advocated by some authors as a very effective, low-mortality technique to manage this neoplasm. In general, this technique is best reserved for cases with disease limited to the nasal cavity and not extending into the maxillary sinus or frontal recess.

REHABILITATION AND FOLLOW-UP

Follow-up of a medial maxillectomy requires frequent debridement of nasal crusts. The patient should be maintained on normal saline irrigations postoperatively and can be weaned off of normal saline irrigations once healing is complete. Close long-term follow-up with endoscopy/examination is recommended due to a substantial recurrence rate. The risk of squamous cell carcinoma is most likely within the first 2 to 5 years. Complications of a medial maxillectomy include cerebrospinal fluid leak, dacryocystitis, epiphora, diplopia, nasocutaneous fistula, nasal collapse, scar, and frontal sinus mucocele.

SUGGESTED READINGS

BECK JC, MCCLATCHEY KD, LESPERANCE MM, et al. Presence of human papilloma virus predicts recurrence of inverted papilloma. *Otol Head Neck Surg.* 1995;113(1):49–55.

BECK JC, MCCLATCHEY KD, LESPERANCE MM, et al. Human papilloma virus types important in progression of inverted papilloma. *Otol Head Neck Surg.* 1995;113(5):558–563.

BLITZER A, LAWSON W. FRIEDMAN WH. Pathology. In: *Surgery of the Paranasal Sinuses.* 2nd ed. Philadelphia, PA: WB Saunders; 1991:429–431.

FRIEDMAN WH. *Surgery of the Paranasal Sinuses.* American Academy of Otolaryngology; 1979.

GLUCKMAN JL. Tumors of the nose and paranasal sinuses. In: *The Sinuses.* Donald PJ, Gluckman JL, Rice DL, eds. New York: Raven Press; 1995:Chapter 28.

KNUDSEN SJ, BAILEY BJ. Midline nasal masses. In: Bailey BJ, Johnson JT, Kohut RL, et al, eds. *Head and Neck Surgery—Otolaryngology.* Philadelphia, PA: JB Lippincott; 1993:329–341.

KRESPEI YP, LEVINE TM. Tumors of the nose and paranasal sinuses. In: Paperella MM, Shumrick DA, Gluckman JL, et al, eds. *Otolaryngology. Vol. Three, Head and Neck.* 3rd ed. Philadelphia, PA: WB Saunders; 1991:1935–1958.

MANIGLIA AJ, PHILLIPS DA. Midfacial degloving for the management of nasal sinus and skull base neoplasms. *Otol Clin North Am.* 1995;28(6):1127–1143.

STANIEVICH JF, LORE JM. Tumors of the nose, paranasal sinuses and nasopharynx. In: Bluestone CD, Stool SE, eds. *Pediatric Otolaryngology.* Philadelphia, PA: WB Saunders; 1990:780–792.

STANKIEWICZ J, GIRIS SJ. Endoscopic surgical treatment of nasal and paranasal sinus inverted papilloma. *Arch Otolaryngol Head Neck Surg.* 1993;109:988–995.

WEYMULLER EA. Neoplasms of the paranasal sinuses. In: Cummings CW, Fredrickson JM, Harker LA, et al, eds. *Otolaryngology—Head and Neck Surgery.* St. Louis, MO: Mosby-Year Book; 1993:941–954.

Case 30

PARAPHARYNGEAL MASS

Jack L. Gluckman, M.D.

HISTORY

A 54-year-old male presents with a 6-month history of snoring, possible sleep apnea, and the recent development of mild obstructive dysphagia. He was otherwise asymptomatic. The only history of consequence was that he had undergone a resection of a benign tumor via an intraoral approach 15 years previously.

Examination revealed slight fullness in the region of the right parotid gland on palpation of his neck. However, on examination of his pharynx, there was significant displacement of the right oropharyngeal wall with evidence of a scar on the soft palate (Fig. 30–1). There was no trismus and no evidence of cranial nerve palsy.

Clinical diagnosis was suggestive of a right parapharyngeal mass.

DIFFERENTIAL DIAGNOSIS— KEY POINTS

1. While the differential diagnosis of a parapharyngeal space mass is considerable, with both benign and malignant tumors arising from the many structures coursing through this space, from the practical point of view, the probabilities are as follows:
   A. Tumors of salivary gland origin. These most commonly arise from the deep lobe of the parotid gland and are usually benign (pleomorphic adenoma). However, minor salivary glands in the lateral pharyngeal wall and ectopic tissue in the pa-

rapharyngeal space may be the source of neoplasms.
   B. Tumors of neurogenic origin, that is, schwannoma, neurofibroma, or even paraganglioma, which in this situation usually arise from the vagus (vagal paraganglioma).
   C. Lymph node enlargement due to lymphoma or metastases from cancer arising in the pharynx.
   D. A large but rare miscellaneous group encompassing a multitude of tumors from various anatomic sites.
2. The patient may have a substantially sized tumor with only minimal symptoms and no external signs. It is only on examination of the oropharynx that the lesion is detected. Both pain and cranial nerve palsy are highly indicative of malignancy but rarely can occur in benign tumors. Unilateral eustachian tube dysfunction may be an early manifestation and all adults undergoing evaluation for unilateral otitis should not only have the nasopharynx evaluated but be suspected of having a parapharyngeal space mass.
3. Further tests are now required to determine diagnosis and develop a therapeutic approach.

TEST INTERPRETATION

All patients who have a suspected parapharyngeal space mass should undergo imaging. A computed tomography (CT) scan is an excellent

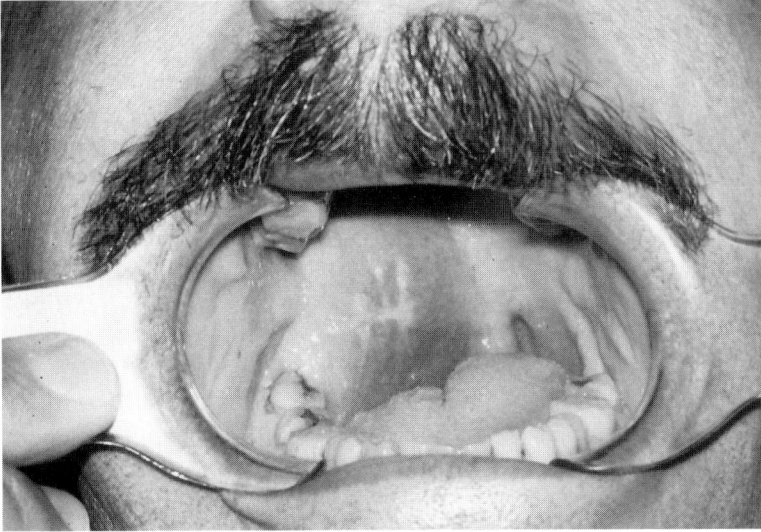

FIGURE 30–1 Distortion of the lateral oropharyngeal wall. Note scar from previous incomplete excision.

first examination although magnetic resonance imaging (MRI) can be requested. CT scan will delineate whether the tumor is prestyloid or poststyloid in origin, whether it arises from the parotid or is extraparotid, and whether there is any base of skull erosion. In this case it was noted that the tumor arose from the deep lobe of the parotid and was prestyloid (Fig. 30–2).

If it appears to be a deep lobe tumor, then no further imaging is required prior to surgery. However, if it appears to be poststyloid, then MRI and even magnetic resonance angiography (MRA) will be needed to determine its extent, whether it is a vascular mass, and its relationship to the great vessels at the skull base. This information is vital in treatment planning. Angiography is indicated if MRA does not give the relevant information or if embolization is being considered and a definitive feeder vessel needs to be identified.

Once imaging has been performed, biopsy is usually not indicated preoperatively except in unusual situations or if malignancy is suspected. This can be performed using fine-needle aspiration, which is CT guided either transorally or externally. Transoral open biopsy should be discouraged because of the danger of vascular injury, seeding of the tumor, and contamination of the operative site, and because in most cases it is unnecessary.

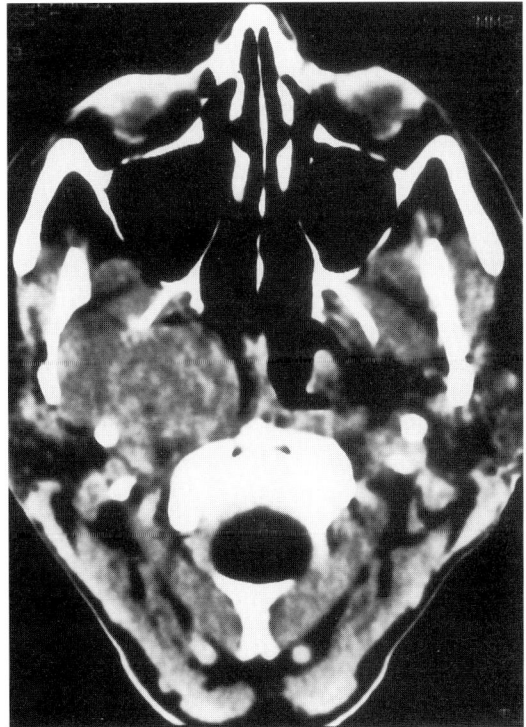

FIGURE 30–2 CT scan demonstrating a large deep lobe pleomorphic adenoma. Note absence of fat plane between deep lobe and tumor.

DIAGNOSIS

Pleomorphic adenoma, deep lobe of parotid.

MEDICAL MANAGEMENT

Other than ensuring that the patient's medical condition is optimized for surgery, there is no nonsurgical therapy indicated for this problem.

SURGICAL MANAGEMENT

The definitive diagnosis is made on surgical exploration. Adequate informed consent should always be obtained preoperatively including the possibility of mandibular osteotomy for improved access. Cranial nerve palsies including VII, IX, X, XI, and XII can occur depending on the pathology encountered, and the consequences of this should be carefully explained to the patient.

A parotidectomy incision is delineated; however, initially only the horizontal limb should be incised and the tail of the parotid elevated. The styloid process is then divided to enable the parapharyngeal space to be entered and the facial artery and vein divided to permit the submandibular gland to be retracted anteriorly to improve exposure to the tumor.

Using finger dissection, it is then possible to determine whether the tumor is arising from the parotid gland or is separate from this gland. If it is arising from the deep lobe, a superficial parotidectomy is performed to permit identification and isolation of the facial nerve. The nerve and its branches are then gently retracted to expose the underlying tumor, which is then delivered. The tumor is then sent for frozen sec-

tion. In this case the diagnosis of a benign pleomorphic adenoma was confirmed.

If the salivary gland tumor is determined to be of extraparotid origin, the facial nerve dissection is unnecessary. In this situation it is necessary to determine if it arises from the pharyngeal wall or from ectopic tissue in the parapharyngeal space. If it arises from the pharyngeal wall, a partial pharyngectomy will be necessary. If it arises from ectopic salivary tissue, then simple blunt dissection without pharyngectomy can be performed.

Indications for mandibular osteotomy to improve exposure would include very large tumors and if direct exposure of the base of skull is needed, particularly if vascular control is essential.

REHABILITATION AND FOLLOW-UP

In most cases of pleomorphic adenoma of the parapharyngeal space, recurrence is not a problem. If injury occurs to cranial nerves during the surgical procedure, then rehabilitation may be required. Thyroplasty for vocal cord paralysis, gastrostomy for dysphagia, and aspiration can both be helpful adjuncts to manage patients who develop multiple cranial neuropathy.

SUGGESTED READINGS

Carrau RL, Myers EN, Johnson JT. Management of tumors arising in the parapharyngeal space. *Laryngoscope*. 1990;100:583–589.

Gluckman JL. Parapharyngeal space. In: Gluckman J, Gullane P, Johnson J, eds. *Practical Approach to Head and Neck Tumors*. New York: Raven Press; 1994.

Olsen KD. Tumors and surgery at the parapharyngeal space. *Laryngoscope*. 1994;104:(suppl 63):1–28.

RECURRENT PLEOMORPHIC ADENOMA

Judith M. Czaja, M.D.
Jack L. Gluckman, M.D.

HISTORY

An 18-year-old white male presents with several small lumps in his right cheek anterior to his ear in the parotid region. The lumps are nontender and have been present for approximately 3 months. He does not think they have changed significantly in size during the 3 months. He denies any facial twitching, history of skin tumors, or pain. His history is significant for an excisional biopsy of a mass in the upper right neck at age 10. Biopsy at that time was positive for pleomorphic adenoma. He was subsequently referred to an otolaryngologist who performed a seventh nerve-sparing partial parotidectomy, removing all gland lateral to the nerve.

On physical exam, he has a well-healed parotidectomy incision in the preauricular sulcus. Discrete subcutaneous nodules are palpable and freely mobile, just beneath the surface of the skin (Fig. 31–1). One measures 9 mm in greatest dimension, the other measures 4 mm or less. They are distinctly separated and are present in the midcheek region. Cranial nerve VII is intact. Intraorally, there is no bulging of the tonsillar fossa. The remainder of the exam is normal.

DIFFERENTIAL DIAGNOSIS— KEY POINTS

1. One should be highly suspicious for parotid pathology in patients with a history of resection of a "lump" in the cheek or high in the neck immediately under the angle of the mandible. Often, patients will state that a small benign tumor was removed and a small scar is present along the edge of the mandibular angle or in the preauricular crease. This is particularly true in patients with recurrent "lumps" many years after the initial surgery.

2. If the pathology slides from the previous resection are available, they should be obtained for review. Old records, including operative reports, may also be helpful, but the tissue itself should be reexamined to confirm a benign tumor. History of facial weakness or paralysis after the initial surgery should be obtained.

3. In cases where pathology is not available, a fine-needle aspiration (FNA) of a nodule should be performed to confirm the diagnosis. This may also be done if the physician's standard of care is to aspirate parotid tumors prior to decisions regarding treatment.

4. The most important factor in the evaluation of patients with recurrent pleomorphic adenoma is the true extent of the recurrence. Typically recurrences occur in three forms: a single nodule of tumor, multiple small nodules, and extensive nodular recurrence peppered throughout the residual parotid gland (deep lobe and superficial bed). One must be careful when assessing tumor extent; what is palpated in the parotid bed may be "the tip of the iceberg" that extends deeply into the parapharyngeal space.

5. Malignant transformation of long-standing recurrent pleomorphic adenoma more commonly occurs in the deep lobe where the symptoms of benign recurrence may be masked for many years until malignancy develops. There have been reports of recurrent pleomorphic adenoma paralyzing the facial nerve, but this is rare and typically facial paralysis heralds malignant transformation. Cranial nerves in the parapharyngeal space may also be involved with malignant transformation, manifesting as symptoms of hoarseness, dysphagia, or dysarthria.

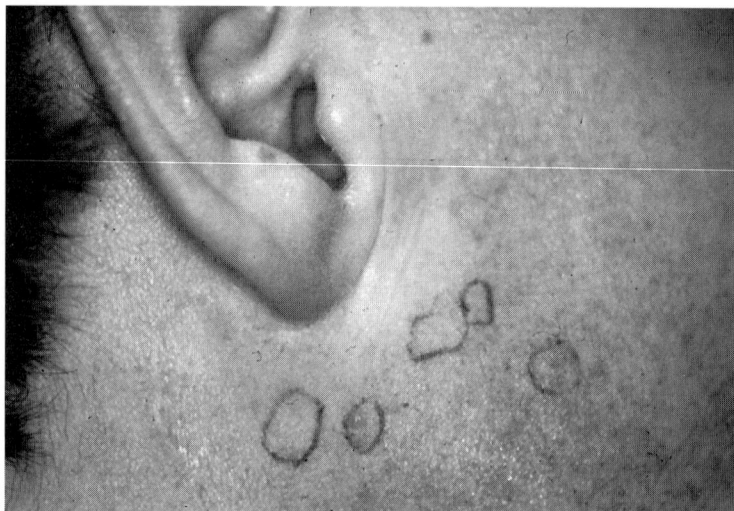

FIGURE 31-1 Discrete subcutaneous nodules, just beneath the surface of the skin, are palpable and freely mobile.

TEST INTERPRETATION

1. *FNA.* Positive for pleomorphic adenoma.

2. *Computed tomography (CT) scan.* This may show extent of tumor involvement in the superficial bed and parapharyneal space.

3. *Magnetic resonance imaging (MRI) scan.* In the evaluation of soft tissue extent of recurrent pleomorphic adenoma, MRI is the test of choice. Extent of tumor invasion is detailed in both the residual parotid bed as well as the parapharyngeal space. Extensive peppering of tumor deep into the neck may be underestimated with CT scan. In the case in question, MRI shows two nodules in the parotidectomy bed with no obvious extension into the parapharyngeal space.

DIAGNOSIS

Recurrent pleomorphic adenoma.

MEDICAL MANAGEMENT

The management of recurrent pleomorphic adenoma of the parotid gland is a difficult problem. Several treatment strategies have been advocated depending on the characteristics of the tumor, number of recurrences, status of the fa-cial nerve, and patient considerations. The controversy stems from the fact that the vast majority of recurrent pleomorphic adenomas are not life-threatening problems because malignant transformation is an extremely rare occurrence. The reported rate of malignant transformation in recurrent pleomorphic adenoma is approximately 0 to 8%. The indications for treatment therefore are cosmetic concerns of the patient and the rare complications of sudden intratumoral hemorrhage with subsequent development of infection and malignant transformation.

One option in the management algorithm is observation. Observation may be reserved for patients unable to undergo surgical removal or for patients who are reluctant to undergo further surgery (particularly after multiple recurrences) because the risk to the facial nerve is considerable. Recurrent tumor masses, especially if small, may be observed. Small incremental changes may be noted by the patient and physician. Significant increases in size of the nodules in patients still unable or unwilling to undergo surgery may continue to be observed if the nodules do not bother the patient, or may be treated with external beam radiotherapy once malignant transformation is ruled out. There are anecdotal reports of arrested growth after radiotherapy for gross recurrent benign pleomorphic adenoma.

SURGICAL MANAGEMENT

The mainstay of treatment for recurrent pleomorphic adenoma is surgical removal with intraoperative facial nerve monitoring. The surgical procedure of choice is total completion parotidectomy with preservation of the facial nerve when possible. The more recurrences and subsequent attempts at surgical removal a patient undergoes, the more obvious risk to the facial nerve. Occasionally, the benign tumor will be intimately associated with branches of the facial nerve that need to be sacrificed for total tumor removal. More commonly, the branches are difficult to dissect from the thick fibrotic scar surrounding the nerve and damage is frequent. The reported incidence of permanent partial facial paralysis is 13% in one series. This is similar to other reports.

There is a role for external beam radiotherapy in patients who undergo gross removal of multifocal recurrent pleomorphic adenoma. Full-course radiotherapy after surgery appears to decrease the rate of recurrence in this high-risk group. Patients with a uniloculated tumor focus do not appear to benefit from radiotherapy after completion parotidectomy and therefore radiation should probably be withheld from this group. Interpretation of statistics from studies of recurrent pleomorphic adenoma must be performed with caution. Because the tumors recur often 15 to 35 years after initial treatment, long-term follow-up is necessary. The duration of the follow-up period may therefore not be sufficient in many studies.

REHABILITATION AND FOLLOW-UP

Second recurrence after treatment of primary recurrent pleomorphic adenoma has an incidence of 15 to 30% within 9 to 14 years. Second recurrence, as one would expect, appears sooner and more commonly in patients treated for multifocal disease than in patients with unifocal disease. The patient should be educated regarding the relatively high likelihood of a further recurrence and increased risk to the facial nerve after multiple recurrences.

There are several theories for the pathogenesis of recurrent pleomorphic adenoma including tumor rupture and subsequent seeding, tumor multicentricity, and pseudocapsular penetration with an inadequate normal parotid margin on enucleation. Studies performed comparing tumor spillage to enucleation or "lumpectomy" show no increased incidence in recurrence in cases where tumor spillage has occurred. Inadequate resection by enucleation accounts for nearly all cases of recurrent pleomorphic adenoma. Masses in or around the parotid region should be considered primary parotid tumors, and partial parotidectomy with facial nerve preservation should be anticipated. Avoidance of inadequate resection, by thorough preoperative evaluation and preparation of the patient for possible parotidectomy, will decrease the incidence of recurrent pleomorphic adenoma and its subsequent problems.

SUGGESTED READINGS

Barton J, Slevin NJ, Gleave EN. Radiotherapy for pleomorphic adenoma of the parotid gland. *Int J Radiat Oncol Biol Phys.* 1992;22:925–928.

Buchman C, Stringer SP, Mendenhall WM, et al. Pleomorphic adenoma: effect of tumor spill and inadequate resection on tumor recurrence. *Laryngoscope.* 1994;104:1231–1234.

Olsen KD, Daube JR. Intraoperative monitoring of the facial nerve: an aid in the management of parotid gland recurrent pleomorphic adenoma. *Laryngoscope.* 1994;104:229–232.

Phillips PP, Olsen KD. Recurrent pleomorphic adenoma of the parotid gland: report of 126 cases and a review of the literature. *Ann Otol Rhinol Laryngol.* 1995;104:100–104.

Renehan A, Gleave EN, McGurk M. An analysis of the treatment of 114 patients with recurrent pleomorphic adenomas of the parotid gland. *Am J Surg.* 1996;172:710–714.

SUBMANDIBULAR GLAND ADENOID CYSTIC CARCINOMA

Judith M. Czaja, M.D.
Jack L. Gluckman, M.D.

HISTORY

A 42-year-old white female saw her family physician 3 weeks earlier for a complaint of a lump under her left jaw. She was diagnosed with chronic sialadenitis and placed on dicloxicillin 500 mg po QID for 14 days. She is referred at this time for persistence of a left submandibular gland infection. The mass has been present for 4½ weeks, is nontender, and has not changed appreciably in size. She denies any paresthesias, dysesthesias, difficulty moving her tongue, slurred speech, weakness of her lower lip, or any other neck masses. She does not have non-healing mouth sores, dysphagia, odynophagia, hoarseness, aspiration, or dyspnea. Her medical history is significant only for a tonsillectomy as a child. She is on oral contraceptive pills and takes occasional aspirin. She is a nonsmoker and drinks alcohol only on occasion. She is a high school teacher. She denies fever, night sweats, nonproductive cough, weight loss, or other systemic symptoms.

On physical examination, her ears, nose, oral cavity, oropharynx, hypopharynx, and larynx are normal. There is no purulent drainage or erythema over Wharton's duct in the floor of the mouth. Palpation of the neck reveals a 3- × 2-cm firm mass in the left submandibular triangle. The remainder of the neck exam is normal. Cranial nerves II through XII are intact.

DIFFERENTIAL DIAGNOSIS— KEY POINTS

1. The differential diagnosis in this case is wide. Infectious, inflammatory, and neoplastic etiologies are most common in this case. These include cervical adenitis and submandibular gland infection secondary to bacterial (strep-tococcus, staphylococcus, syphilis, cat scratch disease, lyme disease, brucellosis, tuberculosis, actinomycosis, atypical mycobacterium, etc.), viral (CMV, EBV, HIV, etc.), and fungal (histoplasmosis, blastomycosis, coccidioidomycosis, etc.) pathogens, granulomatous diseases (sarcoidosis, Wegener's granulomatosis, etc.), benign (pleomorphic adenoma, oncocytoma, monomorphic adenoma, desmoid tumor, etc.) and malignant (adenoid cystic carcinoma, mucoepidermoid carcinoma, metastatic squamous cell carcinoma, adenocarcinoma, lymphoma, acinic cell carcinoma, fibrosarcoma, etc.) tumors, chronic and acute sialadenitis, and sialosis. Congenital abnormalities are less likely in the absence of previous symptoms however can include undiagnosed branchial anomalies or cystic hygroma.

2. In the absence of purulent secretion from Wharton's duct, an acute sialadenitis can probably be ruled out. Most of the time, patients with acute infections of the gland have exquisite tenderness and purulent debris from the duct. A stone may also be palpable in the duct. In this age group, a malignancy should be suspected. In the absence of evidence suggesting an aerodigestive tract malignancy with metastasis to the neck, a primary tumor of the submandibular gland must be considered. A fine-needle aspiration (FNA) should be done to determine if the lesion represents an infectious or inflammatory process or a neoplasm. Atypical infection should be sought on culture, gram stain, and fungal KOH preps.

3. The most common benign tumor of the submandibular gland is pleomorphic adenoma, whereas the most common malignancy is adenoid cystic carcinoma. Symptoms to suggest

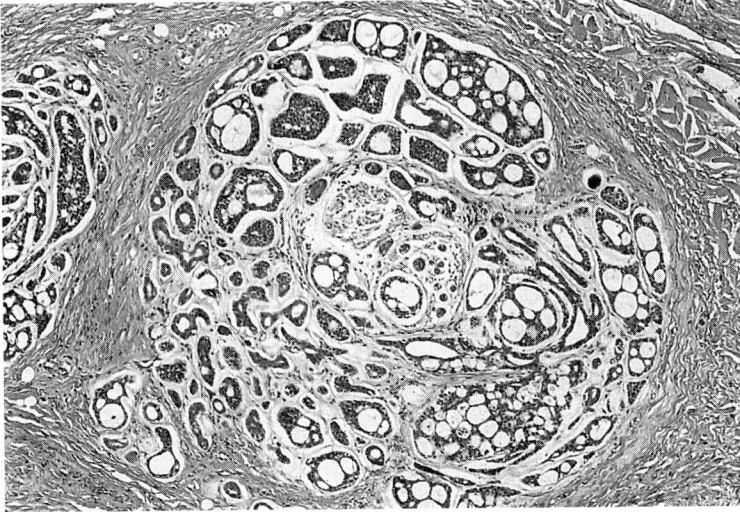

FIGURE 32-1 Histopathologic examination reveals cribiform "Swiss cheese" pattern of adenoid cystic carcinoma.

malignancy include pain, rapid growth, numbness of the tongue (lingual nerve) or slurring of speech (hypoglossal nerve), fixation to the mandible, paralysis of the tongue or marginal mandibular nerve, or other palpable masses in the neck. In cases of suspected adenoid cystic carcinoma, it is important to remember not only the propensity for aggressive perineural spread of this malignancy but also the high incidence of distant metastases in these patients.

TEST INTERPRETATION

1. *Biopsy.* FNA will be diagnostic in most cases. One should refrain from the temptation to do either an incisional or excisional biopsy as the initial diagnostic procedure in this case. In this case presented, an FNA showed aggregates of epithelial and myoepithelial cells surrounding large cystic spaces filled with necrotic debris. At the time of surgical excision, histopathologic examination will reveal the typical cribiform "Swiss cheese" pattern of adenoid cystic carcinoma (Fig. 32–1).

2. *Chest x-ray.* The workup for metastatic disease begins with a chest x-ray. Most patients with adenoid cystic carcinoma metastases present with multiple foci of tumor in the lungs. In addition, metastases to the abdomi-

nal organs, brain, and skin are reported. In the case presented, the chest x-ray was normal.

3. *Computed tomography (CT) scan.* A CT scan gives some indication of the extent of the primary tumor. It may also show widening of the foramina of surrounding nerves, that is, mental foramen, foramen ovale, foramen rotundum, etc., indicating extensive perineural invasion. CT scan in this case shows diffuse enlargement of the left submandibular gland in the submandibular triangle without gross invasion into the surrounding structures (mandible, tongue).

4. *Magnetic resonance imaging (MRI) scan.* In patients with tumors of the skull base, nasopharynx, paranasal sinuses, infratemporal fossa, and orbit, an MRI scan should be obtained to determine the extent, if any, of tumor intracranially. No MRI was obtained in the case presented.

5. Complete blood count, blood chemistries, EKG, and urinalysis were all normal preoperatively.

DIAGNOSIS

Adenoid cystic carcinoma of left submandibular gland. No evidence of metastatic disease.

MEDICAL MANAGEMENT

There is little role for chemotherapy as a first-line treatment in operable adenoid cystic carcinoma. Patients with recurrent or metastatic adenoid cystic carcinoma have been palliated with cytoxan, adriamycin, and cisplatin in some series. In addition, the use of fast neutron therapy as a primary treatment in patients with tumors considered unresectable or recurrent has been successful in certain series.

SURGICAL MANAGEMENT

The mainstay of treatment for patients with resectable adenoid cystic carcinoma is surgical resection, followed by full-course radiotherapy in many series. The extent of the surgical resection is controversial, because the tumor has a propensity to track along nerves for long distances beyond the site of the primary tumor. Most studies of adenoid cystic carcinoma demonstrate that pathologically proven perineural invasion is associated with a higher incidence of local recurrence, and wide resection is therefore advocated. There is no role for elective neck dissection because the incidence of subclinical metastasis is extremely low. Neck dissection is therefore done only in cases of overt cervical metastases.

The reports of adenoid cystic carcinoma in the literature must be studied with caution. Few reports follow patients for extended periods. The natural history of adenoid cystic carcinoma is invariably local recurrence if the patient is followed for a protracted period of time. Comparison of recurrence rates at 5, 10, 15, and 20 years shows a steady increase in local recurrences. Patients should therefore be counseled regarding the high likelihood of a recurrence and should be followed closely for the remainder of their lives. Recurrent tumor can be managed surgically if resectable, or with chemotherapy in the case of palliation. Radiotherapy may be reserved in certain cases for the inevitable recurrence.

REHABILITATION AND FOLLOW-UP

Patients should be followed for the rest of their lives with annual physical examination and chest x-ray. As mentioned, recurrence is often inevitable, either at the primary site or as a pulmonary metastasis.

SUGGESTED READINGS

Anderson JN J, Beenken SW, Crowe R, et al. Prognostic factors in minor salivary gland cancer. *Head Neck.* 1995;17(6):480–486.

Chou C, Zhu G, Luo M, Xue G. Carcinoma of the minor salivary glands: results of surgery and combined therapy. *J Oral Maxillo Surg.* 1996;54(4):448–453.

Garden AS, Weber RS, Ang KK, et al. Postoperative radiation therapy for malignant tumors of minor salivary glands. Outcome and patterns of failure. *Cancer.* 1994;73(10):2563–2569.

Garden AS, Weber RS, Morrison WH, et al. The influence of positive margins and nerve invasion in adenoid cystic carcinoma of the head and neck treated with surgery and radiation. *Int J Radiat Oncol Biol Phys.* 1995;32(3):619–626.

Haddad A, Enepekides DJ, Manolidis S, Black M. Adenoid cystic carcinoma of the head and neck: a clinicopathologic study of 37 cases. *J Otolaryngol.* 1995;24(3):201–205.

Harrison LB, Armstrong JG, Spiro RH, et al. Postoperative radiation therapy for major salivary gland malignancies. *J Surg Oncol.* 1990;45(1):52–55.

Kim KH, Sung MW, Chung PS, et al. Adenoid cystic carcinoma of the head and neck. *Arch Otolaryngol Head Neck Surg.* 1994;120(7):721–726.

Parsons JT, Mendenhall WM, Stringer SP, et al. Management of minor salivary gland carcinomas. *Int J Radiat Oncol Biol Phys.* 1996;35(3):443–454.

Skin

Case 33

BASAL CELL CARCINOMA

Mark J. Abrams, M.D.
Kevin A. Shumrick, M.D.

HISTORY

A 57-year-old white male complains of a lesion on his medial canthal area. He reports its presence for more than 2 years and it has gradually gotten larger and has begun to bleed on occasion. Medical history is significant for athrosclerotic vascular disease, hypertension, and a 20 pack/year cigarette smoking history. He denies allergies or prescribed medications. He also has a history of extensive sun exposure as a former beach vendor.

Physical exam reveals a well-developed, well-nourished middle-aged white male older appearing than stated age. Examination of his face reveals significant photoaging and a 1- × 1.5-cm medial canthal lesion as shown in Figure 33–1. The lesion is nodular with a pearly appearance and a central area of ulceration. There are also areas of telangiectasia. His eye exam reveals normal vision and extraocular muscle movements and there is no evidence of epiphora. There is no cervical adenopathy and the remainder of the physical exam was normal.

DIFFERENTIAL DIAGNOSIS— KEY POINTS

1. *Benign.* Actinic keratoses, seborrheic keratoses, keratoacanthoma, infectious/inflammatory lesion (e.g., chalazion).
2. *Malignant.* Basal cell carcinoma, squamous cell carcinoma, sebacious carcinoma, amelanotic melanoma.

TEST INTERPRETATION

A biopsy is the diagnostic procedure of choice. Biopsy can be preformed either by incisional (punch) biopsy versus excisional biopsy with primary closure. If an incisional biopsy is performed, it is important to include the thickest portion of the nodule and the periphery to show maturation and the deepest area of invasion. The result of the biopsy in this particular case is that of a basal cell carcinoma invading deep into the subcutaneous tissues. Given the invasive nature of this tumor the following additional evaluation should be considered:

1. A complete ophthalmologic exam including the conjunctiva, globe, extraocular muscles, visual acuity, and lacrimal system.
2. Should any signs of orbital or sinus invasion be evident a preoperative high-resolution computed tomography scan of the orbit and perinasal sinuses should be performed up through the skull base to rule out orbital, sinus, or intracranial invasion.

If intracranial invasion is a concern, magnetic resonance imaging may be helpful to evaluate dural invasion. If the tumor is extensive enough to warrant a craniofacial resection and/or orbital exenteration, then a medistatic workup including a chest x-ray and bone and liver serology should be obtained at the minimum. Should any signs or symptoms of distant metastasis be evident then more focal evaluations can be performed at that point.

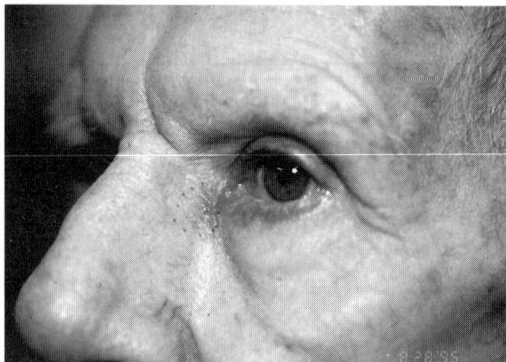

FIGURE 33-1 Photoaging and a medial canthal lesion.

DIAGNOSIS

Basal cell carcinoma of the medial canthas.

MEDICAL MANAGEMENT

This patient has a basal cell carcinoma in a very significant functional and pathologic area. An ophthalmologist should be involved in this patient's care to ensure that optimal treatment with regard to the eye and the lacrimal system be performed throughout the patient's care. In addition, the patient should be examined fully for secondary basal cell carcinomas elsewhere on the body. Note, topical 5-fluorouracil can be used topically to treat noninvasive actinic keratosis and basal cell carcinomas *in situ*.

SURGICAL TREATMENT

Treatment of basal cell carcinomas in the periorbital area is challenging. The various modes of treatment include excision with frozen section control, Moh's micrographic surgery, cryosurgery, and radiation therapy. The cure rates with each of these techniques exceed 90% in most large series. However, the bottom line is that nowhere in the body does a basal cell carcinoma have such significant mortality or functional morbidity than around the eye. There has been quoted a 2 to 11% mortality rate related to periorbital basal cell carcinomas. In addition, mortality rates and recurrence rates increase (to 50% in some series) with the recurrent tumors.

Therefore, aggressive initial treatment is essential.

Excision with frozen section control is the historical standard. This technique has been criticized as not providing adequate control due to the difficulty in obtaining good frozen sections in this functionally crucial area. The concern is that in order to gain adequate frozen section control sacrifice of unnecessary normal tissue may be required. Moh's micrographic surgery has the advantage of using a microscopic sampling technique to enable better preservation of normal tissues. The disadvantages of Moh's surgery is that it is more time consuming and may possibly require two separate sittings for removal and reconstruction. Cryosurgery has also been used significantly in the past but has fallen out of favor near the eye since no tissue sample is obtained with this technique and there is concern that the technique may be less accurate in completely removing the tumor. Finally radiation therapy has a clear advantage of preservation of normal structures. However, in large basal cell carcinomas where this technique would be of significant advantage the cure rates are less than surgical removal. In addition, dry eye, belpharitis, possible cataract formation, and possible cicatricial entropion are possible complications from this technique.

The key point to adequate reconstruction in the medial canthal area is to try to recreate function and cosmesis at the same time. Key functional points to consider include the following:

1. The *vector of pull* should be parallel to the lid but not enough to cause entropion. In addition, it is important to avoid an inferior pull in the lower lid to prevent ectropion.

2. The *function of the lacrimal system* should also be considered. If still present after excision, one should always probe the canaliculi. If the sac or nasolacrimal duct has been occluded or sacrificed, a dacrocystorhinostomy (DCR) should be considered. If both the sac and canaliculi are sacrificed, then a glass Jones tube should be considered.

3. *Lid function* should be restored by an occuloplastic lid repair for both inner and outer lamellar defects. The reconstructive tech-

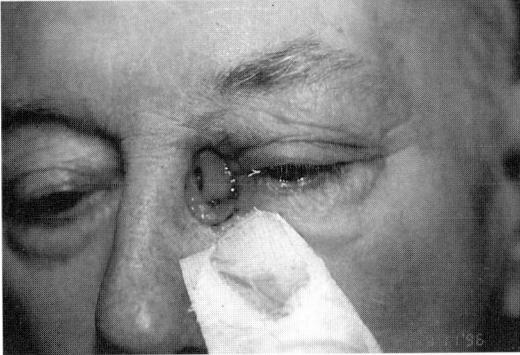

FIGURE 33-2 Basal cell carcinoma.

niques for eyelid reconstruction are well covered elsewhere.

4. *Structural support* for the medial canthal tendon and orbital bone should be restored.

5. In treatment of this type of lesion the *extraocular muscles and globe* may be sacrificed. Note, however, that frozen sections can be made of the bulbar conjunctiva or cornea if necessary to preserve the globe. If the orbit is exenterated prosethic eye reconstruction can be recommended.

To optimize cosmesis, the resultant scars should be lined up in natural skin creases, which are abundant in the medial canthal area.

The options for closure of the defect noted in Figure 33–2 include the following:

1. Healing by secondary intention—or the (Lassez-faire) technique.

2. Primary closure—utilizing elliptical closure or transposition flaps for small defects. (*Key:* Tension should be parallel to lids to prevent asymmetry. *Caution:* Too much tension on lower lid may cause intropion.)

3. Skin graft—full thickness from postauricular area or upper lid donor cites.

4. Local flaps:
   A. *Romboid transposition.* Workhorse flap for medial cauthus. Align the tension to be parallel with the lid margin. The glabellar romboid is ideal for defects at or above the cauthus and the cheek romboid is better for inferior lead located defects.
   B. *V-Y advancement/glabellar transposition.* Has disadvantage of bringing in thicker skin into the medial canthal area, which usually harbors thin skin.
   C. *Bilateral lid myocutaneous advancement.* Rotation of outer lamellar myocutaneous tissue from upper lid to fill upper half of medial canthal defect and a Mustardé-type inferior lid cheek flap to be rotated into the inner half of the medial canthal defect.

Each of these reconstructive techniques has its own advantages and disadvantages and can be used in this particular setting for reconstruction depending on the particular case involved.

REHABILITATION AND FOLLOW-UP

As in any case of a patient with a sun-related cutaneous skin cancer, routine follow-up is important for tumor surveillance. It is especially important in this functionally and oncologically important area. Because the medial canthus lies at embryologic fusion planes it is theorized that the medial canthal region can have a higher likelihood of deep penetration and mortality. As a result, close follow-up of this area is of utmost importance. The earliest sign of recurrence should be biopsied and resected if positive. In addition, the avoidance of sun exposure and the use of sunscreens should be recommended. Routine eye examinations by the ophthalmologist to document eye and lacrimal function should also be recommended.

SUGGESTED READINGS

MONHEIT G, GALLAGHAN A. Moh's micrographic surgery for periorbital skin cancer. *Dermatol Clin.* 1989;7(4):677–97.

PEARLMAN G, HORNBLASS A. Basal cell carcinoma of the eyelid: a review of patients treated by surgical incision. *Ophthal Surg.* 1976;7(4):23–27.

PUTTERMAN A. Reconstruction of the eyelid following resection for carcinoma. *Clin Plast Surg.* 1985;12(3): 393–410.

REALI U, CHIARUGI C, BORGOGNONI L. Reconstruction

of a medial canthal defect with a myocutaneous flap. *Ann Plast Surg.* 1993;30(2):

Shotton F. Optimal closure of medial canthal surgical defects with Romboid flaps: "rules of thumb" for flap and romboid defect orientations. *Ophthal Surg.* 1983;14(1):46–52.

Spinelli H, Gelkas G. Periocular reconstruction: a systematic approach. *Plast Reconstr Surg.* 1993;91(6): 1017–1024.

Tenzel R, Boynton J, Buffan F. Technique of combined lid and medial canthus reconstruction. *Ophthal Surg.* 1976;7(3):25–28.

MALIGNANT MELANOMA

Mark J. Abrams, M.D.
Kevin A. Shumrick, M.D.

HISTORY

A 49-year-old white tobacco farmer was referred with a darkly pigmented scalp lesion that has gradually increased in size during the past year. It is neither painful nor ulcerated. Aside from a 30 pack/year smoking history and chronic sun exposure, the patient has no significant medical history and denies any allergies or prescribed medications. Family history is positive for a paternal grandfather who died of "skin cancer."

Physical exam reveals the lesion shown in the Figure 34–1. Further inspection of the skin of the face and neck reveals evidence of significant photoaging with chronic hyperpigmentation and numerous actinic keratoses. However, no other suspicious lesions are noted on full-body cutaneous examination. There is no palpable cervical or parotid adenopathy.

DIFFERENTIAL DIAGNOSIS— KEY POINTS

1. The differential diagnosis for pigmented skin lesions includes all benign and malignant cutaneous and skin appendage neoplasms. The most significant diagnoses to consider are listed below.

   - **Benign.** Any variety of benign pigmented nevi or lentigo, seborrheic keratosis or pigmented actinic keratosis, squamous papilloma, other chronic inflammatory nodular or ulcerative lesions such as condyloma lata (syphilitic condyloma), cutaneous sarcoid (lupus pernio), cutaneous lupus erythematosus, chronic dermatomycosis, cutaneous tuberculosis, etc.

   - **Malignant.** Malignant melanoma, pigmented basal cell carcinoma or squamous cell carcinoma, other rare cutaneous malig-

nancies (Merkel cell carcinoma, cutaneous metastasis, etc.).

2. *Diagnostic features.* The lesion shown in the figure bears all the hallmarks of malignant melanoma. The ABCD rule is helpful to keep in mind. A, Atypical features (e.g., irregular contour, ulceration, unusual growth); B, irregular Border; C, variegated Color; D, Diameter > 6 mm for acquired nevi. Note that congenital nevi tend to be larger and size is not helpful unless there has been a rapid increase.

   Although the diagnosis is not clear in this patient's grandfather, the positive family history of a lethal skin cancer also goes along with the diagnosis of melanoma in this case.

3. Another key point is the full cutaneous exam of any patient with suspicion of melanoma. Due to the lethal nature of this disease a thorough cutaneous exam is warranted for other atypical nevi or satellite lesions.

4. Finally, the upper neck and parotid are the first echelon levels for metastasis from a temporal scalp melanoma and should be carefully examined for signs of lymphatic spread.

TEST INTERPRETATION

An excisional biopsy, with H&E histology, revealed small melanin rich blue cells invading the superficial dermis to the level of 0.75 mm.

A properly performed biopsy is critical for accurate diagnosis of melanoma. In most cases this will entail an excisional biopsy; however, an incisional biopsy can be performed on large lesions (>2 cm) or for those that would require elaborate reconstruction and planning. An incisional biopsy should entail a biopsy from the most raised and irregular site in the lesion and/or the most melanotic site and should include full thickness skin and subcutaneous fat. The

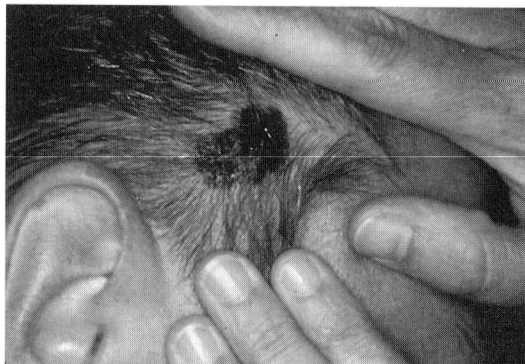

FIGURE 34–1 Presenting lesion.

excisional biopsy should be down to the level of the underlying fascia. A Wood's lamp may be helpful in delineating unclear borders of suspicious lesions. The margin of tissue in the excision is discussed later.

The treatment from that point is then predicted on the depth of invasion. Breslow thickness is the most commonly used depth scale and is measured in millimeters from the thickest part of the tumor. The Clark's level system is older but still quoted commonly in the literature and is measured in terms of histologic invasion of the different levels of the dermis. The tumor in this case has a Breslow thickness of 0.75 mm and a Clark's level of 2 (Table 34–1).

Chest x-ray and liver and bone panel were normal. In large series of head and neck melanoma, the most common site of distant metastasis is the lung (>60%). The central nervous system, liver, and bone are the next most common sites. A head computed tomography scan or magnetic resonance image would be warranted to rule out brain metastases if any neurologic signs or symptoms are present.

DIAGNOSIS

Superficial spreading malignant melanoma.

MEDICAL MANAGEMENT

Although melanoma is a surgical disease, the role of radiation and adjunctive therapy has been a popular source of debate in this area and is covered in the next section.

SURGICAL MANAGEMENT

In this case, the lesion was excised as an ellipse with a 1-cm margin and closed primarily with the patient prepared for a return excision of margins and possible elective neck dissection and superficial parotidectomy if the lesion were of intermediate thickness. One could have taken a 2-cm margin; however, primary closure would have been too difficult with the lack of elasticity in the scalp. A split thickness skin graft with later reconstruction using a scalp tissue expander or scalp flap would probably be required.

There is some controversy in the biopsy and treatment of the primary lesion but based on the latest review of the literature and the NIH Consensus Statement on Early Melanoma the following recommendations are made for treatment of the primary lesion.

For a melanoma *in situ,* a 0.5-cm margin of clinically normal skin is sufficient and should be curative. A 1.0-cm margin is appropriate for superficial melanomas (<1 mm Breslow thickness). For more deeply invading melanomas, a 2.0-cm margin is recommended. The wider margins of the past have not significantly im-

TABLE 34–1 Breslow's and Clark's Method of Melanoma Classification

Histologic Level	Clark's	Breslow's (mm)	Nodal Spread
Epidermis	Level I	0–0.75	Minimal
Basal cell layer	Level II	0.75–1.50	25%
Papillary dermis	Level III	1.50–2.00	57% for 1.5–3.99 mm
Reticular dermis	Level IV	2.00–4.00	
Subcutaneous layer	Level V	>4.00	62%

proved survival or local control and often lead to difficult functional and cosmetic deficits. The Moh's technique has not been adequately studied and is technically difficult because of staining problems and skip lesions in the dermis.

The rationale for taking the 1-cm margin in this case is that it provides a definitive diagnosis and potentially definitive treatment for the lesion in a simple, one-stage procedure. If the lesion is more deeply invading, greater margins and a potentially more difficult reconstruction (as noted above) may be indicated. If a 2-cm margin can be taken simply without significant functional or cosmetic deficit at the outset, then it is reasonable to do so. However, if this extra margin commits the patient to a significant reconstruction, the added morbidity may be incurred without added curative benefit if the lesion proves to be superficial histologically.

In addition, for intermediate thickness lesions, data show that performing elective removal of the primary draining lymph nodes is of benefit for survival and locoregional control. This would entail a superficial parotidectomy and a neck dissection in this case. Because there is a high potential for the need for further surgery, it is reasonable to risk having to go back and take another centimeter of margin as long as the patient is agreeable.

The treatment of the No neck is a topic of debate that is still being investigated. There is some consensus that elective neck dissections are unnecessary in melanoma less than 0.75 mm in thickness due to low risk of metastasis. Also, elective neck dissections are not thought to be worthwhile in deeply invading melanomas (>4.0 mm Breslow thickness) due to the high risk of distant metastases at this point. It is the intermediate lesion that seems to show some benefit. However, conflicting data exist that suget that prognosis is not adversely affected by waiting to treat neck disease until adenopathy is clinically evident. Some centers perform sampling of lymph nodes at highest risk to help guide therapy for lymphatic spread.

If there is clinical lymphatic spread, then a therapeutic neck dissection (and a superficial parotidectomy in this case) is recommended. One is referred to the article by Shah et al. for an excellent review of patterns of lymphatic spread for cutaneous melanoma of the head and neck (which in this case would include the parotid and anterior and posterior neck). Of course, a thorough search for distant metastasis is warranted in this situation because melanoma has often systemically metastasized by the time cervical adenopathy is apparent.

The use of adjuvant therapy has been an area of active research in melanoma. Historically, melanoma has been considered to be radioresistant. However, recent studies with large dose/fraction regimens have shown a benefit for radiotherapy in an elective adjuvant role especially in terms of locoregional control. Chemotherapy has been disappointing in metastatic melanoma. Dacarbazine is the most clinically effective drug with a 20% overall response rate. Immunotherapy has enjoyed significant popularity in melanoma research and several ongoing studies are investigating its effectiveness. Interferon α-2b has been shown recently to prolong disease-free survival and overall survival in an adjuvant role in high risk cases. Other systemic agents such as interleukin-2, lymphocyte-activated killer cells, monoclonal antimelanoma antibodies, and tumor necrosis factor have also been tried in clinical trials with limited benefit. Nonspecific immunoenhancers such as BCG and DNCB and autologous lymphokine preparations have been locally injected in cutaneous metastases. Melanoma vaccines have also been developed and have been used in trial on high-risk patients.

REHABILITATION AND FOLLOW-UP

Routine follow-up examinations (every 6 months) for local, regional, and distant metastases are critical in managing these patients. Patients with high-risk melanomas (>1.0 mm Breslow thickness), positive family history, and multiple atypical nevi should be examined more frequently (every 3 months). Frequent chest x-rays (every 6 months) and blood work (bone and hepatic panels) are useful to screen for distant metastases. In addition, the patient should be placed on a skin protection protocol to minimize ultraviolet light exposure. The use of sunscreens and protective clothing should be advocated. Patients should also be instructed in self-examinations of the skin. Finally, families of melanoma patients should be similarly counseled in self-exams and sun protection and should be enrolled in a regular screening program.

SUGGESTED READINGS

Ang KK et al. Postoperative radiotherapy for cutaneous melanoma of the head and neck region. *Int J Radiat Oncol Biol Phys.* 1994;30(4):795–798.

Conley J. *Melanoma of the Head and Neck.* New York: Thieme; 1990.

Fisher SR. Cutaneous malignant melanoma of the head and neck. *Laryngoscope.* 1989;99:822–836.

Kirkwood JM et al. Interferon α-2b adjuvant therapy of high-risk resected cutaneous melanoma: the Eastern Cooperative Oncology Group Trial EST 1684. *J Clin Oncol.* 1996;14(1):7–17.

National Institutes of Health Consensus Development Conference Statement on Diagnosis and Treatment of Early Melanoma, January 27–29, 1992. *Am J Dermatopathol.* 1993;15(1):34–43.

Seigler HF. Melanoma. In: Sabiston DC, ed. *Textbook of Surgery.* 14th ed. Philadelphia, PA: WB Saunders; 1991:477–484.

Shah JP, Kraus DH, Dubner S, Sarkar S. Patterns of regional lymph node metastasis from cutaneous melanoma of the head and neck. *Am J Surg.* 1991;162:320–323.

GENERAL

Infectious Diseases

Case 35

EPIGLOTTITIS

Allen M. Seiden, M.D.

HISTORY

A 40-year-old white male presented with a severe sore throat he had had for 2 days. The pain had progressed quite rapidly and was particularly pronounced with swallowing so that he was no longer able to tolerate the oral intake of solid food or liquids, and was having difficulty handling his own secretions. He complained of mild shortness of breath but no wheezing.

There was no history of chronic tonsillitis, nor was there a history of foreign body ingestion, trauma, or toxic exposure. The patient denied other significant medical problems and had no history of drug allergy. Medications included only ibuprofen for the pain. He reported smoking one pack of cigarettes per day before these current symptoms began.

On physical examination the patient was clearly uncomfortable and in moderate distress. He was sitting erect and slightly forward, and was noted to be drooling. Although his voice was somewhat muffled, he was not tachypneic or stridorous. His temperature was 102°F and he was tachycardic, but his blood pressure was stable.

Examination of the oral cavity and pharynx was without signifiant erythema or exudate, and was surprisingly benign in view of the severity of the patient's symptoms. Indirect laryngeal examination demonstrated diffuse edema and marked erythema of the supraglottic tissues, including the epiglottis, aryepiglottic folds, false vocal cords, and arytenoids. The vocal cords were not well visualized, and no assessment as to mobility could be determined.

Palpation of the neck revealed bilaterally tender cervical adenopathy. Pain was also elicited by gentle palpation of the larynx.

A lateral soft tissue x-ray of the neck was obtained. The patient was admitted to the hospital and intravenous antibiotic therapy and high-dose corticosteroids were administered.

DIFFERENTIAL DIAGNOSIS— KEY POINTS

1. The severity of this patient's sore throat associated with a high fever would initially suggest the possibility of an acute tonsillitis. However, without significant pharyngeal findings on physical examination, severe odynophagia should immediately raise suspicion for epiglottitis. Sore throat and odynophagia are the most common presenting symptoms, particularly in adults. Such patients are frequently misdiagnosed with a peritonsillar abscess or deep neck infection, but the physical exam would be inconsistent. The history excludes other possibilities such as a foreign body or trauma. While a history of smoking does raise the possibility of malignancy, the rapid progression and physical findings support an inflammatory etiology.

2. Epiglottitis has traditionally been thought of as a childhood illness. However, with the introduction of the Hib vaccine in the late 1980s, the incidence in children has declined from 3.5 cases to 0.6 cases per 100,000 population per year. In adults, the incidence has remained stable or slightly increased to 1.8

127

cases per 100,000 per year. Therefore, a high index of suspicion needs to be maintained, because a delay in diagnosis can lead to increased morbidity. In adults, mortality rates in the range of 6 to 7% are reported.

3. The physical exam is diagnostic, and requires either indirect or fiberoptic laryngoscopy. Whereas in children there is concern that such an exam may precipitate airway obstruction, this would be very unusual in adults and has not occurred in several large studies. Another distinction is that children typically will have a swollen, cherry red epiglottis, while in adults the inflammation tends not to be confined to just the epiglottis but will involve the supraglottis and even occasionally the pharynx and uvula. Hence, it is often referred to as supraglottitis.

4. The patient assumed a position of sitting erect and slightly forward, which helps to reduce obstructive symptoms secondary to supraglottic swelling. A muffled voice is also quite characteristic, as is tenderness to direct palpation over the larynx.

TEST INTERPRETATION

A lateral soft tissue x-ray of the neck has been favored to help make the diagnosis of epiglottitis. However, in adults there is generally little to be gained unless a complete physical examination is not possible. A sensitivity of 38% and specificity of 76% has been reported for such x-rays.

Bacteremia has been reported in anywhere from 23 to 97% of patients with acute epiglotitis, usually associated with *Haemophilus influenzae* type B and *Streptococcus pneumoniae*. Blood cultures should therefore be obtained when indicated. Since the introduction of the Hib vaccine, other causative organisms are being reported with greater frequency and include *β-hemolytic streptococci, Staphylococcus aureus, Klebsiella pneumoniae, Bacteroides melanogenicus,* and *Mycobacterium tuberculosis.* Pharyngeal swab cultures are usually of little benefit because the infection appears to be largely a submucosal cellulitis in adults.

Due to the relatively large proportion of negative cultures in cases of epiglottitis, some

have speculated that the etiology may be viral; one case of herpes simplex epiglottitis has been documented.

DIAGNOSIS

Epiglottitis.

MEDICAL MANAGEMENT

Initial therapy requires intravenous fluid replacement and broad antibiotic coverage to include particularly *H. influenzae, S. pneumoniae,* and β-hemolytic streptococci.

Morbidity in this disease usually relates to the possibility of airway obstruction. Prophylactic airway intervention is usually recommended in children but is not usually necessary in adults. This seems to relate to the size of the airway and not to the causative organism. Some investigators advocate the use of corticosteroids to reduce upper airway edema, although there are no controlled data to support this approach. These patients should be observed closely, usually in an intensive care setting, and appropriate steps taken at the first sign of respiratory distress. Extensive supraglottic swelling often makes intubation difficult (Fig. 35–1), and a tracheotomy set should be available at the bedside.

Tachycardia out of proportion to other symptoms has been suggested to be an early sign of hypoxemia and potential airway compromise. Patients with a respiratory rate greater than 30 breaths/minute or a pCO$_2$ greater than 45 mm Hg generally require immediate airway intervention. In a series of 129 patients, Frantz et al. found that 15% required airway intervention. Predictive factors included sitting erect and stridor, but there was no relationship to age, delayed diagnosis, duration of symptoms, drooling, or positive blood cultures.

SURGICAL MANAGEMENT

The only role for surgery in this disease is to establish an airway if necessary. If the patient cannot be intubated, then a cricothyrotomy is usually the most efficient and recommended approach to secure an airway rather than a formal tracheotomy. The need to convert subsequently

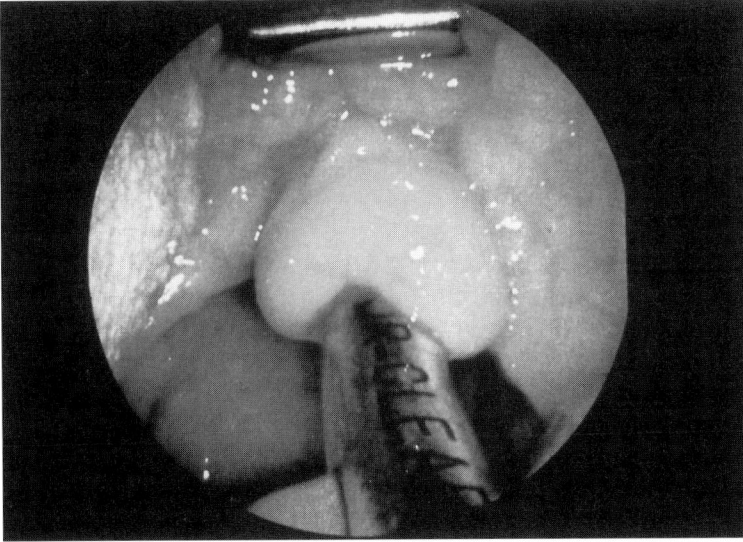

FIGURE 35-1 Endoscopic view in a patient who has been intubated. The epiglottis is markedly swollen and erythematous.

to a tracheostomy is controversial but is favored in the otolaryngology literature due to the potential complications of subglottic stenosis (4%) and vocal dysfunction (15%).

REHABILITATION AND FOLLOW-UP

Recurrence of epiglottitis is rare, but if it does occur the patient should be evaluated for underlying disorders such as collagen vascular disease, sarcoidosis, or even occult malignancy.

The incidence of epiglottitis in children seems to be decreasing as a result of the *Haemophilus* vaccine. Whether a similar decline will occur in adults remains uncertain. Cases of transmission of *Haemophilus* infection from both children to adults and adults to children have been reported, causing epiglottitis and meningitis. Rifampin has been recommended as a prophylaxis against infection after contact, and to eradicate the carrier state, at a dose of 20 mg/

kg/day to a maximum of 600 mg daily for 4 days.

SUGGESTED READINGS

CAREY MJ. Epiglottitis in adults. *Am J Emerg Med.* 1996;14:421–424.

FRANTZ TD, RASGON BM, QUESENBERRY CP. Acute epiglottitis in adults. Analysis of 129 cases. *JAMA.* 1994;272:1358–1360.

GORELICK MH, BAKER MD. Epiglottitis in children, 1979 through 1992. Effects of *Hemophilus influenzae* type b immunization. *Arch Pediatr Adolesc Med.* 1994;148:47–50.

SENIOR BA, RADKOWSKI D, MACARTHUR C, et al. Changing patterns in pediatric supraglottitis: a multi-institutional review, 1980–1992. *Laryngoscope.* 1994;104:1314–1322.

TORKKELI T, RUOPPI P, NUUTINEN J, KARI A. Changed clinical course and current treatment of acute epiglottitis in adults: a 12-year experience. *Laryngoscope.* 1994;104:1503–1506.

DEEP NECK SPACE ABSCESS

Allen M. Seiden, M.D.

HISTORY

A 28-year-old white male presented with a complaint of severe sore throat and dysphagia. He had presented 5 days previously with similar symptoms, had been diagnosed with tonsillitis, and had been placed on oral penicillin. Since then, his symptoms had progressed, with associated fever, poor oral intake, and some neck stiffness. He denied a history of chronic tonsillitis or recent dental work.

His medical history was significant for diabetes mellitus, controlled with insulin. He was taking no other medications and did not smoke.

On physical examination, the patient was febrile to 102°F. He had difficulty speaking because of the pain and was noted to have a *hot potato voice*. He was also noted to have moderate trismus with difficulty handling his secretions. The pharynx was erythematous and diffusely swollen. There appeared to be medial as well as forward displacement of the left tonsil, with fullness of the posterolateral pharyngeal wall. However, the uvula was in the midline and the soft palate was not asymmetrically full. The patient was in no airway distress. A flexible fiberoptic examination confirmed the above findings with fullness and obliteration of the left pyriform sinus, but no significant swelling of the supraglottis. Vocal cord mobility was normal.

Palpation of the neck revealed fullness and tenderness in the left retromandibular and upper cervical region, but no discrete adenopathy and no fluctuance. Although the patient demonstrated some limited mobility when turning his head from side to side, there was no meningismus.

DIFFERENTIAL DIAGNOSIS— KEY POINTS

1. This patient initially presented with tonsillitis and returned several days later with progressive symptoms despite medical therapy. The first concern should be that he might be developing complications from the tonsil infection. The most likely complication would be a peritonsillar abscess, and this is suggested by his persistent fever, trismus, and difficulty handling secretions. However, ordinarily the uvula would be deviated to one side, and asymmetric fullness of the soft palate should be evident.

2. Medial displacement of the left tonsil and pharyngeal wall should alert the clinician to the possibility that the infection has spread deep to the tonsil. Tonsillitis and, in fact, peritonsillar abscess are common causes of deep neck space infection. Other possible sources include dental infection, trauma, sialadenitis, supurative lymphadenitis, or infection of congenital cysts. However, in many instances, no obvious source can be found.

3. Medial displacement of the posterolateral pharyngeal wall, especially just behind the posterior tonsillar pillar, and fullness in the retromandibular region suggest the possibility of a parapharyngeal or lateral pharyngeal abscess. This is the most common of the deep neck space infections, and the most common deep site infected secondarily to tonsillitis. Infection penetrates the buccopharyngeal fascia directly or extends via retrograde thrombophlebitis.

4. Trismus and limitation of neck motion are common signs of deep neck space infection, including the parapharyngeal space. Al-

though neck fullness is present, discrete areas of fluctuance are rarely found due to the deep location of the abscess.

5. The lateral pharyngeal space is pyramidal in shape, with the base lying superiorly along the petrous temporal bone and the apex lying inferiorly at the level of the hyoid bone. It is divided by the styloid process into two compartments. Infection within the anterior compartment more commonly causes pharyngeal wall displacement and trismus. The posterior compartment contains the internal carotid artery; the internal jugular vein; cranial nerves IX, X, and XII; and the cervical sympathetic trunk. Infection within the posterior compartment may therefore spread to the carotid sheath, which in turn may allow extension to the mediastinum. Internal jugular vein thrombosis may occur, with septic thrombophlebitis. Patients may present with cranial nerve deficits involving IX, X, or XII, or a Horner's syndrome may be apparent. Carotid artery rupture, most often involving the internal carotid, has been reported.

6. A history of diabetes mellitus suggests an increased risk to develop infectious complications.

TEST INTERPRETATION

The initial laboratory examination should include a complete blood count with differential, serum electrolyte levels, and blood cultures if there is evidence of sepsis. This patient demonstrated an elevated white blood cell count of 19,500 with 90% polymorphonuclear leukocytes. Serum hyperosmolarity was consistent with dehydration, secondary to both fever and dysphagia.

Imaging is very helpful not only to verify the diagnosis, but to localize the abscess. Computed tomography (CT) is generally preferred, with contrast. Figure 36–1 reveals a large parapharyngeal abscess. This will usually delineate the abscess cavity as a single or multiloculated area of attenuation with contrast enhancement of the abscess wall, with a reported sensitivity of approximately 90%. Cellulitis is suspected when there is only soft tissue swelling with obliteration of regional fat planes.

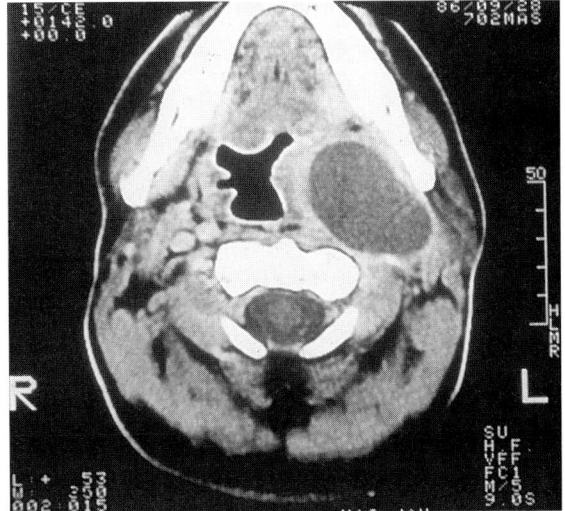

FIGURE 36-1 Large parapharyngeal abscess.

Sometimes it is difficult to distinguish abscess from cellulitis, and ultrasound may be helpful in this regard. Magnetic resonance imaging (MRI) can provide soft tissue definition and perhaps better diagnose vascular complications, but is not usually necessary during the initial evaluation.

DIAGNOSIS

Parapharyngeal space abscess.

MEDICAL MANAGEMENT

In patients with deep neck space infections, it is very important for the physician to make an initial assessment regarding airway stability. Whether or not patients appear to be in respiratory distress, it is essential to visualize the airway either indirectly or with a flexible fiberoptic telescope. If compromise is imminent, then steps need to be taken to secure the airway by intubation or tracheostomy. Otherwise, a tracheotomy set should always be kept by the bedside.

If the airway is stable and the patient appears to be handling secretions, then an initial trial of medical therapy may be warranted. The patient is admitted and placed on appropriate intravenous antibiotic therapy as well as fluid replacement. If there is no improvement within 24 to 48 hours, then a CT scan may be obtained.

However, most of these patients are usually quite toxic when they present, and a more aggressive approach is usually necessary. Although antibiotic coverage is initiated, a CT evaluation is immediately performed and if an abscess is demonstrated, then surgical drainage is planned.

The microbiology of parapharyngeal space infection is generally polymicrobial and reflective of oropharyngeal flora. Therefore, both aerobic and anaerobic coverage is very important. Estimates of β-lactamase production by these organisms range from 17 to 46%, making penicillin a poor choice. Broad coverage is required but will ultimately depend on culture and sensitivity results.

SURGICAL MANAGEMENT

Only 10 to 15% of patients with deep neck space infections will resolve with medical therapy alone. Certainly if there is radiological evidence of an abscess, then surgical drainage is indicated. In addition, if CT or MRI scan suggests only cellulitis but the patient does not improve after 24 to 48 hours of aggressive antibiotic therapy, then again surgical exploration should be considered.

An intraoral approach to the parapharyngeal space is never appropriate since exposure is inadequate and vascular control would be impossible. The external approach is usually through either a submandibular incision, or an incision parallel to the anterior border of the sternocleidomastoid muscle. The dissection proceeds between the tail of the submandibular gland and the anterior border of the sternocleidomastoid muscle, and then in a medial superior direction just medial to the mandible and internal pterygoid muscle.

Other approaches have been suggested, such as needle aspiration with and without CT guidance and CT-guided percutaneous catheter drainage. However, open surgical drainage remains the standard of care.

REHABILITATION AND FOLLOW-UP

Following the successful management of most deep neck abscesses, long-term follow-up and rehabilitation are usually unnecessary. The primary site responsible for the infection such as an oral or dental problem should be addressed either concurrently or immediately following resolution of the deep neck infection.

SUGGESTED READINGS

Gidley PW, Ghorayeb BY, Stiernberg CM. Contemporary management of deep neck space infections. *Otolaryngol Head Neck Surg.* 1997;116:16–22.

Lazor JB, Cunningham MJ, Eavey RD, Weber AL. Comparison of computed tomography and surgical findings in deep neck infections. *Otolaryngol Head Neck Surg.* 1994;111:746–750.

Levitt G. Cervical fascia and deep neck infections. *Otolaryngol Clin North Am.* 1976;9:703–716.

Rabuzzi D, Johnson J. Diagnosis and management of deep neck infections. Self-instructional Package, American Academy of Otolaryngology–Head and Neck Surgery Foundation, Inc., 1978.

Ungkamont K, Yellon RF, Weissman JL, et al. Head and neck space infections in infants and children. *Otolaryngol Head and Neck Surg.* 1995;112:375–382.

STOMATITIS

Allen M. Seiden, M.D.

HISTORY

A 58-year-old white male presented with complaints of burning oral pain, dry mouth, and loss of taste. He had undergone a right lateral pharyngectomy and radical neck dissection for a tonsillar carcinoma 5 months previously, and this was followed by 6 weeks of radiation therapy that had been completed 2 months ago. He received a total of 60 Gray of radiation, and did develop some problems with a sore throat after the third week. He began to notice a loss of taste at that time that as yet had shown little improvement. In addition, his mouth had become quite dry, and this too had not improved. Nevertheless, the soreness seemed to get better until 2 to 3 weeks before presentation, when the burning pain began.

He was tolerating mostly a soft diet but described a particular sensitivity to hot and warm liquids, complaining that they produced a scorched feeling. He denied smoking or use of any tobacco products since the surgery. Appetite was diminished, and he had lost roughly 15 pounds from his preoperative weight. He relied on a rather old pair of dentures, but not having had any mandible resected at the time of surgery, the fit seemed acceptable.

Other medical problems included hypertension, controlled with a diuretic. There was no history of diabetes, heart disease, or other systemic illness.

Physical examination revealed a patient in no acute distress, sitting comfortably, and able to handle his secretions. He appeared thin but not emaciated. He carried a thermos of water and was able to swallow without aspiration.

The lips were somewhat parched and the corners of his mouth somewhat cracked. Intraoral examination did not reveal any significant edema, ulceration, or exudate. However, the dorsal surface of the tongue had a dusky red and smooth appearance (Fig. 37–1). The mucosa over the hard palate also appeared quite red, with a sharply demarcated border that coincided with the patient's denture. The buccal mucosa was very dry but otherwise displayed a normal pink color. Postoperative changes were noted within the oropharynx, which was also quite dry, but normal in color.

DIFFERENTIAL DIAGNOSIS— KEY POINTS

1. The patient's main complaints are burning pain, dry mouth, and taste loss. Initially, it would be logical to consider the impact of his recent surgery and radiation therapy. Mucositis typically begins to develop after 10 Gray (1,000 rads) are delivered, first creating a whitish appearing mucosa that eventually becomes erythematous and sometimes ulcerated. Areas of ulceration will usually be covered by a yellow-white pseudomembrane with a red border. This will cause a sore throat that is sometimes described as burning and may be associated with difficulty swallowing, loss of appetite, weight loss, and general malaise. This patient did describe a sore throat that began after the third week of radiation, after having received approximately 30 Gy, and this very likely did reflect a mucositis. However, this is an acute reaction that begins to heal once radiation is completed, and usually resolves within 3 to 4 weeks. Therefore, although the mucosa may continue to appear somewhat atrophic and dusky red for weeks to months, the fact that this patient experienced a new onset of burning pain suggests an additional problem.

2. Dry mouth, or xerostomia, is a universal result when patients receive more than 60 Gray of radiation, and rarely reverses. This will predispose to irritation and infection, but in and of itself should rarely cause burning pain.

3. Loss of taste is a common occurrence during radiation therapy, and seems to affect sweet, sour, and bitter more so than salt sensitivity. A detectable loss will occur after the first day

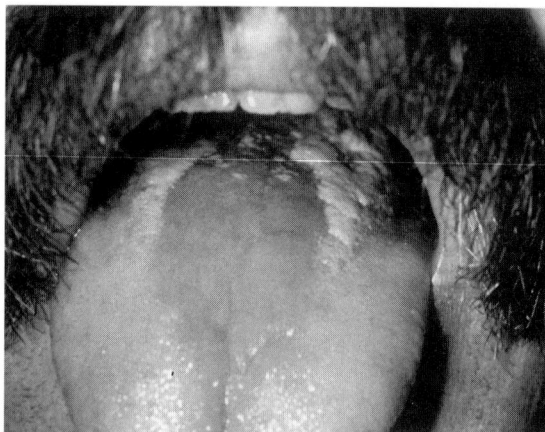

FIGURE 37–1 The central dorsum of the tongue appears smooth. The patient's dentures are in place.

of treatment and will maximize after 30 Gray. The injury seems to involve the taste-cell microvilli, or the taste bud receptor sites, and is not just a consequence of xerostomia. However, regeneration does occur, and recovery will generally begin within 20 to 60 days and be complete by 60 to 120 days.

4. Radiation therapy and its subsequent xerostomia predispose to opportunistic oral infections, and the new onset of symptoms in this patient would suggest that this has occurred. The burning pain and red color is characteristic of a fungal infection, most often due to *Candida albicans*. The patient's sensation of having been scorched after consuming certain foods is also very typical. *C. albicans* is a common inhabitant of the mouth but only becomes pathologic when there has been a reduction of the competitive oral microflora or a compromised resistance on the part of the host such as would occur after radiation.

    When the dorsal surface of the tongue is involved, depapillation generally occurs, giving the tongue a bald or smooth appearance. When the buccal or palatal mucosa is involved, lesions are typically dusky red, flat, and irregular. In the *pseudomembranous* form, profuse yellow-white plaques are present that are likened to milk curds and can be easily dislodged with a tongue blade. In the *erythematous* form, such plaques have largely disappeared.

5. Poorly fitting or improperly cleaned dentures can lead to underlying candidiasis even in noncompromised hosts. It occurs most commonly under a maxillary denture and appears as a red, flat lesion that is sharply demarcated to the outline of the denture. It is frequently asymptomatic but may be associated with mild burning pain.

6. *Candida* may extend to involve the corners of the mouth, particularly when there is a loss of vertical dimension of the jaw as might occur after a variety of head and neck oncologic resections. So-called "angular cheilitis" is characterized by redness and cracking of the angles of the mouth, often with adherent white plaques. It bleeds easily and is usually painful.

TEST INTERPRETATION

The diagnosis of candidiasis is usually based on clinical findings, then confirmed by the patient's response to therapy. However, more definitive confirmation can be obtained by cytologic smears or culture.

A scraping from a suspected lesion may be placed on a glass slide, then spray-fixed and sent to a laboratory for periodic acid–Schiff staining, or simply combined with potassium hydroxide. A search is then made for the presence of typical hyphae. However, a sterile cotton swab may be used to obtain a culture, which will then take 10 days to 2 weeks. However, it is best not to defer antifungal therapy while awaiting such test results.

DIAGNOSIS

1. Oral candidiasis or candidal stomatitis;
2. Radiation-induced xerostomia and transient hypogeusia.

MEDICAL MANAGEMENT

Any patient scheduled to undergo radiation therapy should have a prior dental evaluation, with appropriate treatment of any dental and periodontal disease. Supportive care during therapy is also important. This will help to minimize any secondary infections and complications. Good oral hygiene must be emphasized.

A variety of agents may be used to clean and lubricate the dry, inflamed oral mucosa that results after radiation. Saline, sodium bicarbonate, and hydrogen peroxide solutions help to eradicate dry, sticky mucus and debris. Chlorhexidine gluconate as well as fluoride gels have been shown to help prevent further periodontal disease. Various salivary substitutes or stimulants are also available.

The taste loss is generally reversible, and therefore no specific therapy is necessary.

Several very effective agents are now available to treat oral candidiasis. Nystatin oral suspension at a concentration of 100,000 U/mL may be used four times per day as an oral rinse, to be taken over 2 weeks. Very little is absorbed and it is therefore safe and usually effective. It may be prescribed as an ointment combined with triamcinolone acetonide for use against angular cheilitis and denture candidiasis. Clotrimazole oral troches or lozenges may be taken five times a day and are usually well tolerated, but occasionally will elevate liver enzymes. Systemic agents include ketoconazole, 200 mg/day, and fluconazole, and are reportedly more effective than the topical medications. Again, 2 weeks of therapy is recommended. Rarely would amphotericin B be necessary.

SURGICAL MANAGEMENT

There is no role for surgery in the management of radiation-induced xerostomia and candidiasis.

REHABILITATION AND FOLLOW-UP

Although the fungal infection will resolve with appropriate therapy, this patient will continue to have xerostomia. Therefore, he will remain susceptible to recurring infection and dental disease. Aggressive oral cleansing and lubrication, as described earlier, is important. In addition, it is important to maintain proper care of dental appliances, ensuring proper fit and function.

SUGGESTED READINGS

CARL W. Local radiation and systemic chemotherapy: preventing and managing the oral complications. *JADA.* 1993;124:119–123.

CONGER AD. Loss and recovery of taste acuity in patients irradiated to the oral cavity. *Rad Res.* 1973;53:338–347.

EPSTEIN JB. Antifungal therapy in oropharyngeal mycotic infections. *Oral Surg.* 1990;69:32.

MCDONALD JS. Oral ulcerative diseases. In: Paparella MM, Shumrick DA, Gluckman JL, Meyerhoff WL, eds. *Otolaryngology.* 3rd ed. Philadelphia, PA: WB Saunders; 1991:2003–2019.

ZEGARELLI DJ. Fungal infections of the oral cavity. *Otolaryngol. Clin North Am.* 1993;26:1069–1089.

CERVICAL TUBERCULOSIS

Thomas A. Tami, M.D.

HISTORY

A 25 year-old recent immigrant from Vietnam presented to the ENT clinic complaining of progressive enlargement of a right neck mass. This mass was slightly tender and had grown over the past 6 to 8 weeks from a small 2-cm nodule to its current 8-cm size. He was otherwise healthy and had no other symptoms referable to the head and neck area. He was a nonsmoker and a nondrinker. He had no respiratory symptoms; however, he stated that he lived with his extended family in a small one-room apartment and that his older brother was very ill with some unknown pulmonary condition. He was afebrile at the time of this initial presentation, but described frequent sweats and chills, especially during the night.

On physical examination a slightly tender, rubbery mass was noted in the right submandibular area. He had a few other scattered nodes in the right neck, all less than 1.5 cm. His oral cavity examination was unremarkable except for his poor dentition. His tonsils were present and benign in appearance. The oropharynx, hypopharynx, larynx, and nasopharynx were all unremarkable. The thyroid gland was not enlarged and felt normal.

DIFFERENTIAL DIAGNOSIS— KEY POINTS

1. In evaluating this or any neck mass, an initial assessment should be made to determine whether the mass represents a neoplastic or inflammatory process. In general, inflammatory masses occur in younger patients, tend to be present for a relatively short duration, can be associated with infectious constitutional symptoms, and have local signs of inflammation (redness, edema, tenderness). On the other hand, neoplastic neck masses tend to occur in older patients, usually have a longer time course, and typically have few signs and symptoms of inflammation. In this case, this neck mass appears to have characteristics of both. It has been present for an intermediate period of time (6 weeks); there are some constitutional findings consistent with infection; the mass is slightly tender, but not impressively so; there is little edema and erythema surrounding the mass. Whether the initial impression leads to a workup for neoplasm or inflammation, frequent reassessment of the diagnosis should be ongoing during the workup so that a change in diagnosis can be instituted if necessary.

2. A neck mass in a recent immigrant from southeast Asia should raise the possibility of an unusual infectious process. Of these, fungal or mycobacterial infections should top the list. In fact, the resurgence of tuberculosis (TB) that occurred in the United States in the mid- to late 1980s was due in large part to immigration from central and South America as well as from southeast Asia and Pacific rim countries. The other primary factor responsible for this epidemic was the acquired immunodeficiency syndrome (AIDS) epidemic. Since this patient is at increased risk for TB, he should undergo appropriate testing for this possibility. The family and social history are also factors that tend to support this diagnosis, since it sounds as though his brother may have pulmonary TB.

3. A neoplasm must also be considered. A neck mass is often the first presentation of carcinomas of the upper aerodigestive tract. Although he is a nonsmoker and nondrinker, a careful head and neck examination must be pursued to rule out this possibility. If he were

of Chinese descent, primary nasopharyngeal carcinoma would be a high likelihood. This same association does not appear to occur in other regions of southeast Asia. Other possibilities could include primary lymphoma or metastatic thyroid carcinoma.

TEST INTERPRETATION

- Chest x-ray—normal.
- Purified protein derivative (PPD) skin test—positive (14 mm of induration).
- Computed tomography (CT) scan of the neck—see Figure 38–1.
- Fine-needle aspiration biopsy (FNAB)—cytologic features of granuloma; no acid fast bacilli (AFB) seen.
- AFB culture of FNAB—pending.
- AFB culture of sputum—pending.

The presumptive diagnosis in this case, based on the history and physical examination is cervical tuberculosis. However, the chest x-ray is normal. Of interest, only 10 to 15% of patients who present with cervical tuberculosis will have chest x-ray findings consistent with pulmonary disease. However, despite a normal chest x-ray,

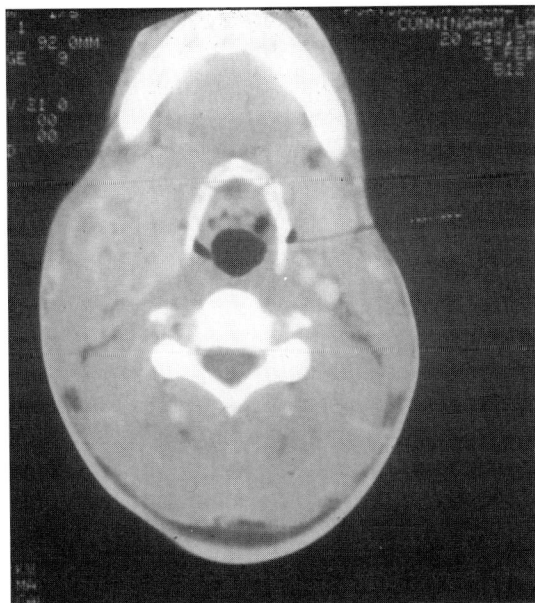

FIGURE 38-1 CT scan of the neck.

some of these patients will have a positive sputum culture for TB. Therefore, even if the radiograph is negative, all patients with suspected cervical TB should have sputum cultures obtained. While the older literature often described cervical TB as a manifestation of disseminated disease, more recent reports describe it as a more localized disease process.

The PPD skin test is integral to making this diagnosis. However, immigrant populations have often had previous exposure to TB or BCG immunization making the use of this test somewhat less helpful. Also, in severely immunodeficient patients, such as patients with AIDS, no skin reaction occurs because of an anergic host. In fact, for patients infected with the human immunodeficiency virus (HIV) a skin reaction of only 5 mm is considered clinically significant (usually a reaction of 10 mm or more is needed for a positive test response).

The CT scan reveals findings consistent with cervical TB. While certainly not pathognomonic, TB typically presents radiographically as lymph node enlargement with central necrosis and multiple loculated abscesses within the node. A CT of the entire upper aerodigestive tract, neck, and nasopharynx would be important to rule out either infectious or neoplastic diseases elsewhere in the head and neck. In this case, these studies were negative except for the single large neck mass.

The increasing use of FNAB for evaluating neck masses has revolutionized our ability to make an early diagnosis, institute appropriate treatment, and in many instances avoid open biopsy. In cervical TB, evidence of granuloma can help in the presumptive diagnosis of this condition. Although there are many conditions other than TB that produce granulomas in the head and neck, a presumptive diagnosis can be made based on the clinical setting even in the absence of a positive AFB stain. Treatment can be instituted while cultures are pending. Cultures for AFB often require up to 6 weeks to identify the mycobacterial organism and obtain antibiotic sensitivities.

DIAGNOSIS

Cervical tuberculosis.

MEDICAL MANAGEMENT

Tuberculosis is primarily a medical disease. If the diagnosis can be established in a timely and accurate manner, the immediate institution of antituberculous chemotherapy can usually produce dramatic resolution. In instances where cultures are pending, but the tentative diagnosis of TB has been made, multidrug therapy is instituted pending positive culture and antibiotic sensitivities. Because of recent emergence of multiple drug-resistant strains of TB, most centers recommend initial four-drug therapy until sensitivities are known. A common regimen would include isoniazid, rifampin, ethambutol hydrochloride, and pyrazinamide. When culture sensitivities return, therapy is usually continued using two effective drugs. Total therapy usually continues for 8 to 12 months. Resistant strains of TB have developed in many instances due to inappropriate or incomplete drug therapy of active TB. To help solve this major public health problem, many agencies have instituted directly observed TB therapy programs to ensure complete and effective medical management of cases of active TB.

Cervical TB is not considered infectious unless there is a concomitant pulmonary infection. In suspected cases of pulmonary TB, patients should be placed in respiratory isolation. Their close personal contacts should also be tested with PPD skin tests. Isolation is continued as long as the patient has infectious sputum.

SURGICAL MANAGEMENT

In the past, surgery has played an important role in both the diagnosis as well as the treatment of cervical TB. The only effective way to make this diagnosis definitively was by performing an open biopsy, and most clinicians emphasized the importance of complete surgical excision of cervical masses in tuberculous lymphadenopathy. With the contemporary use of FNAB a definitive diagnosis can usually be established without a formal open biopsy; and medical management is usually successful in resolving even massive tuberculous cervical infections. Surgery should be reserved for cases in which the diagnosis cannot be otherwise established or for persons who have residual neck masses or draining sinuses despite full-course medical therapy.

REHABILITATION AND FOLLOW-UP

Close follow-up is mandatory to ensure that the entire course of therapy is completed. Subsequently, periodic chest radiographs should be obtained to evaluate for recurrent or persistent infection. As mentioned earlier, evaluation and follow-up of close personal contacts is vital to contain any potential continued spread of the infection within the social environment of the patient.

SUGGESTED READINGS

Centers for Disease Control. Screening for tuberculosis and tuberculosis infection in high risk populations and the use of preventive therapy for tuberculosis. *MMWR.* 1990;39(suppl RR-8):1–12.

Lee KC, Schecter G. Tuberculous infections of the head and neck. *ENT J.* 1995;74(6):395–399.

Lee KC, Tami TA, Lalwani AK, Schecter G. Contemporary management of cervical tuberculosis. *Laryngoscope.* 1992;102:60–64.

ENT MANIFESTATIONS OF HIV DISEASE

Thomas A. Tami, M.D.

HISTORY

A 44-year-old man presents with a left parotid gland mass that has been slowly enlarging for the last year. He has a wasted general appearance and describes a 30-pound weight loss during the past 6 months. He has a chronic productive cough and reports occasional hemoptysis, intermittent fevers, and night sweats nearly every night.

His medical history is significant for many years of IV drug use. He also states that he has developed a sore mouth and gum disease during the past year. He denies other medical problems.

The physical examination reveals a 3-cm soft, nontender mass in the tail of the left parotid gland. He also has generalized bilateral cervical lymphadenopathy. Oral examination reveals erythematous inflamed plaque-like areas of the palate and posterior pharyngeal wall as well as severe periodontal disease and pronounced gingival atrophy. On chest auscultation bilateral diffuse rhonchi and a few bilateral scattered rales are heard.

DIFFERENTIAL DIAGNOSIS— KEY POINTS

1. Although this patient presented with a parotid gland complaint, he appears to have a much more serious problem which must be addressed. Weight loss, generalized lymphadenopathy, chronic cough, and fevers all point to an underlying condition potentially more important than the parotid mass.

2. His pulmonary symptoms suggest an infectious process. Night sweats and hemoptysis in the setting of a chronic cough could be due to community-acquired pneumonia, aspiration pneumonia, tuberculosis (TB) or some other opportunistic infection. Given this differential, which includes active TB, this patient should be placed in respiratory isolation pending an accurate pulmonary diagnosis.

3. Oral thrush is an unusual finding in patients with normal immune function. Chronic antibiotic usage, diabetes mellitus, myelosupression, hematogenous or other malignancies, and acquired or primary immune deficiencies can all be the underlying condition accounting for this finding.

4. His long history of IV drug use should immediately raise the specter of a bloodborne infectious disease such as hepatitis or infection with the human immunodeficiency virus (HIV). Further questioning about needle sharing, sexual habits, etc., should be considered.

TEST INTERPRETATION

A search for the underlying condition accounting for this patient's multiple system problems should include a metabolic evaluation, immunologic testing, and chest imaging. Evaluation of the oral lesions and his sputum are also important. Finally, the parotid mass should also be worked up.

- Chest x-ray—generalized interstitial infiltrates with apical cavitary lesions. The apical lesions and the diffuse miliary pattern are consistent with active TB.
- Electrolytes—normal.
- Fasting glucose—normal.
- Complete blood count:
  Hgb—10.4.
  Hct—31.8.
  White blood cell count—8.8.
- Purified protein derivative skin test—0.5 cm

of reactivity. While normal PPD reactivity is usually considered to be 1.0 cm, 0.5 cm is usually considered as positive in HIV-infected individuals.

- Oral scraping KOH—positive for yeast. While the typical appearance of oral candidiasis is whitish cheese-like plaques with underlying and surrounding erythema, the findings in this patient are consistent with atrophic oral candidiasis

- Sputum AFB stain—few scattered acid-fast bacilli seen.

- Computed tomography scan of the parotid mass—see Figure 39–1. This scan reveals distinct cystic masses within the parotid gland. The surrounding glandular architecture is unremarkable.

- Fine-needle aspiration biopsy of parotid mass—2 cc of fluid containing a mixed population of lymphocytes and epithelial cells.

- HIV test—positive. With a positive test for HIV, further testing should be undertaken to determine the stage of disease in this patient.

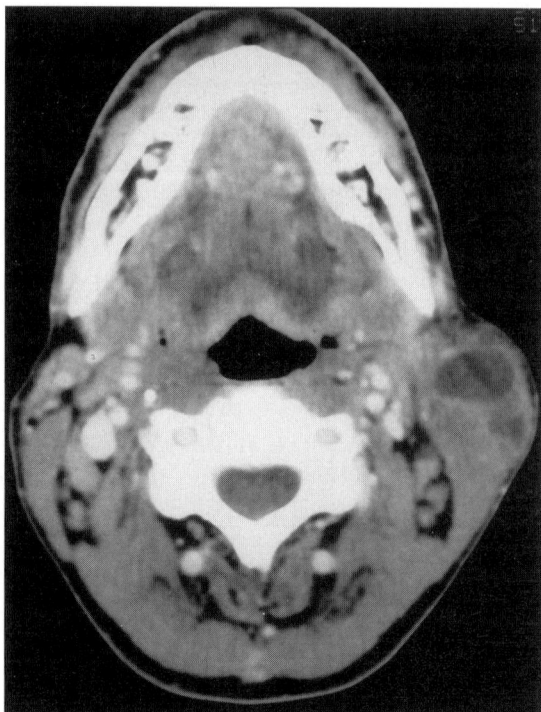

FIGURE 39–1 AIDS—parotid cysts.

The CD:4 lymphocyte level should be determined.

- CD:4 lymphocyte level (T-helper lymphocyte)—87 cells/μL The normal CD:4 level is in the 800–1,000 cells/mL range. Levels below 200 cells/mL represent severe immunodeficiency. The definition of AIDS (acquired immunodeficiency syndrome) now includes a count below 200 as an AIDS defining condition. By definition, this patient has AIDS.

DIAGNOSIS

1. HIV infection—AIDS
2. Active pulmonary tuberculosis
3. Atrophic oral candidiasis
4. Severe chronic periodontal disease
5. Benign lymphothelial cyst of parotid gland

MEDICAL MANAGEMENT

This patient has active TB and must be managed appropriately. Respiratory isolation must be instituted whenever this diagnosis is considered. Hospitalization in a negative pressure ventilation setting is imperative to prevent the spread of this contagious disease. HIV-infected patients with TB often have minimal symptoms, yet are extremely contagious. Given the recent national problem with multiple drug-resistant TB, cultures of this patient's sputum are of extreme importance so that appropriately directed, directly observed, multiple drug therapy can be undertaken.

Oral candidiasis is one of the most common opportunistic infections seen in patients infected with HIV. Topical agents such as Nystatin or clotrimazole are often effective in managing this condition. In recalcitrant cases, oral systemic therapy with fluconizole can often provide an immediate response. Long-term fluconizole is also helpful to prevent recurrence in patients who develop recurrent oral thrush. If severe dysphagia and/or odynophagia is a prominent symptom, esophageal candidiasis, a much more serious problem, must be entertained. Barium swallow can often establish this diagnosis, however, esophagoscopy is also occasionally necessary.

The severe periodontal disease seen in HIV-infected patients can often be difficult to control. Meticulous attention to oral hygiene, frequent oral–dental examinations, and in some cases, systemic antibiotic therapy are all important to minimize this problem.

This patient should be referred to an infectious disease specialist familiar with the management of patients infected with HIV. The use of retroviral agents such as azidothymidine (AZT), prophylactic treatment of opportunistic infections, and the newly available protease inhibitors have augmented our ability to manage this medical condition, improve quality of life, and extend life expectancy in patients with this disease.

SURGICAL MANAGEMENT

Lymphoepithelial cysts, which are commonly seen in these patients, are usually asymptomatic. Occasionally they may enlarge, causing pressure symptoms, or become cosmetically unacceptable. Frequent repeated needle aspirations are usually sufficient to manage these symptoms. Some success has been reported with the use of tetracycline sclerosis of these cysts following needle aspirations. Only rarely is parotidectomy needed to either diagnose or manage this problem.

Any surgical or other invasive procedure undertaken in this HIV-infected patient, or any patient for that matter, should utilize "Universal Precautions" as recommended by the Centers for Disease Control and Prevention.

REHABILITATION AND FOLLOW-UP

This patient will require close monitoring and follow-up by his primary infectious disease physician. When he is treated with multiple drug therapy for pulmonary TB, community nursing will be necessary for directly observed therapy. Evidence has overwhelmingly shown that direct observation of patients to ensure compliance with medications is vital to decrease the incidence of multiple drug-resistant strains of *Mycobacterium* tuberculosis.

SUGGESTED READINGS

Lee KC, Schecter G. Tuberculosis infections of the head and neck. *ENT J.* 1995;74(6):395–399.

Tami TA, ed. Otolaryngologic manifestations of the acquired immunodeficiency syndrome. *Otolaryngol Clin North Am.* 1992;25(6).

Tami TA, Lee KC. AIDS and the otolaryngologist. Self-Instructional Package. American Academy of Otolaryngology—Head and Neck Surgery Foundation, Inc., 1993.

Tami TA, Lee KC. Manifestations of the acquired immunodeficiency syndrome. In: Bailey BJ, ed. *Head & Neck Surgery—Otolaryngology.* Philadelphia, PA: JB Lippincott; 1993:Chapter 60.

CERVICAL NECROTIZING FASCIITIS

Thomas A. Tami, M.D.

HISTORY

A 34-year-old woman with insulin-dependent diabetes mellitus underwent an anterior cervical fusion by a neurosurgeon because of degenerative cervical disk disease. Her immediate postoperative course was uneventful and she was discharged on postoperative day 3. By postoperative day 5 she began to notice swelling and redness at the surgical site. Oral cephalexin was begun; however, the process continued to spread. By day 7 she was readmitted to the hospital and started on intravenous cefazolin. Seropurulent drainage was now noted coming from the wound, so it was reopened at one edge. This also failed to result in any improvement since the process was by now spreading into the lateral neck. The skin around the wound began to necrose (Figure 40–1). She was also beginning to notice numbness over her entire anterior neck. A culture was obtained from the wound and a computed tomography (CT) scan was obtained.

DIFFERENTIAL DIAGNOSIS— KEY POINTS

1. This patient is obviously experiencing a postoperative wound infection. If the usual pathogen, a gram-positive organism such as *Staphylococcus aureus* were the offending agent, the initial antibiotic choice should have been effective.

2. Despite appropriate antibiotic therapy, this infection continued unabated. This patient has diabetes, which places her at increased risk for infections by unusual organisms. Furthermore, she may be unable to mount a normal host response to infection. This fact should be considered early in the course of this infection. Aggressive management must

be instituted immediately when the initial therapy fails to control the process.

3. The finding of hypesthesia or numbness of the skin of the anterior neck is a potentially grim finding because it suggests an underlying necrotizing infectious process. As the skin develops necrosis around the wound site, cervical necrotizing fasciitis must be strongly considered. Although the patient appeared to do well for the first several postoperative days, the possibility of an occult esophageal injury at the time of surgery should be investigated.

4. The metabolic and hematologic status of this patient must be closely monitored. Metabolic acidosis and hypotension in this setting could result in dire, potentially fatal consequences.

5. Patients with cervical necrotizing fasciitis have a high incidence of mediastinal extension even when not immediately clinically detectable. CT scanning should include the neck, mediastinum, and chest.

6. Both aerobic as well as fastidious anaerobic cultures should be obtained immediately so that culture-directed antibiotic therapy can be instituted as quickly as feasible.

TEST INTERPRETATION

- CT scan of neck (Fig. 40–2)–Tremendous soft tissue edema reflects the extensive infection of the anterior neck. The appearance of fluid collections that conform to the fascial planes of the neck is consistent with necrotizing fasciitis. No free air is seen within these fascial planes. Although gas-forming organisms are often part of the clinical picture in necrotizing fasciitis, this is not a constant feature. The mediastinum and chest were both scanned and found to be normal. When CT is performed in patients with suspected necrotizing

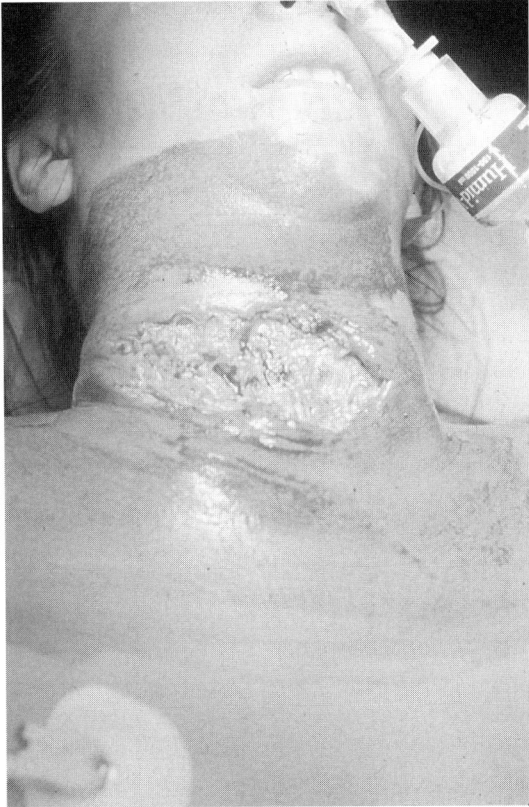

FIGURE 40-1 Necrotizing skin wound.

fasciitis, chest CT should always be done at the same time. Mediastinal extension is often not obvious clinically and can only be detected using CT scanning. Mortality may be increased to nearly 50% in patients with mediastinitis associated with cervical fasciitis. Early detection and appropriate medical and surgical treatment are vital to the successful management of this problem.

- Barium swallow—no evidence of esophageal perforation.
- Serum glucose—335 mg/dL.
- Sodium—133 mg/dL.
- Chloride—103 mg/dL.
- Potassium—3.3 mg/dL.
- Bicarbonate—16 mg/dL.
- White blood cell (WBC) count—22,500 cells/mL.
- Gram stain—many gram-negative rods and gram-positive cocci, many polys.
- Aerobic culture—*Streptococcus viridans, Escherichia coli.*
- Anaerobic culture—*Peptostreptococcus micros, Fusobacterium nucleatum.*

The glucose and electrolytes reveal a fairly hyperglycemic patient. Glucose intolerance of-

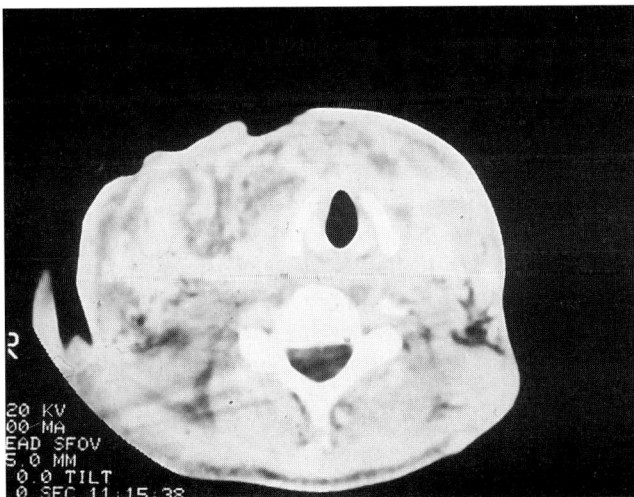

FIGURE 40-2 CT scan of the neck demonstrates soft tissue edema and apparent diffuse fluid collections that conform to the fascial planes of the neck.

ten develops in patients with diabetes during an infection. The low bicarbonate level also suggests a metabolic acidosis. This is a disturbing finding, suggesting that either this patient is in diabetic acidosis or is developing sepsis.

The polymicrobial nature of the culture is typical for necrotizing fasciitis. The aerobes and anaerobes work synergistically to produce an infection that can rapidly extend far beyond its origins.

The elevated WBC is another indication of severe infection. Occasionally, with overwhelming infection and sepsis, the WBC can be normal or low, further confusing the clinical picture.

DIAGNOSIS

Cervical necrotizing fasciitis.

MEDICAL MANAGEMENT

The initial medical management of this patient with antibiotics directed primarily at *S. aureus* was very appropriate. Most surgical wound infections are due to this pathogen. However, the lack of an immediate early response should have resulted in an early aggressive assault on this infection in this young diabetic patient.

Hospitalization for intravenous antibiotics was quite justified. However, instead of continuing treatment with a first-generation cephalosporin, broader coverage should have been considered, possibly including gram-negative therapy. When the initial culture and gram stain was obtained and a mixture of gram-negatives and gram-positives was observed, the possibility of a severe necrotizing soft tissue infection should have been immediately considered in the differential diagnosis. At that time, appropriate antibiotic therapy should include gram-positive, gram-negative, and anaerobic therapy. A reasonable choice might have included a third-generation cephalosporin, clindamycin, and possibly an aminoglycoside.

In this patient, successful therapy will depend in large part on maintaining a normal hemodynamic status as well as controlling her diabetes. A continuous intravenous infusion of insulin is often necessary to control serum glucose adequately. If hemodynamic parameters become difficult to monitor and control due to sepsis, pulmonary artery catheterization using a Swan-Ganz catheter may be a reasonable consideration.

Hyperbaric oxygen (HBO) therapy has been successfully employed in cases of necrotizing fasciitis in other parts of the body as well as in the cervical region. By raising the tissue oxygenation, HBO may inhibit the growth of anaerobic bacteria and improve the killing potential of leukocytes. While most reports of HBO as adjunctive therapy are done without controls, HBO does appear to induce a more rapid control of the infectious process and earlier onset of healing. Most authors recommend its use when the clinical situation allows for its safe administration.

SURGICAL MANAGEMENT

The initial surgical approach to this patient was probably too conservative. While opening the lateral edge of a wound is sufficient for obtaining culture material, it is inadequate as a drainage procedure, especially in this diabetic patient with a rapidly progressing infection. A more formal wound exploration and drainage procedure should have been considered for this patient.

When the diagnosis of necrotizing fasciitis was finally established and the skin around the wound site was showing frank necrosis, a surgical emergency existed. Formal wound exploration and exposure of cervical fascial planes was necessary. Typically, frank purulence is rarely encountered; rather, a thin serosanguinous "dishwater" appearing fluid permeates the entire wound. Debridement of all necrotic tissue, including muscle and skin if necessary, is vital to the success of the surgery and the ultimate survival of the patient. Multiple bedside debridements may be needed over the ensuing week or two, and occasionally return to the operating room may be necessary to delineate the actual extent of debridement necessary.

Throughout this debridement process, the carotid artery must be monitored closely for evidence of necrosis of the vessel wall with potential catastrophic results.

REHABILITATION AND FOLLOW-UP

When extensive debridement has resulted in loss of overlying skin covering, subsequent reconstructive procedures may be necessary. The wound should be kept open with frequent dressing changes. Reconstructive efforts should not be considered until granulation tissue is forming throughout the entire wound bed.

In many cases, the quickest and most effective method to provide immediate wound coverage is via a split thickness skin graft. While this technique does not usually result in an ideal cosmetic appearance, the reliability of this technique often offers great advantage. Other alternatives include regional musculocutaneous flaps, such as the pectoralis major flap, or possibly a free tissue transfer such as a forearm or abdominal free flap.

SUGGESTED REFERENCES

KADDOUR HS, SMELT GJ. Necrotizing fasciitis of the neck. *J Laryngol Otol.* 1992;106(11):1008–1010.

LANGFORD FP, MOON RE, STOLP BW, SCHER RL. Treatment of cervical necrotizing fasciitis with hyperbaric oxygen therapy. *Otolaryngol Head Neck Surg.* 1995;112(2):274–278.

MAISEL RH, KARLEN R. Cervical necrotizing fasciitis. *Laryngoscope.* 1994;104(7):795–798.

MATHIEU D, NEVIERE R, TEILLON C, et al. Cervical necrotizing fasciitis: clinical manifestations and management. *Clin Infect Dis.* 1995;21(1):51–56.

Case 41

ORBITAL COMPLICATION OF SINUSITIS

Thomas A. Tami, M.D.

HISTORY

A 38-year-old man with a long history of allergic rhinitis and nasal obstruction noted the onset of right-sided retro-orbital headache and periorbital swelling. Self medication with over-the-counter cold preparations failed to improve his symptoms, so he presented to the emergency department of a local hospital. Plain sinus x-rays were obtained and interpreted as being normal. Outpatient therapy was initiated with cephalexin for presumed facial cellulitis.

Three days later he began to note bulging of his right eye as well as double vision. By the time he was seen in the emergency department, the vision in his eye was decreased and he was able to move he eye only with difficulty. Diagnostic tests were ordered and otolaryngology was consulted.

DIFFERENTIAL DIAGNOSIS— KEY POINTS

1. While facial cellulitis of a nonsinogenic etiology might have been entertained during this patient's initial emergency room visit, since he had a previous history of substantial sinus symptoms and problems, ethmoid sinusitis should have been high on the initial differential diagnosis.

2. Plain sinus radiographs of the paranasal sinuses were obtained to rule out sinusitis as the primary problem. Although plain sinus x-rays are helpful in determining maxillary or frontal sinusitis, they are notoriously poor for making the diagnosis of ethmoid sinusitis.

The negative plain sinus x-ray series should not have been used to reliably rule out a sinogenic cause of this patient's problem.

3. The initial antibiotic choice was inadequate for the treatment of acute ethmoid sinusitis. Cephalexin has poor *Haemophilus influenzae* coverage and should therefore be avoided for the management of acute sinusitis.

4. When this patient presented to the emergency department for a second time, the diagnosis was clear. He was developing extensive orbital involvement from what should have been previously diagnosed as ethmoid sinusitis. Chandler's staging system of orbital complications of sinusitis has been widely accepted (Table 41–1). This patient is clearly in either Chandler stage III or stage IV. Since his opposite left eye appears not to be involved at this time, he has probably not developed cavernous sinus thrombosis. Appropriate diagnostic testing at this time should include a computed tomography (CT) scan of the sinuses and orbit. Contrast should be used to help in the evaluation of the cavernous sinus.

5. The progressive visual loss that is occurring in this patient makes this an emergent situation. An ophthalmology consultation should be obtained immediately to help in assessing this patient's vision and orbital function.

TEST INTERPRETATION

• *Plain sinus radiographs.* The Caldwell view of the paranasal sinuses is usually used to evaluate the ethmoid sinuses. Even when no abnor-

TABLE 41-1   Chandler's Staging System

Stage I. Preseptal inflammatory edema of the eyelids; minimal to no tenderness; no limitation of ocular movement or visual loss

Stage II. Orbital cellulitis with inflammation and edema of orbital fat and orbital contents; no abscess

Stage III. Subperiosteal abscess; mass displacement of globe away from abscess; proptosis; may begin to experience decreased visual acuity; may have diplopia

Stage IV. Orbital abscess; severe symmetric proptosis; ophthalmoplegia with possible visual loss

Stage V. Cavernous sinus thrombosis; ophthalmoplegia; visual loss; extension to the contralateral eye

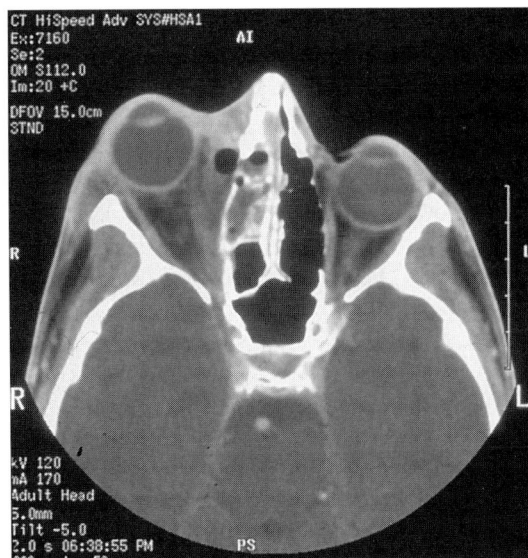

FIGURE 41-1 CT view through the ethmoid sinuses and orbit revealing anterior ethmoid sinusitis and an orbital subperiosteal abcess.

mality is noted on this view, and the radiologist in fact described this film as being essentially normal in this case, ethmoid sinusitis can be easily missed. Plain sinus x-rays are notoriously poor in evaluating the ethmoid sinuses. Given this patient's history, this negative film should have been confirmed with a screening sinus CT scan. In most institutions, the cost of a screening sinus CT (usually consisting of 6 to 8 coronal cuts through the paranasal sinuses) is comparable to that of plain sinus radiography, yet can offer much more meaningful clinical information.

- *CT scan of the paranasal sinuses and orbit.* Figure 41-1 is a CT view through the ethmoid sinuses and orbit. Ethmoid sinusitis can be easily detected on this scan despite its absence in the plain sinus x-rays. Contrast has been used to enhance the inflammatory process in the orbit as well as to assist in visualization of the cavernous sinus. If the cavernous sinus enhanced asymmetrically or failed to show enhancement on the involved side, cavernous sinus thrombosis would be a further consideration in this case.

DIAGNOSIS

Periorbital subperiosteal abscess (Chandler's stage III); ethmoid sinusitis.

MEDICAL MANAGEMENT

The initial medical management of this patient when he presented with an early orbital complication (probably Chandler's stage I, preseptal cellulitis) should have been appropriately selected antibiotics and nasal decongestants/anti-inflammatories. Oral amoxicillin may have been appropriate; however, given the increasing incidence of bacterial resistance to this drug, a better choice may have been amoxicillin/clavulanate, cefuroxime axetil, or clarithromycin. Systemic decongestants such as pseudoephedrine or phenylpropanolamine should also have been included, assuming that the patient had no underlying cardiovascular disease. Topical nasal steroid sprays can also be effective for chronic sinusitis and might have been considered. The role for systemic steroid therapy in acute sinusitis is controversial; however, it is also often included.

As the orbital process progresses, the need for more aggressive therapeutic measures increases. Hospitalization for observation and treatment with intravenous antibiotics is mandatory in this situation. Intravenous ampicillin/sulbactam or the combination of cefuroxime and metronidazole are both good alternatives in this situation to provide good *Streptococcus pneumoniae, H. influenzae, Moraxella catarrhalis,* and *Staphylococcus aureus* coverage. Intravenous systemic steroids might also be considered to decrease the orbital edema that is beginning to produce visual changes.

Although medical interventions will certainly help contain the infection and prevent progression, the definitive emergency therapy for this patient with a periorbital abscess is surgical.

SURGICAL MANAGEMENT

Operative management should be planned to address both the abscess as well as the underlying ethmoid sinusitis. Ophthalmology should, in most instances, be intimately involved in both the surgical planning as well as the operative intervention.

While the endonasal endoscopic approach to the ethmoid sinuses could effectively manage the ethmoid sinusitis, the use of this route to address the orbital abscess is fraught with danger. Excessive bleeding and edema due to the acute infection process make visualization through this route extremely limited. Although the endoscopic approach has been advocated by some for the management of orbital subperiosteal abscess in the region of the lamina papyrecia, its role even in this setting must be questioned. A failure of adequate drainage of an abscess resulting in progressive orbital infection and possible blindness may be difficult to defend if only the endoscopic approach were utilized.

The external ethmoidectomy approach through a medial canthal, Lynch-type incision is generally preferred. The ethmoids can be adequately and appropriately addressed and the orbit entered and drained through this approach. An intimate understanding of the intraorbital anatomic structures and relationships is vital for the safe performance of this drainage procedure.

REHABILITATION AND FOLLOW-UP

During the immediate postoperative period serial visual examination with frequent evaluation of visual acuity as well as fundal findings is extremely important to monitor the resolution of the process. If ocular findings continue to progress despite what should otherwise have been adequate medical and surgical therapy, repeat imaging should be immediately obtained to diagnose persistence or extension of the process. Examination of the opposite eye for changes in ocular motility or visual acuity should also be part of the monitoring process to exclude the progression to cavernous sinus thrombosis.

SUGGESTED READINGS

CHANDLER JR, LANGENBRUNNER DJ, STEVENS ER. The pathogenesis of orbital complications in acute sinusitis. *Laryngoscope.* 1970;80:1414.

CLARY RA, CUNNINGHAM MJ, EAVEY RD. Orbital complications of acute sinusitis: comparison of computed tomography scan and surgical findings. *Ann Otol Rhinol Laryngol.* 1992;101(7):598–600.

LAWSON W. Orbital complications of sinusitis. In: Blitzer A, Lawson W, Friedman, eds. *Surgery of the Paranasal Sinuses.* Philadelphia, PA: WB Saunders; 1985:316–327.

PAGE EL, WIATRAK BJ. Endoscopic vs external drainage of orbital subperiosteal abscess. *Arch Otolaryngol Head Neck Surg.* 1996;122(7):737–740.

PATT BS, MANNING SC. Blindness resulting from orbital complications of sinusitis. *Otolaryngol Head Neck Surg.* 1991;104(6):789–795.

Case 42

CHRONIC SINUSITIS
Thomas A. Tami, M.D.

HISTORY

A 38-year-old woman, who had no previous history of nasal or sinus problems, developed acute sinusitis following an upper respiratory infection. Since her symptoms of headache, facial pain, and nasal purulent drainage persisted for 3 weeks, she was seen by her primary care physician who prescribed 1 week of cephelexin. Her symptoms persisted despite this treatment, so her physician prescribed a 10-day course of erythromycin. Again, she noted only minimal improvement so she was given a 2-week course of ciprofloxacin therapy. Since this regimen also failed to relieve her symptoms, she was referred to an otolaryngolost (now 8 to 10 weeks following her initial illness). Her medical history was unremarkable. She denied nasal allergies, asthma, or previous nasal symptoms.

On physical examination, the head and neck were unremarkable except for the nasal exam. The septum was mildly deviated to the left; however, it did not completely obstruct the nasal airway. Nasal endoscopic examination showed inflammatory changes with edema and purulence emanating from both the left and the right middle meatus. Polypoid changes were noted beneath the middle turbinates and in both sphenoethmoid recesses. There were no masses noted in the nasal cavity or nasopharynx.

DIFFERENTIAL DIAGNOSIS— KEY POINTS

1. This patient developed an acute sinusitis following an otherwise uncomplicated viral upper respiratory infection. This is probably the most common scenario for acute sinusitis. She has no previous history of nasal problem, no symptoms of hay fever or nasal allergy, nasal obstruction, or other respiratory problems such as asthma. This should be an easily treated condition and should not result in chronic sinusitis.

2. The initial treatment by the primary care provider was inappropriate. The three most common bacteria associated with acute sinusitis are *Streptococcus pneumoniae, Haemophilus influenzae,* and *Moraxella catarrhalis.* Cephalexin is commonly chosen in this situation; however, it has poor coverage for both *H. influenzae* and *M. catarrhalis.* A better choice might have been amoxicillin or sulfamethoxizole/trimethoprim. Furthermore, the length of therapy was too short. A minimum of 2 weeks of therapy is usually recommended for acute sinusitis. Also, decongestant therapy is usually an integral part of the therapy for acute sinusitis. The addition of a systemic decongestant (pseudoephedrine or phenylpropanolamine) and possibly 3 to 4 days of a topical decongestant (oxymetazoline) would have improved the likelihood of successful medical management.

3. Following the initial failure of therapy in this case, a second course of antibiotic therapy was recommended. Again, an antibiotic with an inappropriate antibacterial spectrum (erythromycin) was chosen. Decongestants were again neglected from the therapeutic regimen.

4. By the time the patient needed a third antibiotic, the primary care physician chose ciprofloxicin. While this is a very good choice for gram-negative infections, it is a poor alternative for acute sinusitis. Here again, decongestants were not included.

5. At the time this patient was referred for specialty consultation with an otolaryngologist, she had suffered with these nasal and paranasal sinus symptoms for more than 8 weeks. What was initially an acute process had now become a chronic condition. The possibility of immune dysfunction should always be considered in patients who develop chronic sinusitis. In this particular case, it is probably premature to initiate an extensive immune workup since the patient appears to be

149

healthy otherwise and given the inappropriate therapy that has been provided, this probably accounts for her chronic condition.

TEST INTERPRETATION

• Computed tomography (CT) scan—see Figure 42–1

• Culture (endoscopic directed from middle meatus)—*Staphylococcus aureus*

• Nasal smear—numerous polymorphonuclear cells

The CT scan reveals findings consistent with chronic sinusitis. Chronic obstruction of the maxillary infundibulum and osteomeatal complex all contribute to anterior sinusitis (maxillary, anterior ethmoid and frontal) (Fig. 42–1A). The posterior ethmoids and sphenoid sinus also show changes of chronic inflammation, due to obstruction in the area of the sphenoethmoid recess (Fig. 42–1B).

When sinusitis is prolonged, the once-acute infection begins to take on characteristics of a more chronic one. While *S. aureus* is not usually a pathogen associated with acute sinusitis, it is commonly isolated in chronic sinusitis. Anaerobic bacteria are also often encountered; however, routine culture of the middle meatus will rarely allow these organisms to be detected.

Nasal smear is usually performed to determine if the nasal symptoms are due to allergy or infection. While it is fairly clear in this instance that infection is the etiology of this patient's symptoms, a smear was obtained. Findings of inflammatory cells on the smear of nasal secretions only confirms the presumptive diagnosis of sinusitis.

DIAGNOSIS

Chronic sinusitis.

MEDICAL MANAGEMENT

The medical treatment of chronic sinusitis should follow a two-pronged approach: (1) appropriately selected antimicrobials and (2) decongestant/anti-inflammatory therapy.

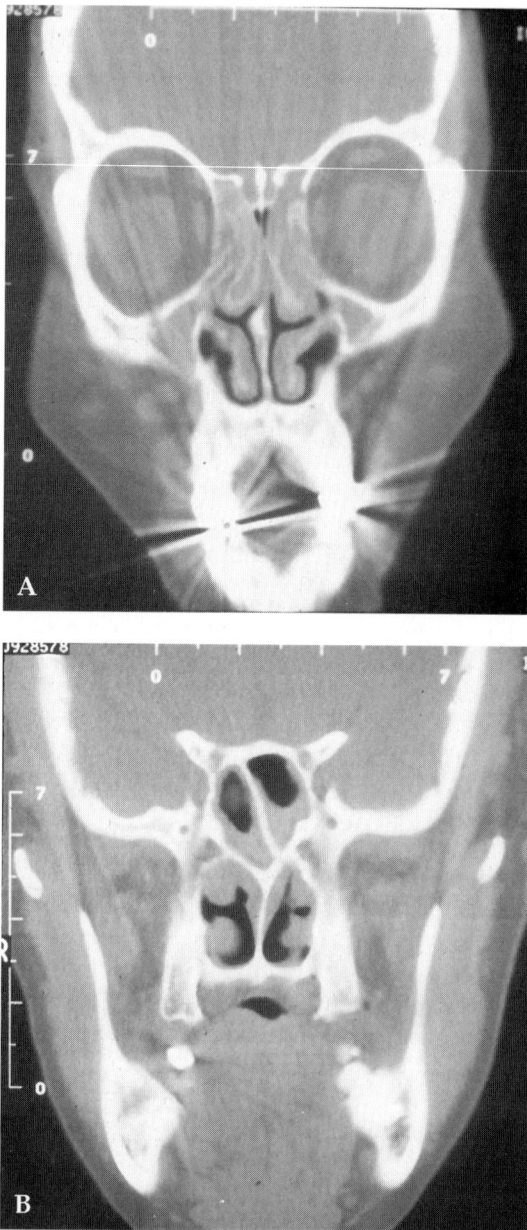

FIGURE 42–1 (A) Chronic obstruction of the maxillary infundibulum and osteomeatal complex. (B) Inflammation of the posterior ethmoids and sphenoid sinus.

This patient has not had adequate or appropriate antibiotic therapy for either her acute sinusitis (as noted above) or for chronic sinusitis. In addition to treating the same bacteria as for acute sinusitis, the antibiotic spectrum for chronic sinusitis must include coverage for both

S. aureus and for anaerobic bacteria. Examples of regimens that would fulfill these requirements include amoxicillin/clavulanate, clarithromycin, and cefuroxime axetil/metronidazole. This antibiotic regimen should be continued for a minimum of 3 weeks, and perhaps for as long as 6 weeks. A culture is extremely helpful if there does not appear to be a response to aggressive medical therapy.

Decongestants can also be helpful in chronic sinusitis. Because the treatment will tend to be prolonged, topical decongestants (such as oxymetazoline) are best avoided. However, systemic agents such as pseudoephedrine or phenylpropanolamine can be very helpful. These agents should be used with caution if the patient has underlying cardiovascular disease.

Mucoevacuants such as guaifenesin are often used for patients with sinusitis. Data to support the efficacy of this agent is anecdotal at best; however, it does appear to help decrease the viscosity and tenacity of nasal mucus in some cases. Since it is a fairly benign drug with very few side effects, it is often combined with other sinus and nasal medications. If guaifenesin is used in this situation, the only dose that has been shown possibly effective is 2,400 mg/day.

Anti-inflammatory agents can be very useful in patients with chronic sinusitis. Topical steroids should be part of the regimen in all patients with this disorder. The safety profile of these agents is extremely good, and there is no evidence to implicate their use in the development of opportunistic nasal infections such as fungal sinusitis. Numerous nasal steroid preparations are available, and there does not appear to be any appreciable difference in efficacy among these agents.

In addition to topical steroid preparations, systemic steroids can often produce a dramatic clinical response in these patients. These powerful anti-inflammatory agents should be avoided in patients with diabetes or other serious immunologic disorders; however, they can be safely employed in most clinical situations. A short (1-week) burst of steroids can often provide a dramatic decrease in local nasal inflammation and thereby increase the effectiveness of the other medical therapeutic agents.

Antihistamines rarely play a role in the medical management of these patients unless there is an underlying allergic component. In these instances, the second-generation antihistamines (terfenedine, astemizole, loratidine, cyterazine) should be chosen. This group of agents is nonsedating and tends to have minimal anticholinergic effects on nasal mucus production, thus avoiding the thick tenacious mucus associated with the first-generation antihistamines.

Topical normal saline mist or nasal irrigations can often provide symptomatic improvement. Nasal hygiene can also be improved since the nasal mucus blanket can remove crusts and other infectious debris more efficiently because of the cleansing effects of normal saline therapy.

SURGICAL MANAGEMENT

This patient is not currently a surgical candidate since she has not undergone adequate medical treatment. If following aggressive medical therapy her symptoms persist, then functional endoscopic sinus surgery should be considered. Since her septum is deviated, a septoplasty will probably be required to provide access to both middle meatus regions. Surgery will probably include endoscopic ethmoidectomy, maxillary antrostomy, and sphenoidotomy. Since this patient has not had long-standing sinus disease (many years), the frontal sinuses will probably respond to ethmoidectomy alone, and frontal sinusotomy may be avoidable.

When discussing this surgical option with the patient, the risks of surgery should be emphasized, including bleeding, infection, eye injury, blindness, brain injury, and cerebrospinal fluid leak. The limitation of sinus surgery should be emphasized and the possible need for a second surgical procedure discussed.

REHABILITATION AND FOLLOW-UP

This patient will probably respond to aggressive medical management. However, if medical therapy is unsuccessful, then the possibility of an underlying immunologic disorder should be investigated. Other possible nasal problems should also be considered, such as granulomatous diseases, autoimmune disorders, or fungal infections. An evaluation by an allergy/immunology specialist can be helpful anytime a chronic infection fails to respond as expected.

Following successful management (either medical or surgical) the use of long-term nasal steroid sprays (4 to 6 months) is usualy safe and often helpful to prevent recurrence.

SUGGESTED READINGS

DRUCE HM, ed. *Sinusitis: Pathophysiology and Treatment.* New York: Marcel Dekker; 1994.

FACER GW, KERN EB. Sinusitis: current concepts and management. In: Bailey BJ, ed. *Head and Neck Surgery—Otolaryngology.* Philadelphia, PA: JB Lippincott; 1993:Chapter 29.

TAMI TA. Try a two-pronged therapy to clear the way for patients with sinusitis. *Mod Med.* 1993;61:30–49.

NASAL GRANULOMATOUS DISEASE

Thomas A. Tami, M.D.

HISTORY

A 23-year-old white woman presented with increasing nasal obstruction and headaches. She was noted to have hypertrophic inferior turbinates and underwent bilateral partial turbinate resections. Despite this, she continued with nasal obstruction and began to develop increasing headaches and intermittent bloody nasal discharge. Over the ensuing 3 to 4 months she noted extreme tenderness of her nasal dorsum and developed a saddle nasal deformity. Her septum was thickened throughout and there was granulation tissue covering much of the nasal mucosa. Her turbinates were still very enlarged and inflamed despite prior turbinate surgery. Even with maximum topical decongestion she had near-complete nasal obstruction.

She also described a chronic productive cough that had begun approximately 6 weeks prior to presentation. Her medical history was otherwise unremarkable.

DIFFERENTIAL DIAGNOSIS— KEY POINTS

1. While this patient's initial problem appeared to be turbinate hypertrophy, she obviously has a more aggressive problem now. Nasal saddling and the persistent intranasal inflammation suggest some type of aggressive local process. The associated productive cough further raises the possibility of a multisystem problem. This patient needs a chest x-ray to assess her pulmonary status.

2. An infectious problem must be considered. This is certainly not typical of a paranasal sinus or nasal infection; however, unusual pathogens such as fungi or mycobacteria could account for this clinical picture. Appropriate diagnostic tissue for both histopathologic examination as well as culture should be obtained to evaluate this possibility. This patient's pulmonary symptoms provide further evidence that this may be an infectious process. Possible infectious etiologies might include rhinoscleroma, tuberculosis, rhinosporidiosis, invasive aspergillus, or other fungal disease. Besides obtaining tissue for culture and histopathologic examination, a purified protein derivative (PPD) skin test should be placed.

3. A chonic granulomatous process such as sarcoidosis, Wegener's granulomatosis, or lethal midline granuloma (polymorphic reticulosis) also must be included in the differential diagnosis. While these diagnoses must be considered in the differential diagnosis of this patient, it is imperative that an infectious process be excluded prior to instituting therapy for any of these conditions.

   A chest x-ray often can be helpful in making the diagnosis of sarcoidosis. Gallium scanning as well as salivary gland biopsy can also assist in this diagnosis. The serum ACE (angiotensin-converting enzyme) is also often elevated in patients with sarcoidosis.

   Wegener's granulomatosis is often a multisystem disease. Both the upper and lower respiratory systems can be affected by this vasculitic process. In systemic Wegener's, renal involvement is usually a component. The c-ANCA (anti-neutrophil cytoplasmic antibody) test is often helpful since it is elevated in many patients with Wegener's granulomatosis.

4. Cocaine abuse has recently also been associated with an often destructive nasal granulomatous process. Although this patient did not volunteer any information in the history to suggest this, specific questions regarding this possibility should be directed to this patient.

5. While atrophic rhinitis and ozoena have been

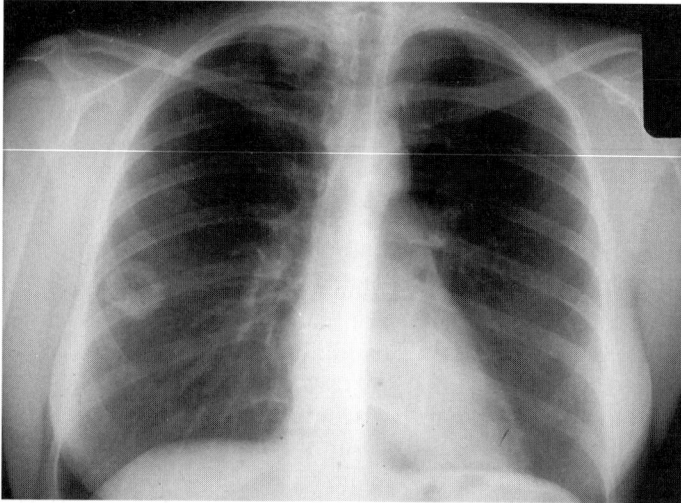

FIGURE 43–1 Chest x-ray revealing multiple cavitary lesions.

described as sequelae of aggressive inferior turbinate surgery, this patient appears to have a condition much more impressive than might be expected from atrophic rhinitis.

TEST INTERPRETATION

- Chest x-ray—see Figure 43–1
- Erythrocyte sedimentation rate (ESR)—54 (normal, less than 20)
- PPD—nonreactive
- Urinalysis—negative
- c-ANCA—elevated
- Serum ACE—normal
- Culture of nasal septal tissue—few *Staphylococcus aureus*
- Nasal turbinate biopsy—nonspecific inflammation and necrosis; both acute and chronic inflammatory infiltration with no obvious evidence of vasculitis; no neoplastic component seen.

The elevated ESR suggests a significant systemic inflammatory process.

The patient's chest x-ray reveals multiple impressive cavitary lesions. Based solely on this x-ray, TB, sarcoidosis, or an invasive fungal infection must be strongly considered. Wegen-

er's granulomatosis can also present with pulmonary lesions that have a cavitary appearance on chest x-ray. The negative PPD and the normal ACE level both tend to argue against either TB or sarcoidosis. Also, patients with sarcoidosis tend to have significant hilar adenopathy, a finding that is not noted on this chest x-ray.

The culture of the nasal tissue failed to reveal a pathologic fungal or mycobacterial organism. *S. aureus* is a common bacterial species causing secondary infection in Wegener's granulomatosis.

The c-ANCA is a fairly specific test for Wegener's granulomatosis. The ANCA test can occur with two patterns; the c-ANCA (cytoplasmic pattern) is predominantly associated with Wegener's while the p-ANCA (perinuclear pattern) is associated with several other vasculitis diseases. While Wegener's is due to a vasculitis, nasal and sinus biopsies are notoriously poor at establishing the pathologic diagnosis in this condition. A microscopic vasculitis is a requirement for the histopathologic diagnosis. Fibrinoid vascular necrosis is a common finding and eosinophils often make up a significant percentage of the inflammatory cells.

The vasculitis of Wegener's appears to be confined to the respiratory tract (both upper and lower). The normal urinalysis suggests that this patient does not have renal involvement (glomerulonephritis) at this time; however, a creatinine clearance may be more accurate in making this assessment. Other sites of systemic involvement can also include the eyes, skin, joints, and heart.

DIAGNOSIS

Wegener's granulomatosis limited to the upper and lower respiratory tracts.

MEDICAL MANAGEMENT

Prior to the availability of effective medical therapy the prognosis for patients with active Wegener's granulomatosis was grim. Most patients who developed renal disease died within 5 months of onset. Still, renal involvement is the most dreaded aspect of this disorder since it is often progressive and irreversible.

The mainstays of treatment for active disease are corticosteroids and cyclophosphamide. Since their introduction for this disease there has been a dramatic improvement in survival, and cures are not unusual. While the pathogenesis of Wegener's is still not known, the most widely held view is that the disease is mediated by immunologic mechanisms inducing an inflammatory response. Therefore the use of these potent immunosuppressives is based entirely on purely empirical thinking. Since the long-term effects of both corticosteroids and cyclophosphamide can be substantial, these drugs are usually titrated according to disease activity. Their use for long-term control of the inflammatory process should be reduced if possible.

The antibiotic combination of trimethoprim sulfamethoxazole was first noted to have activity against Wegener's in the early 1980s and is now frequently used as an adjunct in the management of this disease. The mechanism of action is unknown; however, various theories include antibacterial activity against some as yet unidentified micro-organism; antistaphylococal activity preventing exacerbations due to secondary staphylococcal infections; an intrinsic immunosuppressive property of the combination drug; or perhaps an effect mediated by the folic acid metabolism inhibition induced by

trimethoprim/sulfamethoxazole. Whatever the true mechanism is, this combination agent has an unpredictable response rate. Currently it is often successfully employed for the maintenance of long-term remission and prevention of reactivation.

SURGICAL MANAGEMENT

Except in making or confirming the primary diagnosis, surgery has a very limited role in the management of this disease. The initial diagnosis can occasionally be confirmed with nasal or paranasal sinus biopsy; however, transbronchial lung biopsy is usually a more effective technique.

During the course of the disease, the progressive necrotizing intranasal process often results in tremendous buildup of crusting and debris, which must be constantly debrided. This is usually accomplished in the office setting and can be augmented by a regimen of aggressive home nasal irrigation.

While there is often the temptation to consider nasal reconstructive surgery when loss of septal cartilage has produced a severe cosmetically unacceptable saddle nasal deformity, any attempt at reconstruction should be delayed until assurances can be made that the disease is in complete and, hopefully, long-term remission.

REHABILITATION AND FOLLOW-UP

Long-term management of patients diagnosed with Wegener's granulomatosis should emphasize the early detection and aggressive treatment of remission or flare-up of the underlying process. The c-ANCA test has been successfully used in many instances to monitor disease progression and recurrence. Furthermore, as stated earlier, long-term trimethoprim/sulfamethoxazole can be effective in preventing recurrence and maintaining remission. Since renal disease is often the most devastating aspect of this disease process, any suspicion of recurrence should immediately trigger an evaluation of renal function.

SUGGESTED READINGS

Rao JK, Weinberger M, Oddone EZ, et al. The role of antineutrophil cytoplasmic antibody (c-ANCA) testing in the diagnosis of Wegener's granulomatosis. *Ann Intern Med.* 1995;123:925–932.

Stegeman CA, Tervaert WC, de Jong PE, Kallen- berg GM. Trimethoprim-sulfamethoxazole (cotri- moxazole) for the prevention of relapses of Wegener's granulomatosis. *N Engl J Med.* 1996;335:16–20.

Wegener's granulomatosis and midline (nonhealing) "granuloma." In: Batsakis JG, ed. *Tumors of the Head and Neck.* 2nd ed. Balimore, MD: Williams & Wilkins; 1979: Chapter 24.

Case 44

FUNGAL SINUSITIS
Thomas A. Tami, M.D.

HISTORY

A 39-year-old carpenter presented to an otolaryngologist with nasal congestion and headaches. These symptoms had progressed for the previous 6 months, but were now becoming unbearable. He also described intermittent retroorbital headaches and noted that the bridge of his nose had widened somewhat. His primary care physician had treated him with antibiotics, decongestants, and topical nasal steroids on several occasions during the previous several months, but his symptoms continued to progress.

His medical history was unremarkable. He denied a prior history of nasal allergies, was a nonsmoker, had never worked in a furniture factory, and had no other significant medical problems.

Physical examination revealed massive nasal polyposis with complete bilateral nasal obstruction. He had widening of his glabella and mild hyperteliorism. Ophthalmologic examination revealed full range of motion, but mild bilateral proptosis. The remainder of his head and neck exam was unremarkable. An imaging study of the paranasal sinuses was ordered.

Based on the history, physical examination and radiographic evaluation, an endoscopic polypectomy and partial ethmoidectomy was performed for diagnostic purposes.

DIFFERENTIAL DIAGNOSIS—KEY POINTS

1. New onset nasal obstruction in this 39-year-old man should immediately raise the possibility of a neoplasm. Hyperteliorism and proptosis on physical examination suggest a nasal lesion exerting mass effect. Neoplasms (both benign and malignant), mucocele, or allergic fungal sinusitis could all contribute to such a presentation. A preceding history of head trauma might contribute to consideration of a mucocele. Because woodworkers have an increased incidence of adenocarcinoma of the ethmoids, this should be considered even though he has no direct exposure to this industry. Even though he is a nonsmoker, other neoplasms must also be in the differential diagnosis.

2. Massive nasal polyposis could be interpreted in several ways. Polyps may represent inflammatory changes in the nasal mucosa produced by an underlying obstructing neoplasm. Some neoplasms, such as inverting papilloma, are often misdiagnosed as polyps. Massive polyposis can also be associated with the triad of aspirin sensitivity, asthma, and nasal polyps; however, this is not suggested by the history in this case.

3. Invasive fungal sinusitis can present as ethmoid expansion with associated polyposis. The acute fulminant form is usually associated with a much more rapid progression; however, chronic invasive fungal sinusitis can progress over months and produce these or similar symptoms. Allergic fungal sinusitis can also often display massive nasal polyposis and bony expansion of the paranasal sinuses.

4. A chronic granulomatous process might also produce similar findings, although other systemic symptoms are also usually present. Examples include sarcoidosis, Wegener's granulomatosis, tuberculous sinusitis, and syphilitic infection.

The differential diagnosis should include:

- Nasal/sinus neoplasm
- Ethmoid or frontal sinus mucocele
- Chronic invasive fungal sinusitis
- Allergic fungal sinusitis
- Granulomatous sinusitis (Wegener's or other)

TEST INTERPRETATION

A computed tomography (CT) scan was obtained (Fig. 44–1). This axial scan through the ethmoid sinuses shows complete opacification of the ethmoid and sphenoid sinuses. Expansion through the lamina paparycia is noted producing apparent bilateral proptosis. Intraethmoid bony septation, although attenuated, is still identifiable suggesting a non-neoplastic process. A mucocele would present as more homogeneous expansile lesions with bony expansion and thinning around the periphery of the lesion.

This scan could be consistent with the following possible diagnosis: a neoplasm of the ethmoid labyrinth (*bilateral*); chronic invasive fungal sinusitis; allergic fungal sinusitis; or a chronic granulomatous process. A mucocele is less likely.

Histopathologic evaluation of the biopsied tissue revealed nasal polyposis with abundant eosinophilia. Allergic mucin containing eosinophils, Charcot-Leyden crystals, and a few scattered hyphae were also identified within the specimen. Invasion of fungal elements into the submucosa and bone was not identified. There was no evidence of granulomatous inflammation.

DIAGNOSIS

Allergic fungal sinusitis.

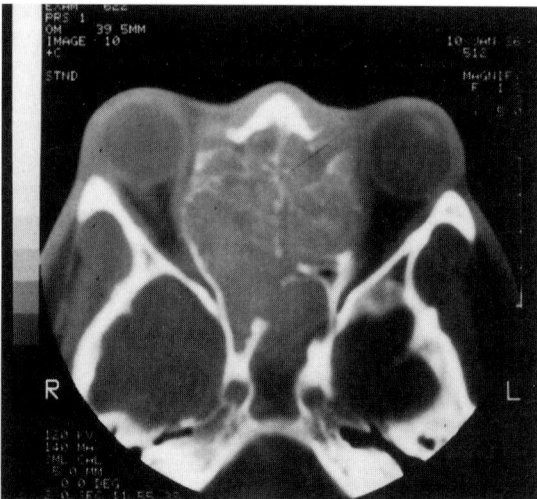

FIGURE 44–1 Allergic fungal sinus. Expansion of the ethmoid sinus is often typical.

MEDICAL MANAGEMENT

Most authors agree that for medical management to be effective, surgical removal of as much of the involved sinus tissue is imperative. While chronic antifungal chemotherapy is occasionally recommended, the mainstay of therapy for this disease is systemic steroids to suppress the active immune response. Steroids can be confidently employed only with assurance that the diagnosis is correct. Painstaking examination of silver stained mucosa, submucosa, and bone to rule out invasive fungal disease must precede the administration of systemic steroids.

SURGICAL MANAGEMENT

While endoscopic management of this problem is certainly possible, most surgeons prefer an open approach given the bony erosion in the region of the lamina papyrecia and possibly other areas (e.g., skull base, sphenoid sinus). Standard external frontoethmoidectomy, sphenoidotomy, and Caldwell Luc would probably be recommended by most authors.

REHABILITATION AND FOLLOW-UP

No studies have evaluated the appropriate role of long-term therapy in this disease. Long-term systemic steroids may be needed to keep the disease in check. One published regimen consisted of daily prednisone (0.5 mg/kg) for 2 weeks, followed by a tapering dose to conclude with an every other day schedule for 3 months. Most agree that topical nasal steroids should be used indefinitely. A potential role for immunotherapy has not been defined.

SUGGESTED READINGS

ENCE BK, GOURLEY DS, JORGENSEN NL, et al. Allergic fungal sinusitis. *Am J Rhinol.* 1990;4:169–178.

KATZENSTEIN A-LA, SALE SR, GREENBERGER PA. Allergic *Aspergillus* sinusitis: a newly-recognized form of sinusitis. *J Allerg Clin Immunol.* 1983;72:89–93.

WASHBURN RG. Chronic fungal sinusitis in the nonimmunocompromised host. In: Druce HM, ed. *Sinusitis Pathophysiology and Treatment.* New York: Marcel Dekker; 1994:205–226.

CEREBROSPINAL FLUID RHINORRHEA

Thomas A. Tami, M.D.

HISTORY

A 47-year-old woman underwent a left medial maxillectomy for inverting papilloma of the middle turbinate and lateral nasal wall. She had no perioperative problems and was discharged from the hospital on the day following surgery. Approximately 2 weeks later she noted increasing clear drainage from her nasal cavity. While initially attributed to the nasal saline irrigation she was using for postoperative nasal care, the nasal discharge soon became an almost constant feature. She also complained of headache, which seemed to improve only when she was recumbent. She described no neck stiffness or photophobia and was afebrile.

On physical examination of the left nasal cavity there was evidence of mild crusting and postoperative inflammation consistent with the surgery she had undergone. Clear fluid seemed to be coming from high in the nasal cavity, but a precise location could not be determined.

DIFFERENTIAL DIAGNOSIS— KEY POINTS

1. Cerebrospinal fluid (CSF) rhinorrhea must be very high on the differential diagnosis for this patient. Although the clear rhinorrhea was noted only after 1 to 2 weeks in the postoperative period, this delay is not unusual. Immediate postoperative edema may prevent immediate detection of CSF; however, as the edema subsided, the leakage of fluid became more obvious. The use of an aggressive irrigation regime in the immediate postoperative period may also have contributed to a delay in diagnosis.

2. Postoperative nasal drainage following extensive intranasal surgery is common. However, when the drainage is due to postoperative inflammatory changes it is usually characterized as thick and mucoid. While occasionally clear, this drainage is usually either yellow, or in some instances dark brown due to retained blood clots. If an infection were responsible for the drainage, greenish or thick yellow drainage would have been noted.

3. While it is always tempting to deny that a complication such as a CSF leak could have occurred following surgery, it is vital that this possibility be entertained and evaluated immediately. The potential consequences of meningitis, which can result from a delayed diagnosis, adds a degree of urgency to the prompt evaluation of this patient for CSF rhinorrhea.

TEST INTERPRETATION

Physical examination is the initial step in the evaluation of this patient. Patients with CSF rhinorrhea can usually easily demonstrate persistent dripping of clear fluid from the nose simply by bending forward. If the leak is a lower volume flow, then the patient often describes a "reservoir sign," which consists of a large volume of clear rhinorrhea in the morning upon awakening. This results from pooling of CSF in the sphenoid or ethmoids during sleep in the recumbent position. This large pooled volume becomes evident as a large volume discharge upon initial arising in the morning.

If fluid is flowing freely from the nasal cavity, the typical "halo" sign can be seen by collecting the fluid on a cloth or paper towel and allowing it to dry.

A better method to establish the correct diagnosis is to collect 1 to 2 cc of fluid in a specimen container and perform laboratory analysis. Glucose levels are usually elevated in CSF, but this test has been replaced by the more specific β-transferrin test. This very sensitive test is almost pathognomonic for CSF rhinorrhea.

Localization of the site of leakage is vital to plan surgical therapy. In this postsurgical case, the defect will undoubtedly be in the ethmoid roof or cribriform plate region. Direct nasal endoscopy may be all that is needed to identify the site. If the site is less clear, contrast cisternogram will be helpful. This test uses a radiopaque dye injected into the CSF to help identify the site of leakage during a CT scan. The leak must usually be fairly brisk during the procedure for this technique to be useful (Fig. 45–1). In this patient, the dural defect appears to have occurred at the junction of the cribriform plate and the fovea ethmoidalis. Because this is the site of attachment of the middle turbinate, this injury probably occurred due to avulsion of the middle turbinate from the skull base.

When the site of leak is more obscure, and when the leak is not a brisk one, nuclear medicine scans can occasionally prove helpful. A protein bound radionucleotide is injected into the

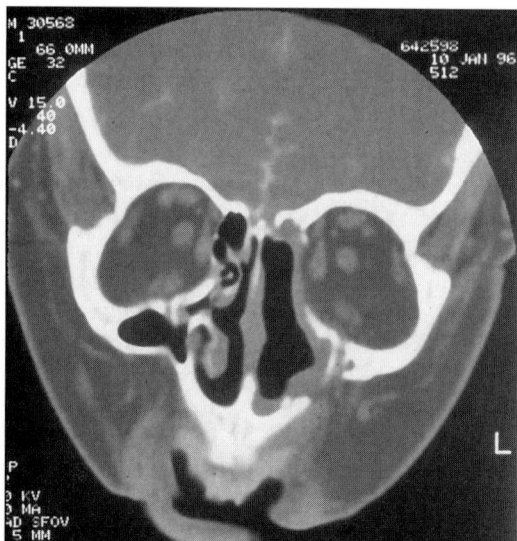

FIGURE 45-1 CT scan demonstrating leak at the junction of the cribriform plate and fovea ethmoidalis.

subarachnoid space. Pledgets are placed at various sites in the nasal cavity (middle meatus, high nasal cavity, sphenoethmoid recess, and eustachian tube) for an adequate length of time before being scanned for radioactivity. The poor sensitivity and specificity of this test make it a less than ideal method for evaluating this problem.

DIAGNOSIS

Postoperative CSF leak, left anterior ethmoid/cribriform plate.

MEDICAL MANAGEMENT

Conservative, nonsurgical therapy can often be successfully used to manage CSF leaks. Bed rest, head elevation, inhibitors of CSF production such as diamox, and the active draining of CSF such as with the use of a lumbar drain are all interventions that can allow small leaks to heal on their own. A lumbar drain can be very effective; however, it must be used with great care. If fluid is drained too rapidly, herniation of the brain stem can result with potentially disastrous consequences. Infection at the site of the drain with subsequent meningitis is also a possibility when a lumbar drain is used. The use of a lumbar drain to decrease CSF pressure is usually limited to 4 to 5 days so as to minimize the infection risk.

The role of prophylactic antibiotics in patients with CSF leak is controversial. Generally, data do not support their use to prevent infection, and they may actually encourage overgrowth and possible subsequent infection by resistant organisms. Nevertheless, prophylactic antibiotics are often used in this situation, perhaps to provide a measure of confidence and peace of mind for both patient and physician.

Vigilance for any signs of meningitis is extremely important throughout the nonsurgical and surgical course of these patients. Early signs of central nervous system infection such as increasing headache, photophobia, nausea, vomiting, fevers, neck stiffness, or personality and mood changes must be taken very seriously and evaluated in an expeditious manner.

SURGICAL MANAGEMENT

If conservative measures fail to result in a permanent cessation of CSF drainage, surgery must be considered. Surgical therapy can be performed either through the endonasal route, extranasally but from below, or alternatively through a formal craniotomy.

Traditional repairs from below are usually performed through an external ethmoidectomy approach or via a lateral rhinotomy. Identification of the site of leakage was followed by using various tissue alternatives such as septal flaps, middle turbinate flaps, or free mucosal grafts. Fibrin glue has also been extensively used via this approach to add support to the repair. In most instances, the nose is packed postoperatively for up to 1 week to allow tissue ingrowth to the grafted region.

With the advent of endoscopic endonasal surgery, successful repairs from below can now often be achieved via this approach. While this method avoids the need for an external incision, the intranasal repair is still essentially unchanged from the open technique. While an onlay graft can be successful in this situation, it is always a better repair if the graft material can be tucked between the dura and the anterior cranial fossae bone. Fascia grafts, cartilage, middle turbinate and free mucosal flaps are but a few of the repair materials employed in this situation.

When the dural defect is too large or inaccessible to be repaired from below, or when an intranasal attempt at closure has been unsuccessful, craniotomy is usually recommended as the definitive repair technique. This technique usually utilizes a fascia lata graft to repair the defect. Since this approach usually requires extensive retraction on the frontal lobes with disruption of the olfactory bulbs, permanent anosmia usually results.

REHABILITATION AND FOLLOW-UP

In the follow-up period, the patient would be closely monitored for any evidence of recurrence. Careful monitoring of the patient for evidence of CSF rhinorrhea or early signs and symptoms of meningitis must be undertaken to make this diagnosis when indicated. With extremely large dural defects, meningoceles or encephaloceles can occur months or years later; however, this is an extremely unusual occurrence with small defects.

While a CSF leak following an otherwise routine intranasal surgical procedure can be an emotion-filled event for both the surgeon and patient, careful and complete preparation of the patient during the consent process in the preoperative period is extremely important. An informed patient who is aware of the potential for serious surgical complications in even a routine case such as a medial maxillectomy forms the basis for trust and understanding when an untoward event such as a CSF leak occurs.

SUGGESTED READINGS

CARMEL PW, KOMISAR A. Cerebrospinal fluid rhinorrhea. In: Blitzer A, Lawson W, Friedman WH, eds. *Surgery of the Paranasal Sinuses.* Philadelphia, PA: WB Saunders; 1985:Chapter 17.

MATTOX DE, KENNEDY DW. Endoscopic management of cerebrospinal fluid leaks and cephaloceles. *Laryngoscope.* 1990;100:857–862.

ROLAND PS, MARPLE BF, MEYERHOFF WL, MICKEY B. Complications of lumbar spinal fluid drainage, *Otolaryngol Head Neck Surg.* 1992;107:564–569.

STANKIEWICZ JA. Cerebrospinal fluid fistula and endoscopic sinus surgery. In: Stankiewicz JA, ed. *Advanced Endoscopic Sinus Surgery.* St. Louis, MO: Mosby–Year Book; 1995:Chapter 10.

Case 46

EPISTAXIS

Thomas A. Tami, M.D.

HISTORY

A 64-year-old man presented following a long history of recurrent epistaxis. These episodes had required management in the emergency department on several occasions using silver nitrate cautery and occasionally with nasal packing. During the past 1 to 2 years the problem seemed to have worsened to the point of having an episode of bleeding on an almost daily basis. He routinely carried a small package of salt pork around with him, since this seemed to be the only method available to easily control the bleeding.

His medical history was significant for a mild transient ischemic attack (TIA) approximately 1 year prior to presentation. He had mild hypertension and was a heavy smoker for 30 years. His brother, who also had frequent nose bleeds, died from a stroke at the age of 38.

On physical examination there were multiple small 2- to 3-mm heaped up hypervascular lesions throughout his nasal cavity. These were very friable and bled freely following even minimal manipulation. He had many small 2- to 3-mm vascular lesions of the oral mucosa (Fig. 46–1), lips, and skin of his face and neck.

DIFFERENTIAL DIAGNOSIS— KEY POINTS

1. The differential diagnosis of recurrent epistaxis is fairly broad. Someone with recurrent epistaxis often has recurrent bleeding from the anterior septum in Kiesselbach's plexus. A deviated nasal septum might contribute to this recurrent bleeding due to the turbulent airflow produced by this deformity. Other considerations must include a septal perforation, a tumor (either benign or malignant),

an underlying coagulopathy, or a possible posterior source of the bleeding.

2. When evaluating epistaxis, whether acutely or in a chronic epistaxis patient, the hematologic and hemodynamic status must be considered. Patients often overestimate the amount of bleeding they have experienced, yet if there has been substantial acute or chronic blood loss, this information must be readily available. The evaluation should include an assessment of hemoglobin and hematocrit, clotting studies, and an examination, which includes orthostatic changes in blood pressure and pulse.

3. Occasionally a systemic disorder such as leukemia or lymphoma can result in chronic epistaxis. Other inflammatory intranasal disorders such as Wegener's granulomatosis, sarcoidosis, or other autoimmune problems can also cause frequent chronic epistaxis.

4. In the case of this patient, given the family history of a similar problem, the mucocutaneous findings on physical examination, and the history of neurologic problems, the diagnosis of hereditary hemorrhagic telangiectasia (HHT) must be considered. This condition results from an autosomal dominant genetic defect that produces abnormalities of vascular structures. The hallmark telangiectases are caused by dilatation of postcapillary venules, which often connect directly to dilated arterioles. These telangiectases are well represented on nasal mucosa accounting for the frequent epistaxis encountered in patients with this condition. Also prominent in patients with this disorder are the frequent occurrence of arteriovenous malformations (AVMs). Their occurrence as pulmonary (PAVM) or cerebral (CAVM) account for many of the transient and/or

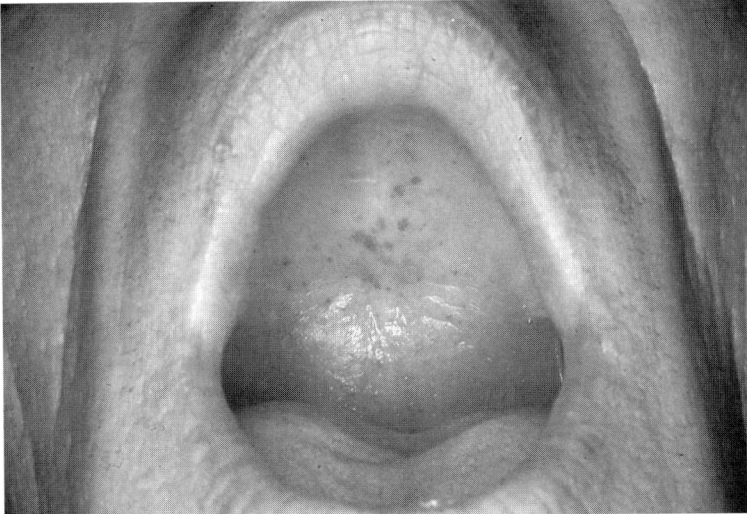

FIGURE 46–1 Vascular lesions of the oral mucosa.

permanent neurologic sequelae of this disorder.

TEST INTERPRETATION

- Hemoglobin—10.2 mg/dL
- Hematocrit—30
- Platelet count—210,000 per dL
- PT/PTT—normal
- Chest x-ray—normal

The low hematocrit and hemoglobin reflect the
chronic blood loss this patient has experienced
due to his chronic recurrent nasal bleeding. As
expected, the platelet count and the coagulation
parameters are normal.

While the chest x-ray is reported as normal,
small PAVMs are often missed with routine
chest radiography. Chest computerized tomography (CT) scanning or angiograpy can often
delineate small otherwise undetectable PAVMs.
Cerebral emboli due to arteriovenous shunting
in PAVMs can cause transient, or occasionally
permanent, neurologic deficits.

DIAGNOSIS

Hereditary hemorrhagic telangiectasia (HHT)
(Osler–Weber–Rendu syndrome).

MEDICAL MANAGEMENT

The most important, and often the most difficult, medical aspect of managing this condition
is making an accurate diagnosis. Although the
diagnosis is relatively straightforward in cases
like the one presented, this is not always the
case. The classical cutaneous and mucosal telangiectases typically become more prominent
with advancing age; however, PAVMs or
CAVMs can occur and cause symptoms before
the development of these telltale clinical stigmata. For this reason, some authors advocate
aggressive screening programs for family members of patients with known HHT. The reported
incidence of PAVMs in HHT patients is from 8
to 20% and for CAVMs may be as high as 10%.
Controversy exists regarding the most cost-
effective screening method for evaluating these
patients and their family members. Chest x-ray
is the minimum screening tool that should be
used to screen for PAVMs. While this technique
is not as sensitive as chest CT or angiography
for detecting small lesions, it is probably adequate for diagnosing clinically important lesions. Recommendations for screening for
CAVMs is less clear. While CT scans, magnetic
resonance imaging, or angiography can all be
highly sensitive to detect CAVMs, the clinical
significance and need for surgical management
of these lesions is uncertain.

Patients with large PAVMs often have significant pulmonary arteriovenous shunting, which can produce relative arterial hypoxemia, especially when the patient is standing. These large lesions are often amenable to surgical resection or arterial embolization. Even when small PAVMs are detected, they deserve close observation because they can be the source of septic or nonseptic cerebral emboli. Patients with known PAVMs should receive prophylactic antibiotic treatment prior to procedures that may produce bacteremia. Also, these small lesions have been observed to enlarge significantly during pregnancy.

The chronic blood loss that can occur due to recurrent epistaxis can be further exacerbated by occult loss secondary to gastrointestinal tract telangiectases. Routine monitoring of hemoglobin, iron replacement therapy, and occasionally blood transfusions are often part of the ongoing medical management of this disorder.

Since this condition is often more pronounced in males, and seems to increase in women following menopause, the role of estrogen therapy has been considered for this problem. While estrogen therapy may play a minor role in decreasing the progression of HHT, this treatment is usually poorly tolerated in adult men because of the accompanying feminizing side effects.

SURGICAL MANAGEMENT

Depending on the extent of the nasal disease, management of epistaxis can range from simple cautery (early in the disease process) to the need for extensive anterior and/or posterior packing to control what can often be extremely brisk bleeding. In advanced HHT, even minor manipulation of the nasal septum can produce profuse bleeding. These patients often present following profuse bleeding that seems resistant to all therapeutic interventions. In these cases, prevention of recurrent bleeding becomes the mainstay of therapy. Arterial embolization of the internal maxillary arteries has no role in the management of this condition since the problem is at the capillary/venule level. Even if this technique affords a temporary decrease in bleeding, it will not provide any long-lasting effect.

Laser treatment of nasal telangiectases using the KTP laser is often successful in controlling recurrent bleeding. While telangiectases can be eliminated using this technique, other new lesions invariably recur. Repeated laser treatment every 3 to 6 months is usually necessary to maintain adequate bleeding control. It is often useful to apply thin silastic nasal septal splints following this procedure. These splints are usually well tolerated by the patient and can provide protection to the septum from mechanical trauma as well as the drying effects of turbulent nasal airflow.

The use of septal dermoplasty as first described by Saunders in 1973 has been widely used to surgically manage patients with severe HHT. In this technique, the anterior intranasal mucosa is removed and replaced by skin grafts. When performed by an experienced surgeon, this technique appears to provide fairly good long-term relief from recurrent epistaxis. It does, however, result in a nasal cavity that tends to be dry and crusted most of the time due to the loss of respiratory mucosa.

REHABILITATION AND FOLLOW-UP

Patients with HHT deserve close long-term follow-up and management. As noted earlier, their hematologic status should be constantly assessed so that anemia can be recognized and treated when appropriate. Known PAVMs or CAVMs should also be serially evaluated for increasing size or clinically significant arteriovenous shunting. When clinically indicated, these serious vascular lesions should be surgically or angiographically treated.

Family members of HHT patients should be screened for the presence of this disease. Since HHT is an autosomal dominant disorder, 50% of offspring and immediate relatives of these patients would be expected to express this disorder. In fact, in one study of family members only 37% were diagnosed with this disease, perhaps reflecting various expression of the genetic defect. The recent discovery of a gene causing HHT encodes a protein that binds transforming growth factor β may help to both further elucidate the pathophysiologic mechanism underlying the vascular abnormalities in this disorder as well as provide a screening tool to identify patients affected by this disease.

SUGGESTED READINGS

GUTTMACHER AE, MARCHUK DA, WHITE RI. Hereditary hemorrhagic telangiectasia. *N Engl J Med.* 1995;333(14):918–924.

HAITJEMA T, DISCH, F, OVERTOOM TTC, et al. Screening family members of patients with hereditary hemorrhagic telangiectasia. *Am J Med.* 1995;99: 519–524.

SAUNDERS WH. Septal dermoplasty for hereditary telangiectasia and other conditions. *Otolaryngol Clin North Am.* 1973;6:745–755.

ANOSMIA

Allen M. Seiden, M.D.

HISTORY

A 46-year-old white male presented with a complaint of both taste and smell loss that had been present for 8 years. The problem began following a severe upper respiratory infection, and was noted when the acute infectious symptoms had resolved. He denied any associated trauma, nor did he describe a history of exposure to toxic chemicals or solvents. He did not have a history of chronic sinus problems, and denied any residual nasal obstruction, postnasal drainage, or recurring bouts of infection except for the occasional cold. There was no history of allergies or asthma.

The patient had no complaints of dysosmia or dysgeusia, and although he complained of a taste loss, he could clearly distinguish salty, sour, sweet, and bitter. When questioned further, he did admit that on occasion he seemed to detect some odors, but these experiences were quite brief, infrequent, and unpredictable. Otherwise, he had no other medical problems, was taking no medications, and did not smoke.

On physical examination, anterior rhinoscopy demonstrated an intact nasal airway, with no erythema, discharge, or evidence of polyps or inflammatory disease. The remainder of his head and neck examination was unremarkable. Olfactory testing was performed (see below), and was consistent with anosmia.

After application of topical anesthesia and decongestion, nasal endoscopy was performed. On the right, although the middle meatus was clear, polypoid disease was seen superiorly within the superior meatus, obstructing the nasal vault (Fig. 47–1). On the left, polypoid disease was seen within the meatus that could not be seen with a nasal speculum.

DIFFERENTIAL DIAGNOSIS— KEY POINTS

1. The most common causes of olfactory loss include an upper respiratory viral infection, head trauma, and nasal or sinus disease. Also, toxic exposure, usually in the workplace, is not uncommon. While other systemic and neoplastic disorders may need to be considered, they are unusual in patients presenting with a primary complaint of olfactory loss. This patient described a loss of smell immediately following an infection, and had no complaints to suggest subsequent sinus disease. Therefore, a presumptive diagnosis of postviral olfactory loss could easily have been made.

   Nasal or sinus pathology is the only etiology to cause an obstructive rather than sensorineural olfactory loss, and therefore some aspects of the history may provide important clues. A history of chronic sinusitis or allergies, for example, may suggest underlying inflammatory disease. A complaint of nasal obstruction is certainly important, but has been noted in only 35% of patients presenting with obstructive olfactory loss. The reason is that the olfactory cleft is located high in the nasal vault, measuring only 1 mm wide on either side. Obstruction can occur high in the nose secondary to inflammation, while the nasal airway remains intact. These patients may present with a primary complaint of olfactory loss, yet have few other nasal symptoms.

   It is important to question whether the loss of smell fluctuates. This would suggest variation with changes in nasal congestion, and only occurs with an obstructive loss. Unfortunately, patients are often vague about this, as in the current example. In addition, only 45% of patients presenting with an obstructive olfactory loss will have a history of fluctuation.

2. This patient complained of both a loss of taste and smell. However, due to the more extensive neural input mediating taste (involving the chorda tympani, glossopharyngeal, and vagus nerves on either side), a true measurable taste loss is quite uncommon. On the other hand, the *flavor* of foods is determined not only by gustatory input, but also by tem-

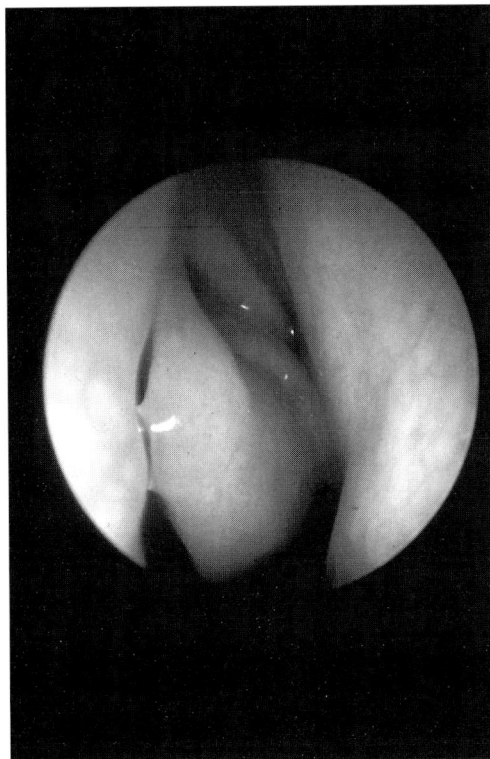

FIGURE 47–1 Nasal endoscopy demonstrates polypoid disease obstructing the nasal vault.

perature, texture, and olfactory information. Without olfactory input, foods tend to taste flat and patients perceive this as a loss of taste. It is more reliable to ask patients whether they can distinguish between the four basic taste qualities of salty, sour, sweet, and bitter.

3. Dysosmia is an abnormal odorant sensation that may be precipitated by an environmental stimulus (parosmia) or may occur spontaneously (phantosmia). It is described more commonly in association with postviral olfactory loss, but may sometimes be associated with purulent sinusitis.

4. Even though the history may suggest a viral etiology, it is very important that a thorough physical examination be performed to rule out the possibility of underlying sinus pathology. In this case, anterior rhinoscopy was unremarkable, and in patients presenting with olfactory loss as their primary complaint, this is not unusual. Nasal endoscopy provides a much more revealing examination, and can detect more subtle pathology that may be limited to the nasal vault, ostiomeatal complex, or sphenoethmoidal recess.

TEST INTERPRETATION

Some form of testing is important to verify a patient's complaint of olfactory loss, but it must be based on psychophysically sound testing procedures and be reproducible. Several such tests have now been developed and are available in a clinical setting. The most widely utilized is the University of Pennsylvania Smell Identification Test (Sensonics, Haddonfield, NJ). This test provides 40 microencapsulated odorants, each on a scratch-and-sniff pad, with four choice alternatives for each odorant. The number correctly identified determines olfactory sensitivity.

If nasal or sinus pathology is suspected based on the history and physical examination, then further radiographic study is helpful. The low sensitivity and specificity of plain x-rays, and their ability to properly delineate the ostiomeatal complex and ethmoid sinuses, make them generally inadequate. Computed tomography (CT) has become the procedure of choice for imaging the paranasal sinuses. Based on nasal endoscopic findings in this case, a CT scan was obtained, demonstrating patchy thickening or inflammatory changes throughout the ethmoid sinus (Fig. 47–2).

Magnetic resonance imaging is the procedure of choice when searching for intracranial causes of olfactory dysfunction. However, when the history and physical examination clearly implicate one of the common causes described earlier, such testing is usually not necessary.

Despite the presence of sinus pathology, it is still possible that this patient experienced a viral infection that resulted in his loss of smell. In the absence of a clear history of fluctuation, it is important to establish the reversibility of this loss in order to support an obstructive and exclude a sensorineural etiology. Systemic steroids may be useful in this regard. By theoretically decreasing mucosal edema, at least a temporary improvement in olfactory sensitivity may be observed. This serves as a useful diagnostic maneuver to help verify the obstructive

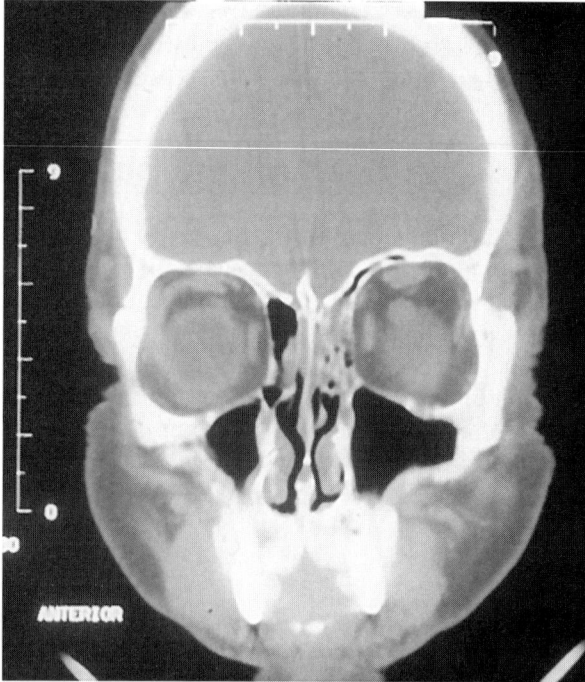

FIGURE 47–2 CT scan demonstrates patchy thickening or inflammatory changes throughout the ethmoid sinus.

nature of an olfactory loss. Topical steroids alone seem to be less effective in the short-term reversal of such a loss. The patient in the current example was placed on a tapering course of systemic steroids and noted a dramatic return of smell function that quickly dissipated once he was off of the medication.

DIAGNOSIS

Obstructive olfactory loss secondary to sinus disease.

MEDICAL MANAGEMENT

As noted earlier, systemic steroids will generally reverse an obstructive olfactory loss. However, due to the risk of long-term side effects, only a short tapering course is usually appropriate. The patient should then be given a topical steroid spray, which may or may not be able to maintain this improvement.

Associated allergies should be evaluated and adequately treated. Antibiotic therapy may be necessary if active infection is found.

SURGICAL MANAGEMENT

Although olfactory loss may be a patient's only complaint, if normal function cannot be maintained medically, then surgical intervention should be considered. The most appropriate surgical approach will depend on the extent of pathology and the experience of the surgeon, but is clearly effective in restoring an obstructive olfactory loss as long as the underlying sinus disease is controlled. Care must be taken to avoid scarring or injury in the area of the olfactory cleft.

REHABILITATION AND FOLLOW-UP

No studies have properly evaluated the long-term stability of olfaction in relation to the treatment of chronic sinusitis. The best recommendation at present would be to maintain regular follow-up to keep any associated infection under control, and avoid restenosis or recurrence. Topical steroids are probably helpful, and control of underlying allergies or other irritant exposures is helpful.

SUGGESTED READINGS

CAIN WS, GOODSPEED RB, GENT JF, LEONARD G. Evaluation of olfactory dysfunction in the Connecticut chemosensory clinical research center. *Laryngoscope.* 1988;98:83–88.

DEEMS DA, DOTY RL, SETTLE RG, et al. Smell and taste disorders, a study of 750 patients from the University of Pennsylvania Smell and Taste Center. *Arch Otolaryngol Head Neck Surg.* 1991;117:519.

DOTY RL, SHAMAN P, DANN M. Development of the University of Pennsylvania Smell Identification Test: a standardized microencapsulated test of olfactory function. *Phys. Behav.* 1984;32:489–502.

SEIDEN AM, ed. *Taste and Smell Disorders.* New York: Thieme; 1997.

SEIDEN AM, DUNCAN HJ, SMITH DV. Office management of taste and smell disorders. *Otolaryngol Clin North Am.* 1992;25:817–835.

VASOMOTOR RHINITIS

Michelle M. Cullen, M.D.
Thomas A. Tami, M.D.

HISTORY

A 25-year-old female presents with complaints of nasal obstruction, watery rhinorrhea, and facial pressure that occurs several times a day. Her symptoms have persisted for many years and she denies fever, weight loss, watery eyes, and itching, but relates occasional sneezing. She has tried over-the-counter nasal sprays, which provide short term relief of the congestion, but her symptoms quickly return. She has also tried oral antihistamines and oral decongestants, which did not provide significant relief. Her symptoms are usually worse in the daytime and seem to be worse overall in the winter season. There is no change with position; however, she states her symptoms do improve for several hours following vigorous exercise but then the symptoms return (sometimes worse).

Her medical history was remarkable for a nasal fracture in a motor vehicle accident 10 years ago and a history of hypertension, which is presently controlled with diet and exercise. There is no family history of atopy or asthma. She takes no medications and denies habitual over-the-counter nasal spray use. The patient denies allergy to medications, including aspirin, denies recreational drug use, and states she is not pregnant. The patient's surgical history includes a turbinate cautery approximately 2 years ago, which initially decreased the symptoms of nasal congestion, but within 1 year her symptoms returned.

Physical exam reveals a normal nasal bridge and external nose with no evidence of infraorbital edema or allergic shiners. The patient frequently sniffles while being examined but does not sound congested. She has chapped lips and mild to moderate mouth breathing. Intranasal examination reveals normal nares and a mildly deviated septum to the right. The turbinates are markedly enlarged, left greater than the right.

The nasal secretions are clear. There is no evidence of polyps, crusting, granulomas, ulcerations, or perforation. A nasal smear is taken from the inferior turbinate and the patient's nose is sprayed with topic oxymetolazine with a marked decrease in inferior turbinate size and a decrease of the patient's symptoms of nasal congestion.

DIFFERENTIAL DIAGNOSIS— KEY POINTS

1. The differential diagnosis of rhinitis is extensive (see Table 48–1).

2. Most allergic rhinitis manifests in childhood and the patient's age (25) is more consistent with a disease process other than allergic rhinitis. The patient's history of symptoms during the last several years should alert the physician to the possibility of a chronic infection or other chronic condition.

3. The patient's symptoms of nasal obstruction and rhinorrhea with a relative absence of sneezing and palatal itching is less consistent with an allergic cause. Nasal congestion is the most common symptom of vasomotor rhinitis.

4. A history of facial pressure should raise the possibility of a paranasal sinus infection. The absence of fever, yellow discharge, and facial tenderness and the patient's healthy appearance make this far less likely.

5. This patient's long-standing and frequent symptoms should alert the physician to look for provocative factors for the patient's condition such as irritants, allergens, environmental factors, or change in temperature. This patient notices that her symptoms are worse in winter and seem to be provoked by changes in temperature or cold temperature.

TABLE 48-1 Causes of Chronic Rhinitis

1. Vasomotor rhinitis
   a. Drug induced (antihypertensives, nose drop, nose spray abuse, cocaine, birth control pills)
   b. Pregnancy induced
   c. Temperature mediated
   d. Irritative rhinitis
   e. End-stage vascular atonia of chronic allergic or inflammatory rhinitis
   f. Recumbency rhinitis
   g. Paradoxical nasal obstruction and nasal cycle
   h. Nonallergic rhinitis and eosinophilia syndrome
2. Allergic rhinitis
3. Inflammatory rhinitis
   a. Bacterial, viral, or fungal
   b. Nasal polyposis
   c. Atrophic rhinitis
   d. Chronic inflammatory disease (sarcoidosis, Wegener's granulomatosis, polyardis nodose, polymorphic reticulosis)
4. Structural abnormalities
   a. Internal or external trauma
   b. Congenital malformation
   c. Neoplasm (benign or malignant)
   d. Foreign body

Some patients have a hypersensitivity to their normal nasal cycle, which is a possibility in this patient, although most patients with this condition notice their symptoms are worse at night. Recumbency rhinitis, or rhinitis with change in positioning, is unlikely due to the daytime symptoms and the patient's job.

6. The decrease in symptoms with topical vasoconstriction and no change in the patient's symptoms with antihistamine or oral decongestant are typical of vasomotor rhinitis.

7. The suspicion of rhinitis medicamentosa should be investigated. The chronic use of topical sympathomimetics causes a semi-ischemic state, which leads to an abundance of the products of metabolism (which are strong vasodilators). Rebound congestion occurs and loss of vascular tone can lead to profound congestion.

8. The patient's improvements in her symptoms with exercise is a normal physiologic response. An increase in sympathetic tone during exercise releases norepinephrine from nerves around the arterial venous sinusoids and seromucinous glands. This constricts the vasculature and shrinks the mucosa with an increased patency in the nose. The effect lasts only 2 to 3 hours.

9. This patient had a history of nasal trauma from a motor vehicle accident many years ago, which raises the possibility of nasal obstruction due to a structural defect. With variation in the nasal cycle, a septal deformity can cause symptoms of nasal obstruction several times a day. Furthermore, there could be a compensatory hypertrophic rhinitis whereby the contralateral turbinate to the side of the structural obstruction hypertrophies.

10. The use of hypertensive medications can cause a drug-induced vasomotor rhinitis due to the depletion of norepinephrine stores resulting in unopposed parasympathetic vasodilatation. Sympathetic blocking agents that can cause drug-induced vasomotor rhinitis include guanethidine, hydralazine, methyldopa, propranolol, and other β-blockers. Reserpine can produce drug-induced vasomotor rhinitis in 8% of patients.

11. Chronic diseases associated with nasal congestion include rhinoscleroma, rhinospherulosis, tuberculosis, syphilis, mucormycosis, histoplasmosis, aspergillosis, lupus, Wegner's granulomatosis, polymorphic reticulosis, and leprosy. Other systemic processes associated with nasal congestion include cirrhosis, uremia, thoracic masses causing superior vena cava syndrome as well as Horner syndrome (secondary to interference with sympathetic innervation resulting in hypersecretion, and nasal congestion due to relative increase in parasympathetic tone of the nasal mucosa).

12. Examination of the external nose in a patient with symptoms of rhinitis is important. Nasal polyposis can cause an enlarged nasal bridge and systemic disease can result in saddle nose deformity (Wegner's granulomatosis, syphilis, sarcoidosis); deviation of the nasal bridge can indicate previous trauma with possible internal nasal deviation. Allergic shiners (darkening of the infraorbital skin with edema) are associated with allergic rhinitis. These develop due to

edema of the mucosa of the nasal and paranasal sinuses, which produces pressure on the venous arcades and interference with venous outflow of the inferior ophthalmic vein into the pterygoid plexus.

13. Notation of the inferior turbinate size is important, as is the consistency of the secretions. Watery secretions are more associated with an irritative rhinitis or allergic rhinitis, whereas thickened secretions are more consistent with bacterial infection or chronic rhinitis. The color of the mucosa is not specific. Acute viral and bacterial infections typically manifest with erythema and edema of the nasal mucosa. Allergic rhinitis usually produces pale, bluish, edematous inferior turbinates with clear secretions. Crusting, ulcers, or granulomas of the inferior turbinates should alert the physician to the possibility of systemic conditions.

14. Cobble-stoning of the posterior pharyngeal wall is a non-specific finding but is consistent with chronic postnasal drip.

TEST INTERPRETATION

1. *Nasal smear.* Vasomotor rhinitis is associated with no or few eosinophils; infectious rhinitis is associated with the finding of polymorphic neutrophils, whereas allergic rhinitis is associated with eosinophils and an increased number of goblet cells.

2. *Topical decongestion.* A vasoconstrictive response of the nasal mucosa helps differentiate a vasomotor rhinitis/allergic/infectious rhinitis (which will constrict) from a structural abnormality or neoplastic process (which will not).

DIAGNOSIS

Tempreature-mediated vasomotor rhinitis.

MEDICAL MANAGEMENT

Vasomotor rhinitis is a disorder that is secondary to a relative imbalance of the autonomic nervous system with a preponderence of action of the parasympathetic nervous system. Congestion of the nose is primarily regulated by the underlying vasculature of the nasal turbinates, which is most prominent in the inferior turbinates. The dilitation or constriction of the venous sinusoids greatly changes their size.

The amount of blood within the venous sinusoids is controlled by the tone of the muscular layer surrounding the veins. Sympathetic innervation (mediated by α-adrenergic receptors) and sympathometic drugs increase the vasoconstrictive tone and decrease the amount of blood in the sinusoids. The parasympathetic system not only controls congestion by increasing blood flow to the sinusoids by a decrease in muscular tone, but also mediates nasal secretion.

Substance P (a neuro peptide parasympathetic transmitter) also induces vasodilitation, hypersecretion, and hyperpermeability of the mucosa. It is released from unmyelinated c fibers secondary to a variety of stimuli.

The following medical regimens can be used for patients with vasomotor rhinitis:

1. Atrovent (ipratoprium bromide) is a topical anticholinergic that blocks the parasympathetic innervation of the submucosal seromucous glands and nasal vasculature. Typical dosage schedule is 80 μg inhaled through the nostril every 6 hours. If nasal dryness develops from utilization of this medication, a twice daily dosage is often efficacious and can cause fewer side effects. As much as 1600 μg a day have been used in patients with severe symptoms.

2. The use of normal saline in the nose can augment mucociliary flow, thin mucus, remove crusts, enhance tissue repair, and improve olfaction.

3. A change in habits to avoid irritants, strong odors, fumes, or other provoking factors should be made, and humidity should be increased to 35 to 50%.

4. Pseudoephedrine, phenylephrine, and phenylpropanolamine can be used to increase sympathetic tone and decrease nasal congestion.

5. A regular and vigorous exercise program to reestablish vasomotor tone and control should be instituted.

SURGICAL MANAGEMENT

Inferior turbinate injection with corticosteroids provides temporary relief of symptoms and should be used only after topical vasoconstrictors have been applied to decrease the chance of intravascular injection. Typically triamcinolone acetonide is utilized by injecting multiple sites of the inferior turbinate with a small-bore needle.

Sclerosing injection of the turbinates has been abandoned secondary to pain and poor short-term results.

Lateral fracture of the inferior turbinate is simple to perform but does not affect the underlying problem of nasal mucosal congestion.

Surface cautery with electrocautery or chemicals results in scabbing, crusting, and possible infection, as well as ciliary dysfunction. It has fair short-term results and poor long-term results.

Submucosal cautery with electric or cryosurgical methods results in crusting and possible infection of underlying bone. It may provide longer relief of symptoms than those mentioned earlier.

Laser vaporization of the inferior turbinate provides significant long-term symptomatic relief with approximately 2% risk of bleeding and osteitis but frequent crusting and postoperative care.

Submucous resection of the inferior turbinate is efficacious in long-term relief of symptoms with less chance of bleeding and maintenance of the physiologically functioning tissue.

Partial resection of the anterior inferior turbinate provides good to excellent long-term results with some short-term crusting and has some risk of bleeding.

Total inferior turbinectomy is associated with initial good results of relief of symptoms but has a high risk of significant daily crusting long term.

Vidian nerve section interrupts the parasympathetic and sympathetic supply of the vidian nerve and is used for those with severe intractable symptoms. Transantral, transpalatal, transeptal, or transnasal and endoscopic approaches have been described. Electrocoagulation is applied most commonly through the transantral route and can provide approximately 90% long-term relief of symptoms.

REHABILITATION AND FOLLOW-UP

Patients treated with conservative medical care should be followed up after a period of 4 to 6 weeks to assess the efficacy of this therapy. Those undergoing turbinectomy or cautery may require monthly or bimonthly debridement during the first year following surgery to remove crusts. A regimen of normal saline douche should be maintained. Overaggressive resection of turbinates may leave the patient with ozena or an atrophic rhinitis-like nasal airway.

SPECIAL SITUATIONS

1. *Vasomotor rhinitis of pregnancy.* Increased estrogen levels during pregnancy are associated with increased parasympathetic tone due to inhibition of acetylcholinesterase from estrogen. Prior to any therapy, consultation with the patient's obstetrician is advisable. Treatment of vasomotor rhinitis of pregnancy can include exercise commensurate with pregnancy and normal saline nasal lavages. Pharmacologic therapy for nasal congestion can safely be accomplished with pseudoephedrine.

2. *Eosinophilic nonallergic rhinitis.* This term, also called "NARES" (nonallergic rhinitis with eosinophilia), applies to patients with a history of allergic nasal symptoms (repetitive sneezing, profuse rhinorrhea, itchy eyes, etc.) in response to environmental stimuli, but with normal skin testing and serum IgE tests. Nasal smear cytology shows eosinophilia, and these patients respond well to nasal steroids but poorly to antihistamines and decongestants.

SUGGESTED READINGS

FAIRBANKS DN, RAPHAEL GD. Nonallergic rhinitis and infection. In: Bailey BJ, Johson JT, Kohut RI, et al, eds. *Otolaryngology—Head and Neck Surgery.* St. Louis, MO: Mosby-Year Book; 1993:Chapter 45.

FINEMAN P. Allergic rhinitis. In: Bluestone CD, Stool SE, eds. *Pediatric Otolaryngology.* Philadelphia, PA: WB Saunders; 1990:793–804.

GOODE RL. Diagnosis and treatment of turbinate dysfunction. Self-instructional package, American Acadmey of Otolaryngology—Head and Neck Surgery, 1977, pp. 12–61.

KNOPS JL, McAFFREY TV, KERN EB. Inflammatory diseases of the sinuses: physiology—clinical applications. *Otolaryngol Clin North Am.* 1993;26(4):517–534.

KOPKE RD, JACKSON RL. Rhinitis. In: Bailey BJ, Johnson JT, Kohut RI, et al, eds. *Head and Neck Surgery—Otolaryngology.* Philadelphia, PA: JB Lippincott; 1993:Chapter 23.

MARKS MB. Stigmata of respiratory tract allergies. Upjohn Company; 1972.

RADFORD ER, BECKER GD. Diagnosis and management of inhalant allergy. Self-instructional package, American Academy of Otolaryngology, Head and Neck Surgery Foundation, Inc., 1988, pp. 35–40.

Laryngology

Case 49

VOCAL CORD PARALYSIS

Keith M. Wilson, M.D.

HISTORY

A 48-year-old woman presents with hoarseness for approximately 3 months. She reports that she underwent recent surgery to remove the entire thyroid gland for papillary carcinoma. Shortly after surgery she developed an upper respiratory infection, which lasted for 1 week. She has difficulty lifting heavy objects and becomes short of breath while talking. She occasionally coughs while drinking liquids. Her medical history is remarkable for hypertension for which she takes a calcium channel blocker.

On physical examination she is found to have an immobile right true vocal cord in the paramedian position. There is inadequate compensation with the left vocal cord, which moves normally. Her voice quality is breathy and raspy. There are no other neurologic signs. On chest auscultation, her lung fields are found to be clear.

DIFFERENTIAL DIAGNOSIS—
KEY POINTS

1. When hoarseness develops after thyroidectomy, it must be assumed that there was injury to either the recurrent laryngeal nerve or the external laryngeal nerve. In this patient, it would be more likely that the recurrent laryngeal nerve is injured since the patient has an immobile vocal cord.

2. This patient may have undergone a difficult intubation at the time of thyroid surgery with resultant arytenoid dislocation.

3. The possibility of a mediastinal mass, including left atrial enlargement, involving the left recurrent laryngeal nerve must be investigated. Apical lung lesions on the right side can involve the right recurrent nerve.

4. This patient could have developed laryngeal edema secondary to an upper respiratory infection. Upper respiratory infections are frequently associated with laryngeal edema and cough, which could lead to granuloma formation on the posterior vocal cords. However, the physical finding of a paralyzed vocal cord without a mass lesion makes this unlikely.

5. If there is no obvious cause, the diagnosis of idiopathic vocal cord paralysis is made.

TEST INTERPRETATION

The patient with a unilateral vocal cord paralysis, especially with significant symptoms such as aspiration and inability to adequately Valsalva, should be evaluated with at least a chest x-ray and a flexible nasolaryngoscopy. Laryngeal electromyography and videostroboscopy can be helpful in that they are diagnostic as well as prognostic. When surgical intervention is planned, these tests, with acoustic analysis, can be helpful and should be used routinely.

- *Chest x-ray.* The chest x-ray was without evidence of active disease. Therefore, we conclude that there is no evidence of aspiration pneumonia or a mediastinal mass.

- *Flexible nasolaryngoscopy.* This reveals a right true vocal cord paralysis in the paramedian position with inadequate compensation by the left true vocal cord. There is mild bowing of the right true vocal cord and the arytenoid is not anteriorly displaced. Therefore, arytenoid dislocation is ruled out (Fig. 49–1).

- *Videostroboscopy.* The patient has difficulty triggering the stroboscopy secondary to the breathy nature of the voice. Intermittently you can see mucosal wave formation that does not fully propagate across the superior surface of the vocal cord. A posterior glottal gap is also evident when the patient attempts to phonate.

- *Laryngeal electromyography.* Shows spontaneous activity in the absence of any voluntary motor units. This is consistent with a flaccid paralysis. Return of function is not likely.

- *Acoustic analysis.* There is a high signal-to-noise ratio and abnormal jitter and shimmer. Maximum phonation time is 6 seconds.

DIAGNOSIS

Right vocal cord paralysis, flaccid, secondary to right recurrent laryngeal nerve injury.

MEDICAL MANAGEMENT

The medical management of vocal cord paralysis is voice therapy. Various maneuvers can be

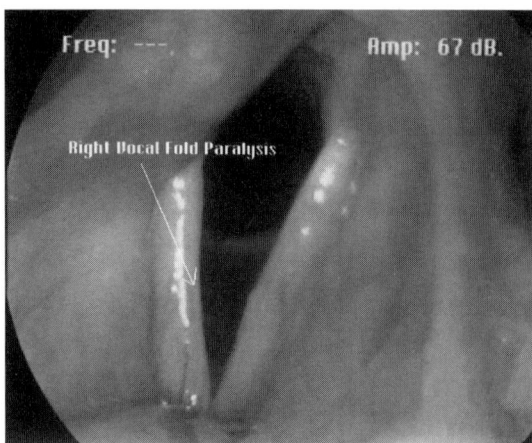

FIGURE 49–I Flexible nasolaryngoscopy reveals a right true vocal cord paralysis. Note the mild bowing of the right true vocal cord. The arytenoid is not anteriorly displaced, ruling out arytenoid dislocation.

utilized to improve glottal competence. These exercises are isometric in nature with the intent of gaining better sphincteric control of the laryngeal introitus. Many patients with unilateral vocal cord paralysis do well with voice therapy alone, provided that the paralyzed vocal cord assumes a midline or slightly paramedian position. There is no effective medical management for bilateral vocal cord paralysis.

SURGICAL MANAGEMENT

The overwhelming concern in the surgical management of vocal cord paralysis is that of balancing airway with voice. In a situation of bilateral vocal cord paralysis, the voice is usually excellent but the airway represents an emergency situation. Tracheotomy is the definitive and quickest treatment. However, arytenoidectomy, cordectomy, and cordotomy are all options that could be utilized in lieu of tracheotomy provided the patient is not in extremis. The usual scenario has a tracheotomy performed first to stabilize the airway. Subsequently, arytenoidectomy, cordectomy, or cordotomy will be performed, depending on the surgeon's preference, in an attempt to obviate the tracheotomy tube. Again, the better the airway the worse the voice, and vice versa.

Unilateral vocal cord paralysis does not present as a medical emergency. Therefore, the surgical treatment of unilateral vocal cord paralysis is based more on the constellation and severity of symptoms. The aim of all surgical procedures is to medialize the paralyzed vocal cord so that the patient will have improved glottal competence. These procedures can be divided into endoscopic procedures or laryngeal framework procedures.

Endoscopic procedures include Teflon, fat, collagen, and Gelfoam injections. Teflon was considered the gold standard for unilateral vocal cord paralysis until recently. Teflon injections, originally described by Arnold in 1962, have been associated with migration and granuloma formation. However, in expert hands Teflon injections are quite effective. The current trend is to use Teflon in terminally ill patients with unilateral vocal cord paralysis. Fat, collagen, and Gelfoam undergo total or near-total absorption and therefore are considered temporary remedies for vocal cord paralysis or atrophy.

The procedure that provides best rotation of the vocal process of the arytenoid cartilage, and therefore the best glottal closure, is the arytenoid adduction procedure. This procedure is not considered reversible and should not be performed if there is reasonable chance for recovery of vocal cord mobility. The arytenoid adduction procedure is often performed in association with or subsequent to the thyroplasty, type I, procedure.

Thyroplasty, type I, or medialization laryngoplasty is becoming the procedure of choice for unilateral vocal cord paralysis that is not well compensated. This procedure has the main advantages of being adjustable and reversible and is performed under local anesthesia usually with intravenous sedation. Additionally, bilateral thyroplasty, type I, procedures can be performed for vocal cord bowing, with and without atrophy. However, long-term results are not overwhelmingly satisfactory.

REHABILITATION AND FOLLOW-UP

Although it is not absolutely necessary to study patients postoperatively with videostroboscopy to determine if surgery was successful, video-stroboscopy and acoustic analysis do offer objective means of analyzing results. Ultimately what matters most is whether the patient is happy with the functional result in terms of voice, airway, and swallowing.

Many patients develop compensatory techniques of vocalizing when they have a paralyzed vocal cord. After the lateralized vocal cord is medialized, there is often need for a brief period of voice therapy to retrain the patient in proper voice technique.

SUGGESTED READINGS

ARNOLD GE. Vocal rehabilitation of paralytic dysphonia. IX. Technique of intracordal injection. *Arch Otol.* 1962;76:358–368.

DEDO HH, URREA RD, LAWSON L. Intracordal injection of Teflon in the treatment of 135 patients with dysphonia. *Ann Otol Rhinol Laryngol.* 1973;82:661–667.

ISSHIKI N, OKAMURA H, ISHIKAWA T. Thyroplasty type I (lateral compression) for dysphonia due to vocal cord paralysis or atrophy. *Arch Otolaryngol.* 1975;80:465–473.

ISSHIKI N, TANABE M, SAWADA M. Arytenoid adduction for unilateral vocal cord paralysis. *Arch Otolaryngol.* 1978;104:555–558.

KOUFMAN JA, ISAACSON G. Laryngoplastic phonosurgery. *Otolaryngol Clin North Am.* 1991;24:5.

MAVES MD, MCCABE BF, GRAY S. Phonosurgery: indications and pitfalls. *Ann Otol Rhinol Laryngol.* 1989;98:577–580.

SPASMODIC DYSPHONIA Keith M. Wilson, M.D.

HISTORY

A 55-year-old white female presents complaining of chronic hoarseness for 3 years. She describes her voice as "choppy" and notes that it is worse at certain times. Her biggest problem is speaking on the telephone. The patient reports being treated with multiple courses of antibiotics and a trial of steroids. She has seen her primary care doctor, two otolaryngologists, and a psychiatrist during the last 3 years with no improvement in her voice. Her medical history is remarkable for anxiety. She takes a benzodiazepine as needed.

Her voice has a strangled quality, which is noticed during the interview. When asked to count to 10, she almost cannot produce any sound with certain words. On indirect examination of her larynx she is found to have normal vocal cord mobility with no evidence of a mass lesion on the vocal cords. A detailed neurologic examination reveals only a mild tremor of the hand with voluntary movements.

DIFFERENTIAL DIAGNOSIS— KEY POINTS

1. Spasmodic dysphonia is the leading diagnosis in a patient with chronic hoarseness characterized by a "choppy" voice quality. Spasmodic dysphonia is a laryngeal dystonia that has two forms. The more common adductor form is characterized by a voice that has a strained or strangled quality. The less common abductor variety is characterized by intermittent breaks in phonation that manifest as periods of absence of voicing. Patients with spasmodic dysphonia are often misdiagnosed for many months, sometimes for many years.

2. This patient appears to have an essential tremor of the hand. It is very important to determine if the patient also has an essential tremor of the laryngeal muscles. Essential tremor involving the larynx is a 4- to 12-Hz tremor seen in the vocal cords during respiration and speech. Distinguishing between essential tremor of the larynx and spasmodic dysphonia is critical because of the treatment implications.

3. Other basal ganglia diseases, that is, Huntington's disease, Parkinson's disease, tardive dyskinesia, should be considered in a patient like this. Although laryngeal manifestations of these diseases could be present in the early stages, it is unlikely that they would be the only signs or symptoms. Articulation and limb movement disorders tend to present early. A thorough neurologic examination that is normal would rule out these diagnoses.

TEST INTERPRETATION

In the evaluation of the hoarse patient with no overt laryngeal pathology, physiologic tests are indicated. Radiologic studies should be utilized only if there is a high index of suspicion for central nervous system pathology.

- *Speech evaluation.* The patient has severe difficulty reading sentences with words that have voiced consonants followed by vowels. She is able to read sentences with words that alternate between voiceless consonants and vowels without significant difficulty. This would imply that this patient has adductor spasmodic dysphonia. If her problem were with words that alternate between voiceless consonants and vowels, then her diagnosis would be abductor spasmodic dysphonia. The idea here is to trigger either adductor or abductor spasms by forcing the patient to close or open the vocal cords repetitively.

- *Acoustic analysis.* Increased jitter and shimmer with a decreased signal-to-noise ratio is noted. A tremor analysis is run which does not reveal a tremor of the larynx. Increased perturbations and a reduced signal-to-noise ratio are seen in spasmodic dysphonia and essential tremor. The signal-to-noise ratio is even lower with abductor spasmodic dysphonia due to the periods of voicelessness. The tremor analysis is a software program that detects repetitive periods of voicelessness. Therefore, with a negative tremor test, essential tremor can be ruled out.

- *Electromyography (EMG).* Bursts of electrical activity at rest and enlarged motor unit action potentials during phonation are noted. While EMG is not necessary for the diagnosis of spasmodic dysphonia, it does provide important information. It also can be used to guide botulinum toxin injections. Therefore, diagnosis confirmation and treatment can be combined into one session.

DIAGNOSIS

Adductor spasmodic dysphonia.

MEDICAL MANAGEMENT

The treatment of choice for spasmodic dysphonia is direct injection of botulinum toxin type A (Botox) into the laryngeal muscles. In treating the adductor form, the injections can be performed either transorally or percutaneously with the Botox being deposited into the thyroarytenoid muscle (Figs. 50 1 and 50 2). In the abductor form, the posterior cricoarytenoid muscle is the target. The dose of Botox can vary from less than 1 mouse unit to as much as 10 mouse units and is given unilaterally or bilaterally. The onset of improvement is usually within 1 to 2 days and lasts 3 to 6 months on average. While the voice result is not totally normal, most patients are sufficiently satisfied that they usually request reinjection after the beneficial effects of Botox wear off. The side effects of Botox injection are mild. Many patients complain of breathiness. Some complain of short-lived episodes of dysphagia and aspiration.

Voice therapy has been used in the treatment of spasmodic dysphonia with little long-term success. Most techniques attempt to reduce the degree of vocal tightness and the incidence of voice breaks. Biofeedback, inverse phonation (speaking during inspiration), and identification and correction of dysfunctional vocal habits have all been utilized with low levels of success.

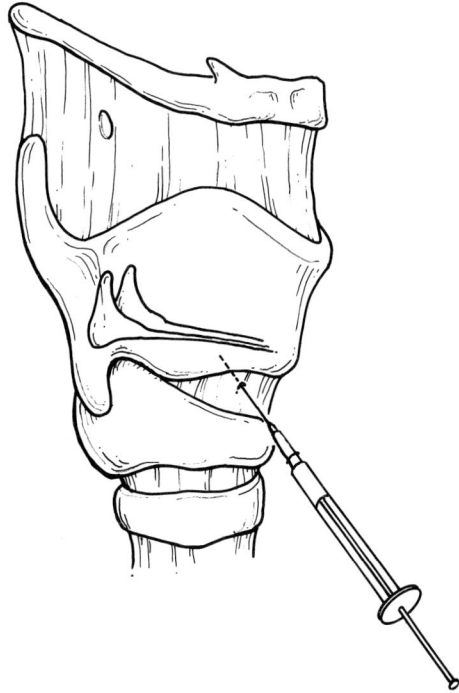

FIGURE 50-1 Schematic diagram showing percutaneous Botox injection technique through cricothyroid membrane into the vocalis muscle for adductor spasmodic dysphonia.

SURGICAL MANAGEMENT

Surgical interruption of the recurrent laryngeal nerve or crush injury of this nerve in the treatment of spasmodic dysphonia has been reported. The initial results for these techniques were reported as high as 92%. Unfortunately long-term results were not favorable. These procedures are no longer recommended. Anterior laryngoplasty is a procedure that was originally developed to treat senile bowing of the vocal cords by relocating the anterior commissure more anteriorly such that there would be more tension on the vocal cords. Tucker modified the procedure

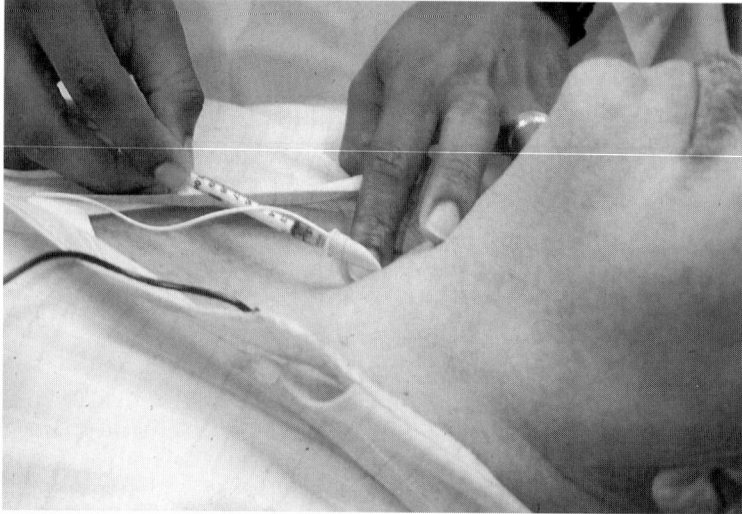

FIGURE 50-2 Botox percutaneous injection for adductor spasmodic dysphonia with EMG guidance.

such that the anterior commissure would be posteriorly displaced resulting in less tension on the vocal cords. Initial results were promising, recurrence rates were high. No surgical procedure is available today that is recommended for the treatment of spasmodic dysphonia.

REHABILITATION AND FOLLOW-UP

Patients with spasmodic dysphonia will need repeat injection, on average, every 3 to 6 months. There is usually only a minor role, if any, for voice therapy. Most patients adjust well after the Botox takes effect.

SUGGESTED READINGS

ARONSON AE, DESANTO LW. Adductor spastic dysphonia: three years after recurrent laryngeal nerve resection. *Laryngoscope.* 1983;93:1–8.

BILLER HF, SOM M, LAWSON W. Laryngeal nerve crush for spastic dysphonia. *Ann Otol Rhinol Laryngol.* 1983;92:469.

BLITZER A, BRIN MF, FAHN, S, LOVELACE RE. Localized injections of botulinum toxin for the treatment of focal laryngeal dystonia. *Laryngoscope.* 1988;98:193–197.

LUDLOW C, NAUNTON RF, SEDORY SE, et al. Effect of botulinum toxin injections on speech in adductor spasmodic dysphonia. *Neurology.* 1990;38:1220–1225.

REFLUX LARYNGITIS

Michelle M. Cullen, M.D.
Keith M. Wilson, M.D.

HISTORY

A 42-year-old female presents with complaints of 4 years of hoarseness and feeling of a "lump in her throat." The patient states that the hoarseness is worse in the morning and slowly lessens as the course of the day goes on but never completely resolves. The patient denies hemoptysis, hematemesis, and weight loss, but does complain of a chronic nonproductive cough. Medical history is noncontributory. She is a nonsmoker but quit only 3 years ago after a 20 pack/year history.

The physical examination reveals an obese female with a low-pitched, hoarse voice. Flexible nasopharyngoscopy reveals dysphonia plicae ventricularis, thickening of the true vocal folds and an exophytic, fleshy mass of the middle and the posterior third of the left vocal cord (Fig. 51–1). The patient's otolaryngology head and neck exam is otherwise unremarkable.

DIFFERENTIAL DIAGNOSIS—KEY POINTS

1. The patient's many years of symptoms point toward a chronic condition. Dysphonia plicae ventricularis is a condition in which the false cords become edematous or hypertrophied so that they override the true vocal cords. Instead of the true vocal cords vibrating, the false cords begin to vibrate, producing a ventricular voice that is harsh. Usually the causative factor is vocal abuse.

2. Vocal fold granulomas may be due to vocal abuse, hyperacid environment or endotracheal intubation. Trauma and denuding of the overlying mucosa of the vocal process may result in perichondritis and overgrowth of granulation tissue. With the finding of a unilateral abnormality, a malignant or premalignant condition must be ruled out.

3. Reflux laryngitis may appear as
   a. Erythema and edema of arytenoid and interarytenoid mucosa
   b. Reinke's edema without significant erythema
   c. Diffuse erythema with friable mucosa of supraglottic larynx
   d. Vocal process granulomas with or without edema and erythema.

4. The term *globus hystericus* is defined as a choking sensation or lump in the throat. This may be due to the edema of the mucosa surrounding the upper esophageal sphincter at the level of the cricopharyngeus or spasm of the cricopharyngeus, secondary to gastroesophageal reflux. Another consideration includes Zenker's diverticulum or other cause of upper esophageal inflammation, is esophageal candidiasis.

5. Hoarseness, chronic cough, and constant throat clearing are symptoms frequently noted with reflux laryngitis. A majority of patients with reflux laryngitis do not have heartburn. Others symptoms include regurgitation of acid contents into the throat causing choking, burning or laryngospasm, cervical odynophagia, cervical dysphagia, excess salivation, and repeated swallowing. Otalgia may be described by patients with reflux and can be explained by the common sensory innervation of both the esophagus, hypopharynx, and the external auditory meatus through the vagus nerve.

6. Classic symptoms of gastroesophageal reflux include heartburn and a feeling of regurgitation, as well as excessive belching or spasmodic chest pain in the epigastric and substernal region.

7. Common conditions that predispose patients to gastroesophageal reflux include obesity, straining, the supine position, prolonged intubation, nasogastric tube placement, and foods that increase acid production such as fats, chocolate, carminatives (peppermint,

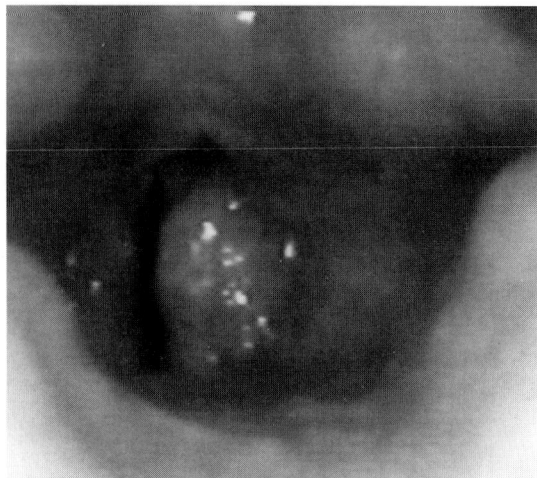

FIGURE 51–1 Flexible nasopharyngoscopy reveals dysphonia plicae ventricularis, thickening of the true vocal folds, and an exophytic, fleshy mass of the middle and posterior third of the left vocal cord.

spearmint, cinnamon, garlic, onions), milk, beer, orange juice, and tomato juice. Nicotine and caffeine have a similar effect. Medications that have been associated with gastroesophageal reflux include antidepressant medications, progestrone, β-blockers, calcium channel blockers, α-blockers, valium, and morphine. These foods and medications act primarily by reducing the lower esophageal sphincter pressure.

8. Other more unusual causes of reflux include multiple sclerosis, amyotrophic lateral sclerosis, Guillain–Barré, diabetes, myasthenia gravis, scleroderma, esophageal gastric carcinoma, caustic burn, cervical osteophytes, Zenker's diverticulum, myoma or other benign tumor of the esophagus, esophageal web, and/or Plummer–Vinson syndrome and previous radiation.

9. Severe gastroesophageal reflux can be associated with development of subglottic stenosis and cricoarytenoid fixation.

TEST INTERPRETATION

The diagnosis of reflux laryngitis can be made with a history and physical exam consistent with the disease process. The patient may then be treated with conservative or medical thera-

pies. However, if the history or physical exam is not classic for the condition or if medical therapy fails and surgical therapy is contemplated, several tests can be useful in confirming the diagnosis of gastroesophageal reflux.

1. *Barium swallow.* This test provides useful information concerning esophageal motility, lumen integrity, aspiration, and intrinsic and extrinsic masses. The patient's position can be modified during the test to look for reflux with change in position.

2. *Computed tomography (CT) scan—magnetic resonance imaging (MRI).* CT scan or MRI can be useful in identifying a mass causing intrinsic or extrinsic compression.

3. *Esophageal manometry.* This test measures the duration, amplitude, and velocity of the peristaltic wave, as well as the upper and lower esophageal sphincter pressure.

4. *pH monitoring.* A 24-hour pH probe measuring the pH at the site of the upper and lower esophageal sphincter can be performed on an outpatient or 23-hour observation inpatient basis. With this technique, reflux is defined as a pH of less than 4.0.

5. *Endoscopy.* Endoscopic evaluation is via direct laryngoscopy, direct esophagoscopy, or flexible esophagoscopy. Direct laryngoscopy should be performed if asymmetric laryngeal findings are encountered, if there is a suspicion of malignancy, or if medical management fails to resolve a persistent suspicious abnormality of the larynx. Rigid esophagoscopy provides better visualization of the pharynx and upper esophageal sphincter than can be obtained with flexible endoscopy. On the other hand, flexible esophagoscopy can be performed under local anesthesia with sedation, allows for the concurrent examination of the stomach and duodenum, and allows for closer examination of mucosal lesions.

6. *Bronchoalveolar lavage.* Lipid laden macrophages have been shown to be consistent with and highly sensitive for gastroesophageal reflux.

DIAGNOSIS

Gastroesophageal reflux disease with vocal fold granuloma.

MEDICAL MANAGEMENT

Medical management begins with lifestyle modification, which includes weight reduction if applicable, elevation of the head of the bed 6 to 8 inches while sleeping to decrease reflux, avoidance of tight-fitting clothing, and smoking cessation. Dietary changes that are advocated include avoidance of fat, caffeine, chocolate, mints, and carbonated drinks, which reduce lower esophageal sphincter pressure. Avoiding alcohol, overeating, and ingestion of food or drink 3 hours before bedtime can reduce gastroesophageal reflux. Over-the-counter liquid antacids (15 cc after meals and 30 cc before bedtime) are simple first-line measures that can be tried. An empiric trial of H_2 blockers such as cimetidine (Tagamet), ranitidine (Zantac), and famotidine (Pepsid) can be utilized, as can other drugs that have been found to be helpful, including the prokenetic drugs metoclopramide (Reglan) and cisapride (Propulsid), as well as cytoprotective agents such as sucralfate (Carafate). In severe or recalcitrant cases the proton pump inhibitor omeprazole can be trialed initially. These medications or lifestyle changes should be instituted for a period of 6 weeks and then the patient is reevaluated. The chronic laryngeal changes associated with reflux laryngitis may take months for resolution.

SURGICAL MANAGEMENT

Contact ulceration will typically spontaneously heal although if it persists direct laryngoscopy and biopsy should be performed. Contact granulomas may require direct laryngoscopy and microlaryngoscopy or laser ablation for removal. Dysphonia plicae ventricularis may require voice therapy for reversal and resolution.

In cases of severe gastroesophageal reflux, Nissen fundoplication or vagotomy may be performed.

REHABILITATION AND FOLLOW-UP

Following adequate medical or surgical therapy, the patient may require lifelong antireflux medication. Although controversial, the development of carcinoma in the setting of any chronic condition including gastroesophageal reflux is possible and the patient should be followed on a yearly basis following symptomatic and pathologic reversal to ensure adequate treatment and compliance of the patient's condition.

SUGGESTED READINGS

FEEHS RS, KOUFMAN JA. Laryngitis. In: Bailey BJ, Johnson JT, Kohut RL, et al, eds. *Head and Neck Surgery—Otolaryngology.* Philadelphia, PA: JB Lippincott; 1993:612–619.

JOHNSON JT, HERSHENSON LM, BOGDASARIAN RS. Head and neck manifestations of gastroesophageal reflux. Self-instructional package. American Academy of Otolaryngology—Head and Neck Surgery; 1988.

OLSON NR. The problem of gastroesophageal reflux. In: *Special Topics in Otolaryngology, Otolaryngol Clin North Am.* 1996;19(1):119–133.

PASSY V. Hoarseness evaluation and treatment. In: *Common Problems in the Head and Neck Region. A Manual and Guide for Management of Diseases and Injuries, Otolaryngology—Head and Neck Surgery, 1986–87 version.* American Academy of Otolaryngology, Head and Neck Surgery, pp. 79–96.

SHOCHLEY WW. Esophageal disorders. In: Bailey BJ, Johnson JT, Kohut RL, et al, eds. *Head and Neck Surgery—Otolaryngology.* Philadelphia, PA: JB Lippincott; 1993:690–710.

Case 52

SUBGLOTTIC STENOSIS

Douglas B. Villaret, M.D.
Keith M. Wilson, M.D.

HISTORY

A 48-year-old black male with a history of smoking, insulin-dependent diabetes, and myocardial infarction underwent a coronary artery bypass graft (CABG) for three-vessel occlusion. Postoperatively his course was complicated by wound breakdown and prolonged ventilator dependence. He eventually was extubated on postoperative day 11. At that time, he had mild dyspnea with exertion and a small oxygen requirement, but no hoarseness or stridor. He was soon discharged to home after his pulmonary status improved.

During the next few months, the patient began having progressive dyspnea, now occurring while at rest. A mild inspiratory stridor was also present. He denied dysphagia, chest pain, and chronic cough, but did complain of nocturia.

The physical exam revealed biphasic stridor and mild retractions with breathing. His wounds had completely healed. Heart sounds were unremarkable and no rales or rhonchi were auscultated in the lungs.

DIFFERENTIAL DIAGNOSIS— KEY POINTS

1. Dyspnea and nocturia in a patient who has undergone a CABG requires that cardiac function be evaluated to rule out fluid overload. In this case, no abnormalities were found postoperatively except for an inferior area of ischemia on the thallium scan, unchanged from the preoperative scan.

2. Vocal fold paralysis is also a consideration after cardiac surgery, because the left recurrent laryngeal nerve is at risk. However, unilateral paralysis will usually result in a hoarse voice with an adequate airway. The unusual event of diabetes-associated ischemic neuropathy of the recurrent laryngeal nerve is also possible.

3. Vocal fold fixation from arytenoid dislocation could have occurred, but his symptoms should not be progressive. Rarely, cricoarytenoid joint fixation can occur associated with collagen-vascular disease.

4. The possibility of a laryngeal tumor needs to be evaluated, especially with his history of smoking.

5. Inflammatory or infectious disorders may also cause airway obstruction. Wegener's (subglottic), sarcoid (supraglottic), and tuberculosis are potential causes.

6. Laryngotracheal stenosis, most commonly subglottic, is the most likely diagnosis. Endotracheal tube trauma to the airway has become the most common cause of subglottic stenosis.

TEST INTERPRETATION

A thallium scan was obtained, showing inferior ischemia. Cardiac output was also evaluated and shown to be normal.

A purified protein derivative (PPD) skin test was placed and was negative. The chest x-ray showed no airspace disease, nodules, or adenopathy. Acetylcholinesterase and calcium levels were normal (for sarcoid). The autoimmune workup for Wegener's included erythrocyte sedimentation rate, antinuclear antibody, and anti-neutrophil cytoplasmic antibody (C-ANCA), and was similarly negative.

Flexible nasopharyngoscopy showed a normal endolarynx. There were no mucosal abnormalities indicative of laryngeal granulomas or neoplasms. Additionally, both vocal folds moved symmetrically with no limitations. The arytenoids showed moderate erythema. Subglottic narrowing was suspected.

No pulmonary function tests or computed tomography scans were ordered. The patient was scheduled for a microlaryngoscopy and bronchoscopy with possible tracheostomy. A rigid 4-mm Hopkins rod telescopic unit was used for evaluation. Again, the larynx appeared normal. In the immediate subglottis, 1 cm distal to the vocal folds, a circumferential, firm narrowing of the airway was encountered (Fig. 52–1). The total length was evaluated at 2 cm. The lumen just admitted the telescope, indicating a 4-mm airway. Distally, the tracheobronchial tree was normal. Decadron, 10 mg IV, was given and a tracheotomy was not performed.

DIAGNOSIS

Subglottic stenosis.

MEDICAL MANAGEMENT

If the stenosis had been due to sarcoid, long-term steroids would be indicated. With Wegener's, appropriate treatment includes cytoxan or trimethoprim–sulfamethoxazole. A positive PPD would prompt assessing the sputum for active tuberculosis and starting appropriate antituberculous therapy. Extensive workups for these infrequent conditions are not routinely performed unless other indications are found during the history and physical exam.

Soft, immature stenosis sometimes responds to inhaled, intravenous, or intralesional steroids. A firm stenosis is a surgical problem.

In children, a 24-hour pH probe is always obtained to evaluate gastroesophageal reflux disease. Appropriate H_2 blockers or proton pump inhibitors are started. A positive history or signs such as posterior glottic edema or erythema are used as indicators to begin treatment in adults.

SURGICAL MANAGEMENT

1. *Endoscopic.*
   a. *Laser.* The CO_2 laser is useful in immature (soft) stenoses that are less than 1 cm in length. If it does not meet these criteria or if the stricture is circumferential or if there is loss of cartilage support, then an open approach will yield better results.

   Using the CO_2 laser at a 5-W pulse is generally safe. Radial, vertical incisions through the stenosis, leaving mucosa between the cuts, is used for larger stenoses. For smaller lesions, a mucosal flap may be raised, followed by laser ablation of the stenosis.

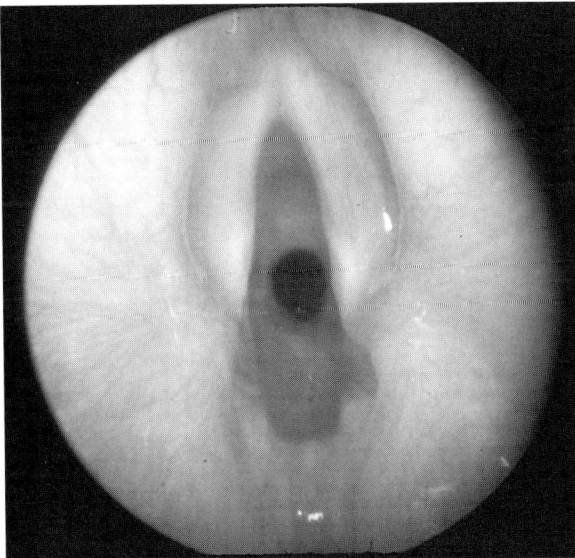

FIGURE 52–1 Bronchoscopy demonstrates a circumferential, firm narrowing of the airway.

b. *Stents.* Indwelling, expandable intraluminal stents are under investigation, but for now are mostly used for palliation in advanced tumors of the trachea.

2. *Open.*

a. *Cricotracheal resection.* Long stenotic segments with total or near total occlusion of the airway often need complete excision to allow an adequate airway. The posterior half of the cricoid can be left in place, with only mucosal advancement of this portion of the airway. This will help protect the recurrent laryngeal nerves.

b. *Stents.* Anterior and posterior splits of the cricoid cartilage, or four-quadrant splits, are expanded with different stents (such as an Aboulker). These require a tracheostomy tube to be placed distal to the stent, and usually stay in place for 6 weeks to 3 months. Alternatively, a Montgomery T-tube may be used for stenting.

c. *Grafts.* More severe stenoses benefit from having grafts placed to reduce the amount of time a stent needs to be in place and to improve the decannulation rate. In children and young adults, costochondral grafts work very well with minimal morbidity. In adults, hyoid interposition grafts with or without a muscular pedicle work well. Everything from nasal septal cartilage grafts with mucosa to sternohyoid rotary door flaps with skin have been used successfully. Important points are to manipulate the airway/graft cartilage as little as possible and place as few sutures as possible. In children, stenting with an endotracheal or T-tube is needed for at least 7 to 10 days except for moderate anterior lesions where only the anterior cricoid ring has been widened. Adults will usually have a stent sutured in place for 6 weeks.

REHABILITATION AND FOLLOW-UP

For complete (Cotton grade IV) stenoses, multiple resections may be needed. After successful stent removal or decannulation, the patient should be followed every 3 months with endoscopic evaluation to remove granulation tissue and evaluate for scarring or malacia for the first few years.

SUGGESTED READINGS

COLEMAN JA, DUNCAUAGE JA, eds. Management of lower airway obstruction. *Otolaryngol Clin North Am.* 1995;28(4).

COTTON RT. The problem of pediatric laryngotracheal stenosis: a clinical and experimental study on the efficacy of autogenous cartilage grafts placed between the vertically directed halves of the posterior lamina of the cricoid cartilage. *Laryngoscope.* 1991;101(suppl 56):1–34.

MYER CM, VILLARET DB. Subglottic stenosis. In: Hotaling AJ, Stankiewicz JA, eds. *Pediatric Otolaryngology for the General Otolaryngologist.* New York: Ieaku-Shoin Medical Publishers; 1996:49–59.

LARYNGEAL TRAUMA

Douglas B. Villaret, M.D.
Keith M. Wilson, M.D.

HISTORY

A 34-year-old obese male was brought to the emergency department via AirCare after a motor vehicle accident. During transport, his airway was tenuous but he was able to be mask ventilated. Upon arrival at the hospital, the trauma service judged his condition as worsening and subsequently performed a cricothyrotomy with establishment of a secure airway. Further resuscitation efforts were limited to administration of lactated Ringer's fluid at this time.

Examination revealed an obese, black male with an irregular 5-cm midline neck wound contiguous with the cricothyrotomy site. There was significant subcutaneous emphysema and the individual thyroid cartilage fragments were easily palpated. Additionally, he sustained a left parasymphaseal mandible fracture and multiple facial lacerations. Auscultation of the left lung yielded decreased breath sounds. A portable chest x-ray revealed a left pneumothorax from a fractured rib, and a chest tube was inserted. Peritoneal lavage was negative for abdominal bleeding. Radiographic analysis confirmed a normal cervical spine. The patient's hemodynamic profile was labile in the surgical intensive care unit and he was judged medically unfit to undergo general anesthesia for 48 hours.

DIFFERENTIAL DIAGNOSIS— KEY POINTS

1. Resuscitative measures following the ATLS guidelines are implemented for all serious injuries.
2. Presenting symptoms of blunt laryngeal trauma include dyspnea, hoarseness, tenderness, cough, hemoptysis, and dysphagia. Signs of laryngeal trauma are edema, crepitance, subcutaneous emphysema, and flattening of the laryngeal prominence. Laryngotracheal separation can also present in this manner.
3. A grading system for laryngeal trauma and management of the acute airway is reviewed in Table 53–1.
4. *Patient assessment.* A complete history of the mechanism of injury should be obtained, as well as any preexisting medical conditions. A thorough physical exam includes both palpation of the neck and a flexible fiber optic laryngoscopy to evaluate endolaryngeal trauma.
5. *Concomitant injuries.* Cervical spine injuries have been reported in up to 50% in patients with blunt laryngeal trauma. Recurrent laryngeal nerve palsies suggest a possible cricoid crush fracture. Pharyngoesophageal tears must also be evaluated.

TEST INTERPRETATION

The chest x-ray showed a fractured left seventh rib and associated pneumothorax. Hgb/Hct were 9.3 and 36.2, respectively.

A computed tomography (CT) scan was obtained, showing comminution of the thyroid cartilage and obvious subcutaneous emphysema (Fig. 53–1). Patients who meet the grade 2 requirements are good candidates for CT. Airway compromise usually dictates that a tracheotomy be performed, but open neck exploration is not always indicated. If the CT scan shows only edema, then the patient can expect a good recovery without surgical intervention. Should a displaced laryngeal fracture be revealed, which was not diagnosed on physical exam, then open reduction and internal fixation should be performed.

DIAGNOSIS

Grade 4 blunt laryngeal fracture.

TABLE 53-1 Grading Laryngeal Trauma and Managing the Acute Airway

Group	Features	Management
1	Minimal or no airway compromise; minor endolaryngeal hematomas or lacerations	Conservative: humidified oxygen, 24-hour observation
2	Moderate edema, hematomas, and airway compromise; minor mucosal lacerations without cartilage exposure and nondisplaced laryngeal cartilage fracture	Tracheotomy under local anesthesia to prevent further damage to the airway by either endotracheal intubation or cricothyrotomy
3	Massive edema, exposed cartilage with large mucosal lacerations and vocal fold immobility with displaced fractures	Same as group 2
4	Similar findings to group 3, plus more than two fracture lines and a disrupted anterior larynx or an unstable laryngeal skeleton	Same as group 2
5	Full cricotracheal separation	Endotracheal intubation; the distal airway usually retracts into the chest, so tracheotomy may compound the problem

MEDICAL MANAGEMENT

Conservative management is only appropriate for patients in group 1: minor hematomas or lacerations. These patients should be hospitalized for at least 24 hours in a monitored setting because the edema may progress, especially in the 6- to 12-hour period. Humidified air or oxygen is supplied and voice rest is instituted. The patient can expect a good result in both vocal quality and airway.

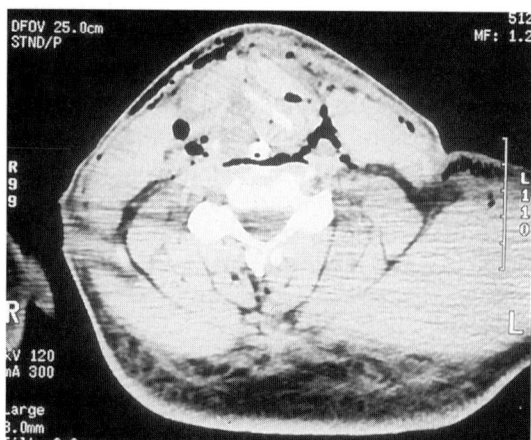

FIGURE 53-1 CT scan demonstrates comminution of the thyroid cartilage and subcutaneous emphysema.

SURGICAL MANAGEMENT

When he was stabilized, the patient was taken to the operating room. The cricothyrotomy was converted to a formal, low tracheostomy. Midline exploration revealed a severely comminuted thyroid cartilage as well as an anteriorly fractured cricoid cartilage (Fig. 53–2). Surgical exploration of the comminuted fragments allowed a paramedian laryngofissure approach to the airway. Partially healed mucosal lacerations were seen.

Surgical repair consisted of irrigating the endolarynx and repairing the mucosal lacerations. The true vocal folds were sutured to the external perichondrium with 5-0 Vicryl sutures, and a modified (Poretex) endotracheal tube stent was placed. The cartilage fragments were repaired with 4-0 Vicryl sutures and the stent was sewn in place with a 2-0 Prolene suture extended out to the skin. The mandible fracture was also repaired at this time.

Group 3 or 4 patients should undergo tracheotomy and surgical exploration; group 5 should have immediate exploration and primary repair of the trachea. Indications for open exploration in group 2 patients are as follows:

1. Severe upper airway obstructions not from edema or hematoma

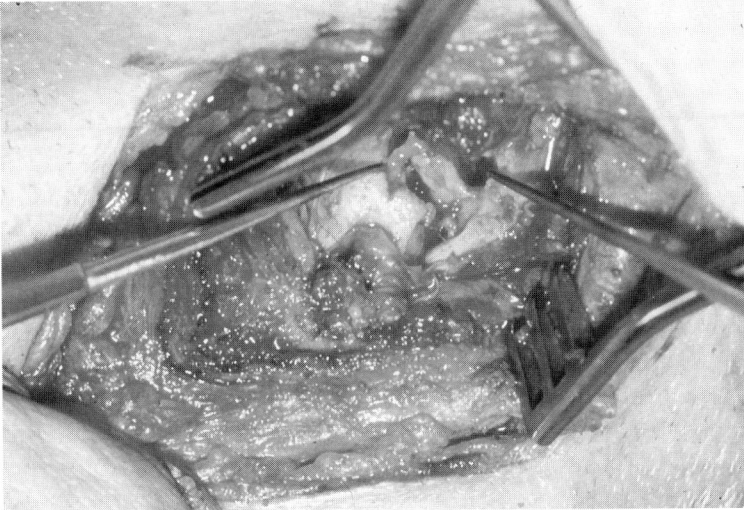

FIGURE 53-2 Surgical exploration reveals a severely comminuted thyroid cartilage and anteriorly fractured cricoid cartilage.

2. Displaced laryngeal skeleton fracture

3. Internal (endolaryngeal) derangement and/or exposed cartilage

4. Active hemorrhage

5. Increasing subcutaneous emphysema

• *Tracheotomy.* Tracheotomy is preferred to reduce the exacerbation of intubating an injured larynx and to provide a more stable airway. For those patients who need general anesthesia and have mild to moderate trauma to the larynx (group 2), but no significant airway distress, tracheotomy is still the preferred method to prevent long-term edema and subsequent airway compromise.

• *Laryngofissure.* When the thyroid cartilage or endolaryngeal mucosa has been severely disrupted or cartilage is exposed, a laryngofissure is needed to gain access to repair the injury. Anterior commissure lacerations and disruption of the free edge of the vocal fold should be approached similarly and repaired primarily. Often, a keel is used to prevent blunting of the anterior commissure.

   Minor mucosal lacerations and non-comminuted thyroid cartilage fractures do not need a laryngofissure for repair.

• *Stenting.* Stenting is necessary for comminuted thyroid cartilage fractures that are unstable even after open reduction and internal fixation. It is also needed to prevent adhesions in massive endolaryngeal lacerations and to act as a keel in trauma resulting in a disrupted anterior commissure. Stents are maintained for a period of 2 to 3 weeks.

REHABILITATION AND FOLLOW-UP

In mild (group 1) injuries, normal voice and airway is the standard outcome. With increasing severity of trauma and a delay greater than 24 to 48 hours for operative intervention, the vocal results suffer more than the airway: Group 4 patients have a 33% chance of a "fair" voice and a small, but real, possibility of a poor airway.

   Long-term follow-up is needed to assist patients who have not returned to their pretraumatic status. Speech therapy, thyroplasty, and laryngotracheoplasty are all possibilities for improving a less than adequate outcome.

SUGGESTED READINGS

BENT JP, PORULOSKY ES. The management of blunt fractures of the thyroid cartilage. *Otolaryngol Head Neck Surg.* 1994;110:195–202.

FRIED MP, ed. Laryngeal trauma. In: *The Larynx*. St. Louis, MO: Mosby–Year Book; 1996:387–396.

PAPARELLA MM, SHUMRICK DA, GLUCKMAN JL, MEYERHOFF WL, eds. Laryngeal trauma. In: *Otolaryngology*. Philadelphia, PA: WB Saunders; 1991:2231–2244.

SCHAEFER SD. The acute management of external laryngeal trauma: a 27 year experience. *Arch Otolaryngol Head Neck Surg*. 1992;118:598–604.

SNOW JB Jr. Diagnosis and therapy for acute laryngeal and tracheal trauma. *Otolaryngol Clin North Am*. 1984;17:101.

Case 54

SNORING AND OBSTRUCTIVE SLEEP APNEA

Thomas A. Tami, M.D.

HISTORY

A 57-year-old man has been forced to sleep in the guest room because of loud sonorous snoring. His wife and other family members who are continuously complaining about this problem have not noticed obvious struggling for breath during his sleep. The patient does, however, complain of daytime sleepiness and was recently reprimanded by his employer for falling asleep on the job. His medical history is unremarkable except for mild systemic hypertension, which is well controlled with hydrochlorothiazide. He is moderately obese, but his general physical examination is otherwise unremarkable. His nasal septum is deviated, causing mild to moderate right-sided nasal airway obstruction. He is interested in treatment for his snoring.

DIFFERENTIAL DIAGNOSIS— KEY POINTS

1. This patient, while primarily complaining of snoring, is at high risk for obstructive sleep apnea (OSA). Despite the lack of observed struggling for breath during sleep or observed apneic events, he does appear to have daytime somnolence, he is overweight, and he has systemic hypertension, all risk factors for OSA. Before any attention is given to his primary complaint (i.e., snoring), he should undergo a polysomnogram (sleep study).

2. Even though he has a severely deviated nasal septum, which is producing marked nasal airway obstruction, the temptation to address this problem surgically should be resisted until the results of a polysomnograph are available. While an occasional patient will respond favorably to septoplasty, both with regard to snoring and to OSA, addressing the nasal problem rarely is sufficient to completely ameliorate the underlying problem.

3. Polysomnographic examinations can be performed in various ways. A level I polysomnogram is the typical in-house overnight or two-night study performed by most sleep laboratories. This study evaluates not only cardiorespiratory parameters (airflow, chest movement, oxygen saturation, EKG, etc.), but in addition obtains neurophysiologic EEG data to evaluate sleep stages and detect arousals. These studies are considered the gold standard for evaluating these patients; however, they often provide information that may not be immediately relevant to the patient's underlying problem. A level II study measures essentially the same physiologic parameters as level I, but it is performed on an ambulatory basis in the patient's home.

   Level III polysomnography is beginning to play a much greater role in evaluation of patients with possible OSA. These systems are equipped to measure all of the important physiologic parameters to establish the diagnosis of OSA, but not to evaluate EEG-generated data regarding sleep. These studies are in general much more cost effective; however, they do run the risk of leaving undiagnosed other potential sleep disorders, such as narcolepsy.

Level IV studies usually consist of the measurement and recording of a single physiologic parameter, such as oxygen saturation, and use these data to screen for possible clinically significant OSA. While this method is widely used in Europe and is certainly cost effective, the sensitivity and specificity of this technique are such that its use as a screen for OSA is usually not helpful.

TEST INTERPRETATION

A level III polysomnograph was obtained for this patient. A sampling of the raw data is shown in Figure 54–1. The overall results of the study were as follows:

Total sleep time	6 hours, 32 minutes (392 minutes)
Total apneas (A)	138
Total hypopneas (H)	104
Total respiratory events (A + H)	242
Apnea index (AI)	21 per hour
Respiratory disturbance index (RDI)	37 per hour

In most laboratories, a normal RDI is considered to be less than 10. Clearly, this patient has severe OSA with an RDI of 37 per hour. Hypopneas are often defined differently between laboratories, but they are generally defined as a substantial reduction in airflow in an obstructed pattern resulting in an oxygen desaturation of at least 4% from baseline. Even if hypopneas are not considered in the diagnosis of this patient, an AI of 21 per hour is at a level that has been associated with increased mortality and morbidity.

DIAGNOSIS

Obstructive sleep apnea—severe.

MEDICAL MANAGEMENT

The initial medical management of OSA is to eliminate associated risk factors. Patients who take sedatives or use alcohol should be encouraged to stop since their use is often associated with OSA. Overweight patients should try to lose weight since a positive correlation between obesity and OSA has also been described. Although weight reduction alone may benefit some patients, the success of weight loss in OSA has been limited, and weight loss alone is rarely adequate. Other noninvasive therapeutic measures such as the use of a nasopharyngeal airway or conditioning the patient to avoid sleep positions that exacerbate the breathing problem

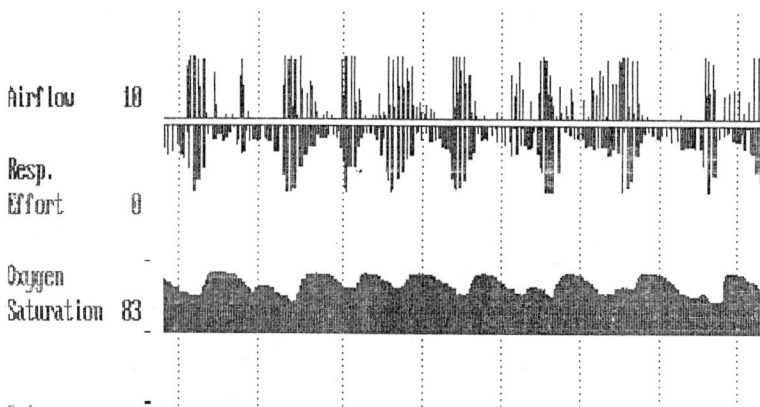

FIGURE 54–1 Level III polysomnograph.

have also been attempted with variable, but generally dismal, success.

The effectiveness of pharmacologic agents to treat this syndrome has also been disappointing. The tricyclic antidepressant protriptyline was the most widely studied of these agents. This drug seemed to have a positive effect in patients with mild OSA by increasing upper airway muscle tone during sleep; however, its use has been abandoned in most circles due to severe anticholinergic side effects.

Orthodontic devices have been developed to alter the upper airway by changing the tongue-jaw relationship. Little controlled data support the efficacy of these devices for OSA, yet their use is fairly widespread. Snoring is usually improved or eliminated in nearly all patients fitted with these devices, but OSA is rarely cured. Many patients also often experience orodental discomfort with these devices.

Nasal continuous positive airway pressure (CPAP) was first introduced in 1981 as a nonsurgical treatment of OSA and has become widely used for this condition. Nasal CPAP delivers positive airway pressure through a tightly sealed and fitting nasal mask. When the pressure delivered to the patient is titrated appropriately, a constant pneumatic pressure is maintained in the upper airway and collapse during nocturnal respiration is prevented. Excessive daytime somnolence and other symptoms associated with OSA are often quickly reversed using nasal CPAP and the cardiovascular sequelae and mortality associated with this disorder can be dramatically reduced.

The effectiveness of nasal CPAP for OSA is often overshadowed by poor patient compliance. Studies that have looked objectively at patient compliance with nasal CPAP have found that as many as 20% of patients stop using the device within 1 month, and in those who continued, the compliance rate is usually less than 50%. Patient compliance with nasal CPAP correlates with increased educational level and professional job status. This finding underscores the need for patient education about OSA and the use of nasal CPAP to motivate patients to accept the inconvenience associated with this therapy.

SURGICAL MANAGEMENT

Prior to the development of nasal CPAP, severely affected patients were usually managed with formal tracheotomy. Since tracheotomy was associated with both patient and physician resistance, only the most severely affected patients with severe daytime somnolence or cardiovascular sequelae were offered this option.

Uvulopalatopharyngoplasty (UPPP), introduced by Fujita in 1981, was the first specialized surgical procedure for OSA. This procedure was quickly adapted by otolaryngologists and offered to all patients with OSA; however, no consideration was usually given to the site of obstruction. Although the area of upper airway obstruction is often the region of the oropharynx and velum, anatomic narrowing in the hypopharynx, larynx and tongue base can also contribute to OSA. Predictably, the success of UPPP alone in all patients with OSA was only in the range of 50%. However, if patients were grouped according to the site of narrowing, UPPP seems to be much more successful when applied only to those patients with narrowing or collapse in the region of the oropharynx and velum. The sites of potential anatomic airway collapse are defined as follows:

- Type I obstruction occurs primarily in the retropalatal airway.

- Type II obstruction has narrowing in the retropalatal and retrolingual regions.

- Type III narrowing occurs in patients with the retrolingual region as the primary site of narrowing or collapse.

If surgical success is defined as a reduction in the AI by 50%, the success rate for UPPP in patients with type I obstruction is 83% However, if success is defined as a postoperative RDI less than 20 or an AI less than 10 and a reduction in the AHI by 50%, the postoperative success using UPPP is only 52%. Patients with type II and III airway narrowing and collapse have only a 5% surgical success rate using UPPP if the more stringent criteria for success were used. If UPPP is used to manage this condition, judicious patient selection is an important factor to optimize the success rate following surgery.

Patients with type II and type III obstruction are candidates for other surgical procedures. The most common adjunctive procedure for obstruction in the hypopharynx and tongue base is the mandibular osteotomy/genioglossus advancement with hyoid myotomy/suspension (GAHM). This procedure expands the hypopharyngeal region at the tongue base by advancing the genial tubercle and hyoid bone. Riley and his group at Stanford University use extensive preoperative data analysis including physical examination, fiber optic nasopharyngoscopy with the Mueller's maneuver, and lateral cephalometric analysis to determine the anatomic site of obstruction. Based on these studies, they recommend either UPPP, GAHM, or a combination UPPP/GAHM. Using these carefully defined preoperative selection criteria, they reported a 61% success rate, as defined by a postoperative reduction of the AHI to less than 20. They concluded that by carefully evaluating patients and directing the surgical therapy at the appropriate pharyngeal region, the surgical success rate could be significantly improved.

For patients who fail this initial surgical protocol, the Stanford group recommends phase II surgical management consisting of formal orthognathic surgery with maxillary and mandibular osteotomies (MMO) to advance the midface and mandible and increase the pharyngeal airway. Riley has reported an overall 97% success rate for surgical management of OSA when phase I failures are referred for the more extensive phase II surgical option.

Recent excitement in the otolaryngology community has accompanied the introduction of laser-assisted uvulopalatoplasty (LAUP). This procedure was initially introduced as an outpatient surgical alternative for snoring, but its similarity to the widely used UPPP has made it an enticing alternative for managing OSA. LAUP appears to be highly successful in decreasing or eliminating socially unacceptable snoring; however, there is only limited data to support its use for OSA. Several recent studies have suggested that LAUP may improve OSA in certain mild cases if patients are properly selected; however, the efficacy of LAUP has not

been clearly established in this setting. At best, LAUP may provide a degree of surgical success similar to the more traditional UPPP. At the present time, LAUP must be considered a good alternative for snoring, but cannot be recommended for most cases of OSA.

REHABILITATION AND FOLLOW-UP

Obstructive sleep apnea has substantial long-term health implications such as systemic hypertension, increased incidence of stroke, heart failure, pulmonary hypertension, and daytime somnolence with resultant industrial and automobile accidents. It is essential that these patients be monitored and followed closely to ensure the effectiveness of therapeutic intervention. For patients treated with nasal CPAP, an ongoing measure of compliance is warranted. Currently available CPAP devices often have built-in microchip monitors to measure patient usage to guide therapy.

Patients who elect surgical intervention should always have a postoperative polysomnogram. Since surgical intervention is very effective in eliminating snoring, these patients often continue to experience "silent apnea." Because the primary motivation to seek medical attention is in many instances the socially unacceptable snoring, these patients often have little or no motivation to seek further medical evaluation or care. Patient education is essential to convince these individuals to undergo a postoperative sleep study with the possible need for further therapy.

SUGGESTED READINGS

FINDLEY LJ, UNVERZAGT ME, SURATT PM. Automobile accidents involving patients with obstructive sleep apnea. *Am Rev Respir Dis.* 1988;138:337–340.

HE J, KRYGER MH, ZORICK FJ, et al. Mortality and apnea index in obstructive sleep apnea. *Chest.* 1988;94:9–14.

RILEY RW, POWELL NB, GUILLEMINAULT C. Obstructive sleep apnea syndrome: a review of 306 consecutively treated surgical patients. *Otolaryngol Head Neck Surg.* 1993;108:117–125.

SCHER AE, SCHECHTMAN KB, PICCIRILLO JE. The efficacy of surgical modifications of the upper airway in adults with obstructive sleep apnea syndrome. *Sleep.* 1996;19:156–177.

SCHMIDT-NOWARA W, LOWE A, WIEGAND L, et al. Oral appliances for the treatment of snoring and obstructive sleep apnea: a review. *Sleep.* 1995;18:501–510.

SERIES F, ST PIERRE S, CARRIER G. Effects of surgical correction of nasal obstruction in the treatment of obstructive sleep apnea. *Am Rev Respir Dis.* 1992; 146:1261–1265.

SHEPARD JWJ. Hypertension, cardiac arrhythmias, myocardial infarction, and stroke in relation to obstructive sleep apnea. *Clin Chest Med.* 1992;13: 437–458.

STROLLO PJ, ROGERS RM. Current concepts: obstructive sleep apnea. *N Engl J Med.* 1996;334:99–104.

YOUNG T, PALTA M, DEMPSEY J, et al. The occurrence of sleep-disordered breathing among middle-aged adults [see comments]. *N Engl J Med.* 1993;328:1230–1235.

NEUROMUSCULAR DISORDER OF THE HEAD AND NECK

Thomas A. Tami, M.D.

HISTORY

A 37-year-old woman has had a sense of chronic imbalance during the past 1 to 2 months. She has experienced no true vertigo and has had no other aural symptoms, but seems to have difficulty maintaining her balance with frequent falls, especially in the dark. In addition, she has recently noted the onset of a mild intention tremor and feels like her speech is somewhat thickened and occasionally difficult to understand. She has no diplopia at this time; however, she has noted fleeting episodes of double vision during the last several months. Each episode has lasted for several days, only to resolve completely. She describes no dysphagia and her voice is strong. She has had no other neurologic complaints except for several episodes of left cheek numbness during the past several months. Each episode has resolved spontaneously.

On physical examination she has a normal general head and neck examination. Her cranial nerve function is normal including no hypesthesia of the face. Extraocular muscle movement is normal throughout with no obvious nystagmus. She has a slight intention tremor and her speech, while intelligible does seem somewhat dysarthric. The patient also displays some emotional lability during parts of the examination when her speech difficulty was discussed. The remainder of the general physical examination is normal.

DIFFERENTIAL DIAGNOSIS— KEY POINTS

1. While chronic imbalance is a common complaint in the practice of otolaryngology, it is somewhat unusual in an otherwise healthy young person. Therefore, this symptom deserves particular attention to rule out an underlying neurologic problem. Imbalance can be produced from defects in either the vestibular system, the visual system, the cerebellum, or the dorsal column pathways. Because this patient does not describe true vertigo, a deficit of one or more of the nonvestibular pathways should be considered. Vestibular testing with an electronystagmography (ENG) might be helpful; however, this situation is ideally suited to posture platform testing. Balance systems other than the vestibuloocular reflex can be evaluated with this test.

2. Several chronic neurologic disorders can present as symptoms in the head and neck region. One of these, amyotrophic lateral sclerosis (ALS) is a disorder that primarily affects the upper and lower motor neurons to produce muscle atrophy and spasticity. Usually occurring during the fifth or sixth decades of life, this disease affects men twice as often as women and is characterized by progressive muscle weakness, cramping, and fasiculations. Dysarthria can be a primary component of ALS due to the involvement of orofacial and laryngeal musculature. Sensory deficits are rare in these patients. Cranial nerve involvement is frequent and usually becomes clinically important when deglutition is affected. The extraocular muscles are almost uniformly spared in this progressive neuromuscular degenerative disease.

3. Another neuromuscular disorder that also often presents with head and neck manifestations is myasthenia gravis (MG). This degenerative disorder is confined exclusively to striated muscles and is characterized by muscle weakness, easy fatigability, and prolongation of return of muscle strength following

exercise. Antibodies produced and directed against striated muscle motor endplates is the pathophysiologic etiology of MG. Women are affected twice as often as men, and the onset is usually during the third decade for women and the sixth decade for men. Ptosis and diplopia are common presenting symptoms in the head and neck region and almost all patients with MG will develop ocular findings at some point during the course of their illness. Dysarthria can occur when the articulatory and laryngeal muscles are affected and is usually noted to worsen as speech is prolonged. Sensory and balance symptoms are generally not features of MG. Since edrophonium chloride (Tensilon) given intramuscularly will restore muscle strength for several minutes following administration, this is often used as a diagnostic test for this disorder. Various treatments for MG include steroids, plasmapheresis, and thymectomy.

4. Multiple sclerosis (MS) is another fairly common degenerative neurologic disorder that produces symptoms in the head and neck area. This progressive neurologic disease is characterized by primary demyelination of the white matter with resultant impairment of axonal nerve conduction. This disease occurs primarily in the second and third decades of life and affects women twice as often as men. The classic triad of symptoms (described by Charcot in 1877) includes nystagmus, intention tremor, and dysarthria. While these often present at different periods during the illness, they rarely all present initially. In the head and neck region, virtually every cranial nerve can be affected by MS. Optic neuritis is a frequent ocular finding that can ultimately result in permanent visual impairment. Bilateral internuclear ophthalmoplegia due to demyelination of the medial longitudinal fasciculus is a common presentation of extraocular muscle involvement and is virtually pathognomonic of this disorder. Both muscular symptoms as well as sensory manifestations are often encountered. The imbalance or "dizziness" often described by these patients can occur as a result of vestibular pathology or secondary to cerebellar and/or dorsal column demyelination. Numbness in

the distribution of the trigeminal nerve is a frequent finding and is often fleeting. Emotional lability is also often encountered in patients with MS.

5. An MRI scan should be considered to detect possible focal neurologic abnormalities which might account for this patient's symptoms. An evaluation of cerebrospinal fluid (CSF) would also be very helpful, especially if an inflammatory process were being considered.

TEST INTERPRETATION

- Magnetic resonance imaging (MRI) of brain—Figures 55–1A and B
- CSF analysis
  glucose—normal
  total protein—normal
  cells—1 to 2 mononuclear cells
- CSF protein electrophoresis—elevated immunoglobulin G fraction
- ENG—normal
- Platform posturography—visual and proprioceptive balance deficits
- Audiogram—normal

These test results, in particular the MRI, reveal findings consistent with MS. Central nervous system imaging using MRI is currently the most sensitive and specific test available to establish this diagnosis. Plaques of demyelination in the white matter (Fig. 55–1A) and at the cerebellopontine area (Fig. 55–1B) can be easily identified, and correlate with this patient's clinical symptom complex.

The findings on the examination of CSF are also completely consistent with this diagnosis. Prior to MRI, this was the most common definitive laboratory test available to aid in diagnosing MS.

While the ENG is normal, this is often the case in MS. The classic finding of internuclear ophthalmoplegia is usually only seen during periods where ocular symptoms such as diplopia are manifested. On the other hand, the abnormal results of the platform posturography probably explain the imbalance this patient has been experiencing. These findings are

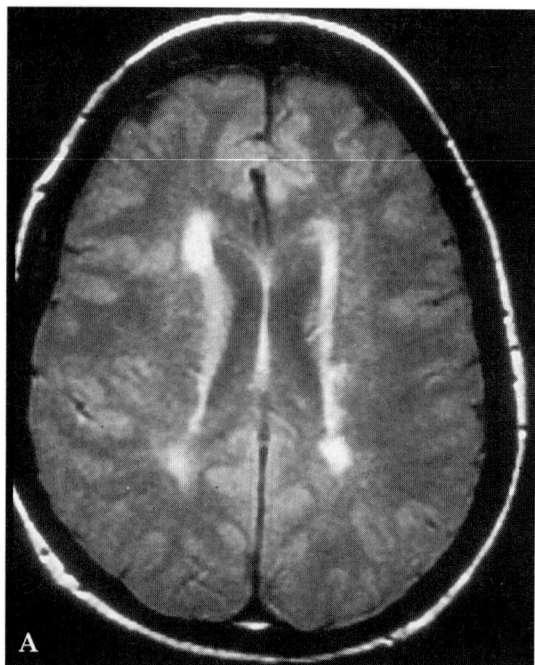

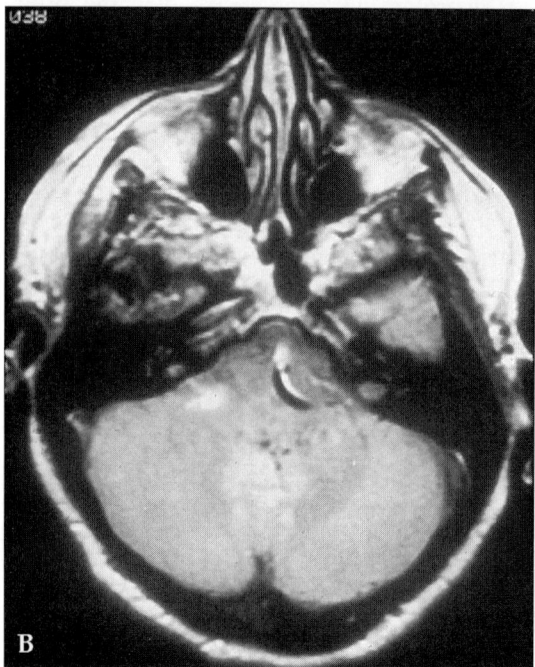

FIGURE 55-1 MRI demonstrates plaques of demyelination in the white matter (A) and at the cerebellopontine area (B).

completely consistent with the diagnosis of MS.

Although the audiogram is normal and this patient does not complain of auditory symptoms, auditory brain stem response testing can be abnormal in these patients. An even more sensitive evoked response test that if often performed on these patients is the visual evoked response, which can be abnormal in a high proportion of patients with active MS.

DIAGNOSIS

Multiple sclerosis.

MEDICAL MANAGEMENT

The medical management of MS is primarily symptomatic. While drugs have generally not been successful in reversing or slowing the progress of this disorder, interferon β-1b has been used experimentally and may show some promise in reducing the frequency or severity of exacerbations. Muscular spasticity, dysphagia, and respiratory compromise can all ultimately result from MS progression and deserve individual management as indicated. Loss of bladder control with the need for chronic or intermittent catheterization can ultimately lead to urinary sepsis.

Due to the progressive nature of this disease, often occurring in an otherwise healthy young adult, the social and psychologic aspects of the disease can be profound. Patients with MS often display emotional lability, depression, and occasionally frank psychosis. These aspects of their condition must always be kept in mind during the evaluation and management so that the patient's emotional status can be understood and effectively managed when appropriate.

SURGICAL MANAGEMENT

Other than in the long-term supportive care of these patients, surgery plays little role. When laryngotracheal aspiration begins to result from dysphagia and poor laryngeal protective reflexes, tracheotomy may be necessary. While often not able to prevent aspiration, it can provide a means to maximize pulmonary toilet. In severe end-stage disease when aspiration becomes massive and uncontrollable, laryngotracheal separation may become an important surgical alternative.

REHABILITATION AND FOLLOW-UP

While the initial diagnosis is often entertained and established by the otolaryngologist, the long-term care and management of these patients is usually best provided by internal medicine or rehabilitative medicine specialists.

SUGGESTED READINGS

BOUCHER RM, HENDRIX RA. The otolaryngic manifestations of multiple sclerosis. *ENT J.* 1991; 70(4):224–233.

GARFINKEL TJ, KIMMELMAN CP. Neurologic disorders: amyotrophic lateral sclerosis, myasthenia gravis, multiple sclerosis, and poliomyelitis. *Am J Otolaryngol.* 1982;3:204–212.

LUBLIN FD, WHITAKER JN, EIDELMAN BH, et al. Management of patients receiving interferon beta-1b for multiple sclerosis: report of a consensus conference. *Neurology.* 1996;46(1):12–18.

NEAL GD, CLARK LR. Neuromuscular disorders. *Otolaryngol Clin North Am.* 1987;20(1):195–201.

Case 56

SJÖGREN'S SYNDROME

Thomas A. Tami, M.D.

HISTORY

A 62-year-old woman complains of difficulty swallowing for the past 12 to 15 months. She notes that her mouth always seems very dry and that certain foods such as soda crackers and dry bread stick in her throat requiring large amounts of water to complete the swallow. She has no voice symptoms, no aspiration, and no symptoms of gastroesophageal reflux.

During the review of systems she also describes a very dry nose and dry eyes, and has been using moisturizing eye drops for the past year. She has severe arthritic pain in her hands, fingers, and knees which has been controlled with high dose ibuprofen. She also has mild hypertension, which is controlled with hydrochlorothiazide.

On physical examination, the upper aerodigestive tract is unremarkable except that her oral and pharyngeal mucous membranes are dry and atrophic and she has several untreated dental caries. Her parotid glands are mildly hypertrophic, but symmetric. Shirmer's tests are performed, blood work is ordered, and a tissue biopsy is obtained.

DIFFERENTIAL DIAGNOSIS— KEY POINTS

1. This patient's primary symptom, dysphagia, seems to be secondary to xerostomia. There is no clinical evidence of other problems, such as an underlying neurologic disorder, an obstructive lesion of the pharynx or esophagus, or gastroesophageal reflux disease.

2. Any of the following are possible etiologies of xerostomia:
   a. Primary disorders of the salivary glands can produce this disorder. These include chronic sialoadenitis, granulomatous disorders such as sarcoidosis, radiation-induced inflammation, HIV infection, and Sjogren's syndrome.

   b. Fluid and electrolyte disorders such as those induced by diabetes, dehydration, and diuretics can also produce xerostomia.
   c. Certain other medications have also been implicated. These include antihistamines, decongestants, antidepressants, and antihypertensives.
   d. Systemic disorders such as hypothyroidism, anorexia/bulimia, alcoholism, and malnutrition can also be associated with xerostomia.
   e. External beam radiation therapy to the head and neck is a common etiology of this problem.

3. In this case, several of the above possible etiologies should be considered. Her symptoms could be secondary to the use of hydrochlorothiazide. Also, the possibility of diabetes should be pursued by obtaining a fasting blood glucose. While HIV-related xerostomia might be reasonably excluded given her low-risk profile, an HIV test might be considered. Primary salivary gland disorders such as sarcoidosis and Sjögren's must also be included and could be diagnosed by salivary glands biopsy.

4. Associated arthritis symptoms makes Sjögren's syndrome a distinct possibility in this case. The average age of onset of Sjögren's is approximately 50 years, occurring much more commonly in women than men (10:1). Primary Sjögren's syndrome is defined as xerostomia and xerophthalmia due to primary chronic inflammation of the salivary and lacrimal glands. Secondary Sjögren's syndrome refers to inflammation of these glands, in association with another rheumatologic or autoimmune disorder, most commonly rheumatoid arthritis.

TEST INTERPRETATION

Laboratory tests should be used to exclude other etiologies of this patient's sicca symptoms. Standard electrolyte values and a fasting glucose will exclude diabetes, dehydration, or diuretic effects. Thyroid function testing, specifically thyroid stimulating hormone (TSH) levels, can exclude hypothyroidism. A basic rheumatologic battery including rheumatoid factor (RF), antinuclear antibody, and erythrocyte sedimentation rate (ESR) can help establish this process as either primary or secondary Sjögren's syndrome. Anti-SS-A and anti SS-B are serum autoantibodies to nuclear antigens Ro and La. While the presence of these circulating autoantibodies is not specific to Sjögren's disease, they can be detected in the serum of most patients with this disorder. In this case the following results were obtained:

- Electrolytes (Na$^+$, Cl$^-$, K$^+$, CO$_2^-$, BUN)— normal
- Fasting glucose—normal
- TSH—normal
- ESR—51 mm/sec (normal <20 mm/sec)
- RF—positive
- ANA—negative
- SS-A autoantibody—positive
- SS-B autoantibody—positive

A minor salivary gland biopsy was performed (Fig. 56–1). This is an easy in-office procedure that can often definitively establish the diagnosis of Sjögren's sialoadenitis. Classic findings include lymphocytic inflammation, ductal hyperplasia, and acinar destruction with fibrosis. By counting the number of lymphocytic foci contained in a 4-mm^2 field, the diagnosis of Sjögren's can be established (greater than one per field is characteristic of this disease compared to other sicca-like syndromes). The figure reveals both a low powered as well as a high powered view of a typical minor salivary gland from a patient with Sjögren's. Note the chronic inflammatory infiltrate, especially in the periductal region as seen in the high-powered view (Fig. 56–1B).

DIAGNOSIS

Secondary Sjögren's syndrome.

MEDICAL MANAGEMENT

Initial management of Sjögren's syndrome is based on the presence or absence remaining salivary flow reserve. This can be assessed by performing a formal salivary flow test or by placing citric acid or other acidic stimuli in the mouth and observing the presence or absence of saliva. When reserve flow exists, treatment can be directed at stimulating the remaining tissue to produce endogenous saliva.

Sialagogues such as acid or bitter tasting substances can help stimulate residual saliva production. Mechanical stimulation such as gum chewing can also be a potent stimulus. Pharmacologic sialogogues are also available. Pilocarpine has been used successfully in patients with xerostomia and although objective improvement has not been demonstrated, sub-

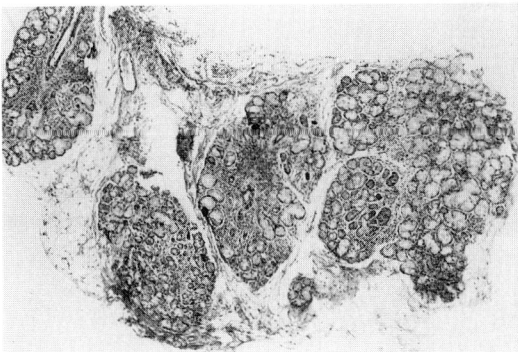
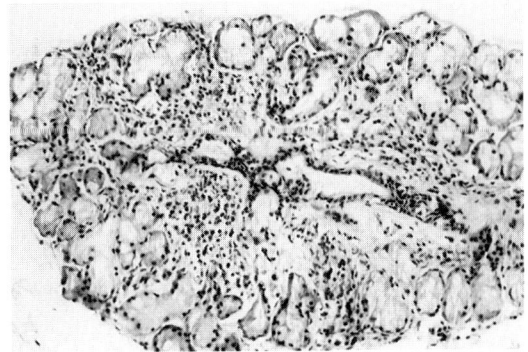

A   B

FIGURE 56–1 A minor salivary gland biopsy. (A) Low power. (B) High power.

jective improvement in the sensation of dryness is usually reported.

SURGICAL MANAGEMENT

Other than to perform a biopsy to diagnose Sjögren's syndrome, surgery rarely plays a role in this disease. Occasionally patients will develop massive enlargement of the parotid glands (Mikulicz syndrome). In these instances, superficial parotidectomy is occasionally considered, primarily for cosmetic reasons. Since some reports describe as much as 5% incidence of lymphoproliferative disorders in Sjögren's patients who have persistently enlarged parotid glands, surgical excision may be indicated if a suspicious sudden enlargement or change of the parotid glands occurs.

REHABILIATION AND FOLLOW-UP

Xerostomia is a life long problem for patients with Sjögren's syndrome. In addition to being tremendously inconvenient, other long-term sequelae must also be considered. Because prolonged xerostomia can produce severe dental and periodontal disease, good dental hygiene with frequent oral examinations is important. Custom trays for fluoride application are often useful for maximal dental protection.

Xerophthalmia is an even more important feature in these patients. Liberal use of saline eye drops or other moisturizing techniques can prevent exposure keratitis. Frequent ophthalmologic evaluations should be scheduled to monitor for sicca induced keratitis.

Since secondary Sjögren's syndrome is often part of another rheumatologic disorder, a search for an underlying disease process such as rheumatoid arthritis or systemic lupus erythematosus is extremely important, even if not immediately obvious. A rheumatologist is often a valuable resource for the medical evaluation and management of the underlying disease.

SUGGESTED READINGS

Atkinson JC, Wu AJ. Salivary gland dysfunction: causes, symptoms, treatment. *J Am Dent Assoc.* 1994;125(4):409–416.

Batsakis JG. The pathology of head and neck tumors: the lymphoepithelial lesions and Sjögren's syndrome, part 16. *Head Neck Surg.* 1982;2:150.

Daniels TE. Benign lymphoepithelial lesions and Sjögren's syndrome. In: Ellis GL, Auclair PL, Gnepp DR, eds. *Surgical Pathology of the Salivary Glands.* Philadelphia, PA: WB Saunders; 1991:Chapter 6.

Johnson JT, Pitman. Xerostomia: current management and treatment. *Curr Opin Otolaryngol Head Neck Surg.* 1996;4(3):200–204.

St. Clair E, St. Clair EW. New developments in Sjögren's syndrome. *Curr Opin Rheumatol.* 1993; 5(5):604–612.

Wise CM, Woodruff RD. Minor salivary gland biopsies in patients investigated for primary Sjögren's syndrome. A review of 187 patients. *J Rheumatol.* 1993;20(9):1515–1518.

PEDIATRIC

AIRWAY FOREIGN BODY   J. Paul Willging, M.D.

HISTORY

An 18-month-old child was noted to choke and gag when playing behind the family couch. He was not directly under observation at the time of the choking spell. The family immediately came to the aid of the child. There was no cyanosis or stridor noted by the family, but they took him to an emergency room for evaluation. No abnormalities were noted on physical examination, and the child was released. No studies were obtained. Thirty-six hours later, the child developed stridor, and presented to a different hospital for further evaluation. A neck x-ray was obtained that showed a metalic laryngeal foreign body (Fig. 57–1).

The child was examined and found to have audible biphasic stridor. His respirations were regular, and his skin color was pink. He was in no acute distress, but was restless. Breath sounds were equal in all lung fields. His airway symptoms worsened when he was placed in a supine position. The remainder of his examination was not contributory.

DIFFERENTIAL DIAGNOSIS— KEY POINTS

1. Stridor in a child that occurs suddenly may be of an acute infectious nature such as epiglottitis. If a prodrome is present where there is gradual worsening of symptoms, croup or bacterial tracheitis must be considered.

2. Foreign bodies must always be considered in the pediatric population, and stridor is common in fixed obstructions on the larynx or trachea. Foreign bodies of the larynx and trachea have the ability to obstruct the airway completely, and are associated with the highest morbidity. Chronic esophageal foreign bodies may also cause airway compression by irritating the common wall between the trachea and esophagus. The ingestion need not be witnessed, frequently the object is placed into the mouth out of sight of the caregivers. The mortality rate for foreign bodies in the upper aerodigestive tract is approximately 2%, accounting for 3,000 deaths per year in the United States. The mortality rate varies with the site of impaction, as well as the duration the foreign body has been in place. Laryngeal foreign bodies have the highest mortality rate, approaching 45%.

3. Stridor that begins suddenly at the age of 18 months is unlikely to be an intrinsic structural problem associated with the larynx.

TEST INTERPRETATION

Findings on physical examination reflect the location of the object within the tracheobronchial tree. Most signs are subtle. Differences in the breath sounds heard on each side of the chest are the most significant physical finding and suggest a bronchial foreign body. Chest auscultation will often show unilateral wheezing, cough, and ipsilateral decreased breath sounds, but this will occur in less than 50% of the cases. A prolonged inspiratory or expiratory phase of respiration is also consistent with a distal airway foreign body.

The initial evaluation of the airway is a high KV PA/LAT neck and chest x-ray. This allows identification of the structural elements of the airway and identification of radioopaque foreign bodies in the airway. The lung fields can also be evaluated for signs of postobstructive emphysema. If a foreign body is ballvalving into the left mainstem bronchus, there could be airtrapping and hyperinflation of the lung field on that side, and mediastinal structures will shift to the right. Conversely, a completely obstructed left mainstem bronchus could lead to widespread atelectasis and col-

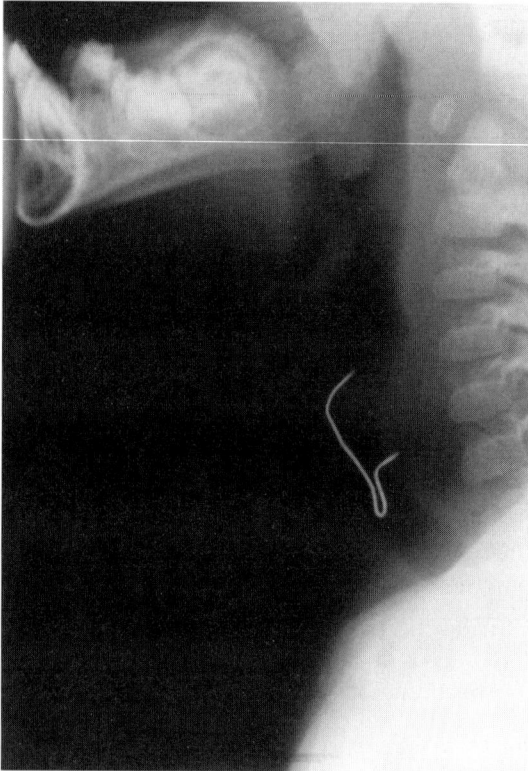

FIGURE 57-1 Lateral neck x-ray with metallic foreign body within the larynx.

lapse of the left lung, with mediastinal shift to the left.

When doubt arises as to the presence of a radiolucent foreign body in the distal airway, decubitus films and airway fluoroscopy can be of assistance in determining the presence of an object in the airway. In a left lateral decubitus view, one expects the left (down) lung volume to be compressed. If the lung remains inflated, this suggests a foreign body within the mainstem bronchus, which is obstructing free airflow. Fluoroscopy allows the movements of the diaphram and mediastinum to be visualized. Asymmetric motion of the diaphram and lung fields suggests obstruction to airflow within that lung field.

The definitive test with respect to the identification of an aerodigestive tract foreign body is direct endoscopy. Endoscopic evaluation with rigid telescopes allows proper evaluation of the entire aerodigestive system and the means of removal of any foreign body that may be present. There is no substitution for evaluation of

the airway under general anesthesia anytime the question of a foreign body has been raised. The onus of proof is on the surgeon to prove there is no foreign body in the airway.

DIAGNOSIS

Bronchial foreign body, identified by the family as a carpet staple.

MEDICAL MANAGEMENT

While in the emergency room the child was spontaneously breathing and able to maintain respiration without intervention. In the transportation of the child to the operating room suite, all equipment necessary to establish an artificial airway must be immediately available. Great care must be exercised to prevent undue agitation of the child, which may significantly compromise his airway. When general anesthesia is induced, the airway may be unstable and mask ventilation or intubation may not be possible. Endoscopic equipment as well as tracheotomy instruments needed to be opened and immediately available for use. Emergent tracheotomy would be used if needed to secure the airway distal to the laryngeal obstruction.

SURGICAL MANAGEMENT

The ability to extract the staple from the larynx endoscopically was a concern due to the double points of the object. Optical foreign body forceps were used to practice on a similarly shaped object prior to the induction of anesthesia to gain familiarization with the best means of manipulating the object for removal from the larynx.

This child underwent mask induction of general anesthesia. Endoscopic evaluation of the larynx demonstrated one tip of the staple resting on the posterior aspect of the left vocal cord (Fig. 57–2), while the other end of the staple was embedded in the common wall between the trachea and the esophagus (Fig. 57–3). Manipulation of the staple could not allow the lower point to be removed from the posterior tracheal wall. Due to the potential of inducing laryngeal edema secondary to the manipula-

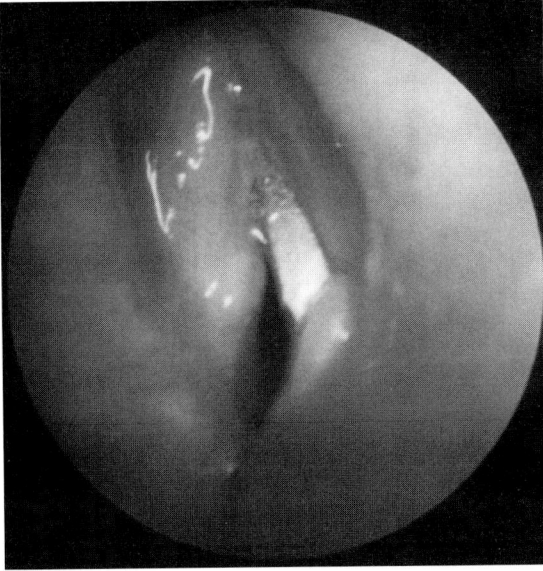

FIGURE 57-2 Endoscopic view of the larynx with a foreign body seen between the vocal folds.

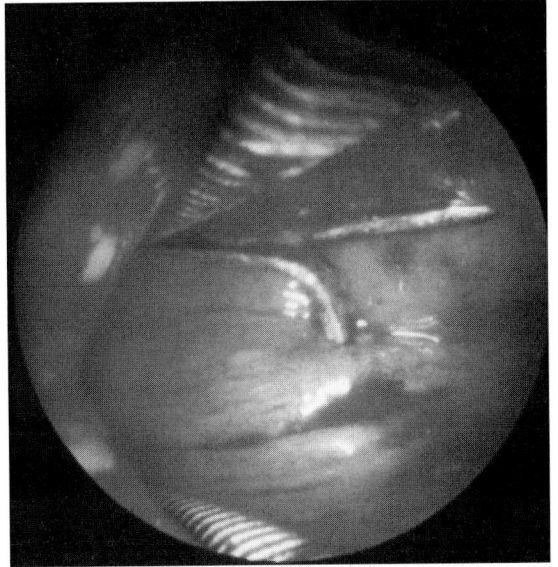

FIGURE 57-4 View of the carpet staple through an incision in the anterior trachea wall. The staple has embedded into the posterior tracheal wall.

tions of the laryngeal foreign body, a 2.0 endotracheal tube was passed around the staple to secure the airway. A tracheotomy was then performed which provided access for extraction of the object from the airway (Fig. 57–4). The cricoid cartilage did not need to be divided. The endotracheal tube was then changed to one of

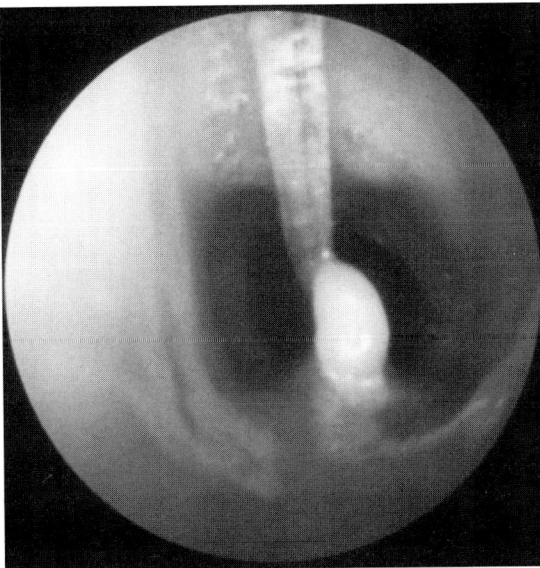

FIGURE 57-3 Inferior extent of the foreign body within the trachea.

an appropriate size for the child's age, and the trachea was closed. The child was left intubated for 48 hours after which the child was observed for an additional 72 hours prior to discharge home. No complications developed postoperatively.

Airway foreign bodies post a challenge to the surgeon. All equipment must be assembled and ready for use before induction so as to be able to intervene should airway difficulties develop. Foreign bodies may be impacted at the level of the larynx, trachea, or bronchus. Complete airway obstruction is possible in all these areas. Extraction techniques often vary according to the site of obstruction.

Rigid ventilating telescopic bronchoscopes are the current standard of care for pediatric airway foreign body extraction. Optical extraction forceps are used to manipulate and extract the foreign body. An assortment of instruments must be available to allow optimal control of a variety of aspirated objects. Occasionally a foreign body may be impacted in a bronchus and it may not be possible to pass the extraction forceps around the object. Fogarty embolectomy catheters are small enough to be passed alongside the foreign body. The balloon can then be inflated (carefully so as not to overdistend the bronchus) and the foreign body can then be pulled into the foreign body forceps.

A foreign body may be encountered that cannot be extracted from the airway due to either the size or the shape of the object. Some objects cannot be grasped, others are too large to be pulled through the glottis with foreign body forceps engaged. In these cases, one must not hesitate to perform a tracheotomy to gain adequate access to the airway for its removal. Impacted distal foreign bodies or chronic foreign bodies that have generated much granulation tissue in the airway may require a thoracotomy for their removal.

The key to successful management of airway foreign bodies is a high index of suspicion. The difficulty of extraction and the complication rates associated with airway foreign bodies increase dramatically when their duration extends beyond 72 hours. Early diagnosis and timely removal are essential to satisfactory resolution of these life-threatening events.

REHABILITATION AND FOLLOW-UP

When the airway problem has been adequately addressed and successfully managed, no long-term follow-up is necessary. Parent education is an important component of preventing recurrent airway aspirations.

SUGGESTED READINGS

BANERJEE A, RAO KS, KHANNA SK, et al. Laryngo-tracheo-bronchial foreign bodies in children. *J Laryngol Otol.* 1988;102:1029–1032.

HOLINGER LD. Management of sharp and penetrating foreign bodies of the upper aerodigestive tract. *Ann Otol Rhinol Laryngol.* 1990;99:684–688.

LIMA JA. Laryngeal foreign bodies in children: a persistent, life-threatening problem. *Laryngoscope.* 1989; 99:415–420.

McGUIRT WF, HOLMES KD, FEEHS R, BROWNE JD. Tracheobronchial foreign bodies. *Laryngoscope.* 1988; 98:615–618.

MOFENSON HC, GREENSHER J. Management of the choking child. *Pediatr Clin North Am.* 1985;32:183–192.

MU L, HE P, SUN D. Inhalation of foreign bodies in Chinese children: a review of 400 cases. *Laryngoscope.* 1991;101:657–660.

MU LC, SUN DQ, HE P. Radiological diagnosis of aspirated foreign bodies in children: review of 343 cases. *J Laryngol Otol.* 1990;104:778–782.

REILLY JS. Prevention of aspiration in infants and young children: federal regulations. *Ann Otol Rhinol Laryngol.* 1990;99:273–276.

SVEDSTROM E, PUHAKKA H, KERO P. How accurate is chest radiography in the diagnosis of tracheobronchial foreign bodies in children? *Pediatr Radiol.* 1989;19:520–522.

SVENSSON G. Foreign bodies in the tracheobronchial tree. Special references to experience in 97 children. *Int J Pediatr Otorhinolaryngol.* 1985;8:243–251.

BRANCHIAL ARCH ANOMALY

Mark E. Gerber, M.D.
J. Paul Willging, M.D.

HISTORY

A 5-year-old female presented to an otolaryngologist with intermittent drainage from a pit in her left neck that would occur simultaneously with drainage from the left ear. There was no history of previous otitis media, hearing loss, or other systemic illness.

Physical examination revealed two pits in the skin. One anterior to the left sternocleidomastoid at the level of the angle of the mandible, and a second in the anteroinferior aspect of the cartilaginous external auditory canal. Digital pressure between the two caused the release of mucoid material from both orifices. Facial nerve function was intact and symmetric. The ipsilateral tympanic membrane and the remainder of her head and neck examination were normal.

DIFFERENTIAL DIAGNOSIS— KEY POINTS

1. Branchial anomalies are a common cause of congenital neck masses. Anomalies related to branchial arch development include cysts, sinuses, and fistulae. Cysts have a mucosal or epithelial lining and no external opening, and arise from embryologic rests trapped within developing tissue. Sinuses and fistulae arise from incomplete closure of branchial pouches and clefts, with a sinus having one communication, and a fistula tract having two openings.

2. In 1972, Work classified first branchial anomalies into types I and II based on their histology and location. Type I first branchial anomalies are ectoderm-derived duplications of the membranous external auditory canal that are lined by squamous epithelium. The sinus or fistula tracts are usually located lateral to the facial nerve in the postauricular region

and can extend medial and anterior to the external auditory canal. Type II first branchial anomalies are ectoderm- and mesoderm-derived duplications of the external auditory canal and auricle that can contain adenexa and cartilage in addition to a squamous epithelial lining. These lesions are more common, and often present with sinus or fistula tracts opening into the concha or external auditory canal, with an additional opening along the lower border of the mandible at the anterior border of the sternocleidomastoid muscle (Fig. 58–1). Their tract can pass medial or lateral to the facial nerve (Fig. 58–2).

3. The vast majority of branchial anomalies are classified as second branchial anomalies. Second branchial sinus or fistula tracts begin anterior to the sternocleidomastoid muscle and course between the internal and external carotid arteries, above both the glossopharyngeal and hypoglossal nerves and enter the pharynx in the region of the tonsillar fossa. A second branchial anomaly is three times more likely to be a cyst than a sinus or fistula, and can be located anywhere along its course.

4. Third branchial anomalies are rare. They are located along the anterior border of the sternocleidomastoid muscle and pass posterior to the great vessels and inferior to the glossopharyngeal nerve and superior to the hypoglossal nerves. Third branchial sinus or fistula tracts may enter the pharynx at the level of the pyriform sinus.

5. Theoretically, a fourth branchial anomaly would course from the apex of the pyriform sinus, inferior to the superior laryngeal nerve, loop around the subclavian artery on the right (the aortic arch on the left), and continue superiorly in the neck just posterior to the common carotid artery to end along the anterior border of the sternocleidomastoid mus-

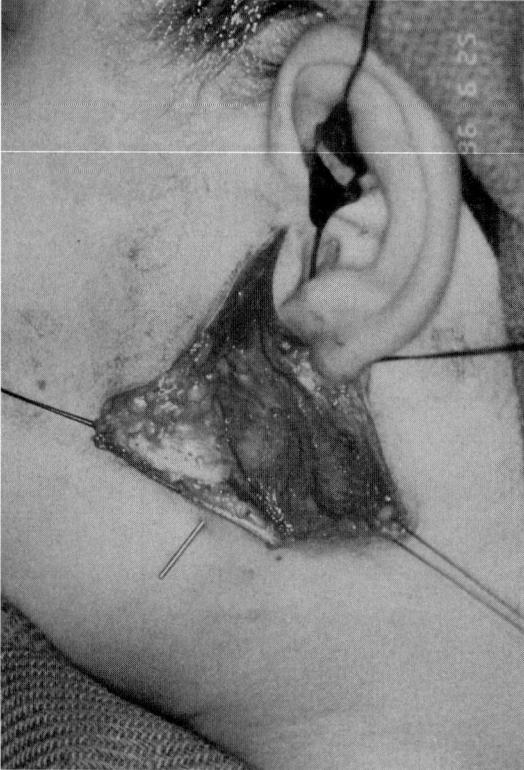

FIGURE 58-1 Skin flap is elevated up to the ramus of the mandible until the facial nerve is identified.

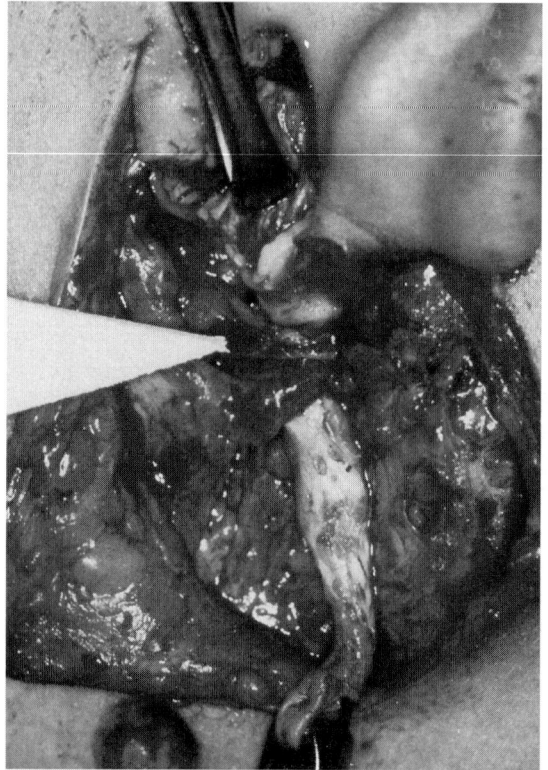

FIGURE 58-2 The facial nerve (white arrow) is lying superficial to the fistula tract.

cle. Fourth branchial anomalies can terminate in the perithyroid space or cervical esophagus, causing perithyroid space abscesses or recurrent lateral or retropharyngeal space abscesses. No true fourth branchial fistulae have been documented.

TEST INTERPRETATION

Radiographic evaluation of a lateral neck mass suspected of being a branchial anomaly is not always required. However, computed tomography (CT) or magnetic resonance imaging (MRI) may assist in the evaluation of lateral neck masses. On CT, a branchial cyst will be homogeneous with low attenuation in the central region with a smooth enhancing rim, and intravenous contrast will aid in identifying its course in relation to the great vessels. MRI will demonstrate a low T1- and high T2-weighted signal. A barium esophagram can be used to look for a possible

branchial sinus or fistula in the evaluation of recurrent pharyngeal or perithyroid abscesses.

DIAGNOSIS

First branchial anomaly, Work's type II.

MEDICAL MANAGEMENT

When there is evidence of acute infection, surgical excision is delayed and antimicrobial therapy that includes coverage against *Staphylococcus aureus* is initiated. Needle aspiration and possibly incision and drainage need to be considered when there is evidence of suppuration. Surgical excision should proceed shortly after resolution of an acute infection to avoid the increased scarring and fibrosis that occur with repeated infections, making the surgical approach more difficult.

SURGICAL MANAGEMENT

Management of a first branchial fistula requires complete surgical excision. Because of the close association of the tract and the facial nerve, the surgical approach needs to include preparation for facial nerve identification and protection. In adults, the mastoid tip, styloid process, cartilaginous pointer, and tympanomastoid suture line are the principal guides to the main trunk of the facial nerve. However, in children, the extra-temporal facial nerve is more superficially located, and while the same surgical landmarks for locating the nerve are present as in the adult, they are much less developed. Therefore, the approach to identification of the facial nerve is altered in children. Instead of the modified face-life incision that is used in adults, a curvilinear incision is made 1.5 to 2.0 cm below the mandible, extending in a skin crease over the mastoid and ending 1.0 to 2.0 cm behind the postauricular crease. The skin flap is elevated in a subplatysmal plane only up to the ramus of the mandible until the facial nerve trunk is identified (Fig. 58–1). The facial nerve is found in the triangular space formed by the anterior border of the sternocleidomastoid muscle, the cartilaginous ear canal, and posterior belly of the digastric muscle. (Fig. 58–2).

Because of the differences in the facial nerve anatomic landmarks used in infants, there is some controversy as to timing of excision of first branchial arch anomalies that are identified in infants. Some have argued that waiting until there is enough growth to utilize the adult landmarks will make identification of the nerve easier. However, the trade-off is that observation for a long period increases the risk of infection with subsequent fibrosis, making dissection more difficult. In general, it is prudent to wait until approximately age 2 when the mastoid tip and the facial nerve will both be larger, allowing for easier identification. However, at this age the facial nerve is still more superficial necessitating the approach given earlier as described by Farrior and Santini in 1985.

When the tract involves the cartilaginous external auditory canal, the cartilage and overlying skin are excised along with the tract. Any portion of the tract that enters the temporal bone or middle ear through the tympanic membrane can be amputated and resected separately with curettage of the bone if needed. If there is significant involvement of the external auditory canal, packing for 3 to 4 weeks may be needed to avoid subsequent stenosis.

REHABILITATION AND FOLLOW-UP

The rate of recurrence for resection of branchial anomalies is less than 5% when there is no history of prior surgery or infection. When the procedure is complicated by prior surgery or infection, the recurrence rate can be as high as 20%. Permanent injury to the facial nerve is rare when first branchial anomalies are approached in a systematic fashion.

SUGGESTED READINGS

FARRIOR JB, SANTINI H. Facial nerve identification in children. *Otolaryngol Head Neck Surg.* 1985;93:173–176.

FINN DG, BUCHALTER IH, SARTI E, ROMO T, CHODOSH P. First branchial cleft cysts: clinical update. *Laryngoscope.* 1987;97:136–140.

MYER CM III. Congenital neck masses. In: Shumrick DA, Gluckman JL, Myerhoff WL, eds. *Otolaryngology.* Philadelphia, PA: WB Saunders; 1991:2535–2543.

WORK W. Newer concepts of first branchial cleft defects. *Laryngoscope.* 1974;82:1581–1593

LYMPHANGIOMA

J. Paul Willging, M.D.

HISTORY

A 23-year-old $P_1G_1A_0$ woman in her 38th week of pregnancy, is in spontaneous labor that cannot be arrested. A previous neonatal ultrasound shows a fetus with a large cervicofacial mass, estimated to be 30% of the fetal weight (Fig. 59–1). Polyhydramnios is also present. The obstetrician is planning to deliver the baby through a cesarean section and would like to have otolaryngology present in the delivery room should any problem develop at the time of delivery. The mass on ultrasound extends from the skull base to the upper mediastinum and is partially compressing the trachea.

DIFFERENTIAL DIAGNOSIS— KEY POINTS

1. The differential diagnosis of a congenital cervicofacial mass is limited to teratoma, neuroblastoma, lymphangioma, and arteriovenous malformation. Regardless of the precise diagnosis of the mass, the initial approach to the airway will be the same for all tumors.

2. The mother and neonate have specific needs in the obstetrical facility that must be met. While the mother's medical condition and associated complication risk are standard, one must be prepared to deal with the potential catastrophic complication that may develop in association with any delivery. A medical team that will not become distracted with events developing in the care of the newborn must be dedicated to the management of the mother.

3. The newborn has the potential for complete airway obstruction, necessitating the mechanical securing of the airway. The infant can be maintained with the umbilical cord attached to the mother to prolong oxygenation of the neonate. Because the length of the umbilical

cord is short, all procedures would then need to be performed across the legs of the mother.

4. The anesthetic techniques for delivery should avoid inhalational agents, narcotics, and benzodiazapines, all of which will physiologically depress the neonate as well as the mother. At the time of delivery, the infant should be vigorous with an intact respiratory drive. Many neonates are able to maintain themselves with a marginal airway, but have an uncontrollable airway when sedated or under general anesthesia. An epidural approach to the anesthetic needs of the mother is ideal for maintaining the respiratory drive of the neonate and fulfilling the anesthetic requirements of the mother.

5. The approach to the compromised newborn's aiway must be orderly. If a newborn is spontaneously breathing, an assessment of the degree of airway obstruction needs to be made to determine the need for elective intubation in the delivery room. If the airway is compromised, endotracheal intubation should be attempted. If the endotracheal tube cannot be passed due to a mass compressing the lumen of the trachea (most of these can be overcome with gentle pressure on the endotracheal tube) a rigid bronchoscope can be passed into the airway to offer a method of ventilation. With a bronchoscope in place, a tracheotomy can then be performed in a controlled fashion. If a bronchoscope cannot be passed, a tracheotomy must be immediately performed. If the cervical component of the mass precludes access to the anterior base of the neck, a thoracotomy must be performed to access the mediastinal trachea.

6. The first component of the team required for the management of the neonatal airway includes the otolaryngologist and surgical nurse to handle the endoscopic equipment. Should a tracheotomy be required, a second

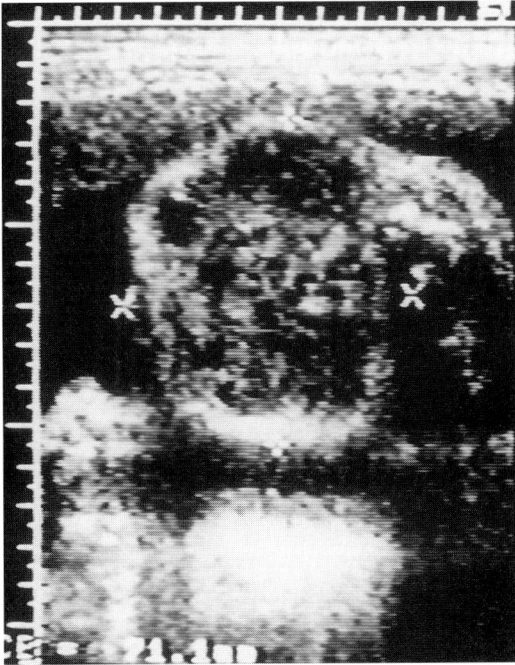

FIGURE 59-1 *In utero* ultrasound of cervicofacial mass. The mass is delineated by the cursors.

surgical nurse should be available to assist with that procedure. A pediatric anesthesiologist should be in attendance to provide for the anesthetic needs of the child. A pediatric surgeon should also be available if concern exists for the need to obtain access to the mediastinal trachea. The team needs to be assembled before the delivery, and all should have their tasks outlined for the intervention of the airway (Figs. 59–2 and 59–3).

TEST INTERPRETATION

Visualization of the mass preoperatively will allow precise surgical planning for excision of the tumor. Ultrasound, computed tomography, or magnetic resonance imaging (MRI) will provide information on the physical characteristics of the mass. An MRI was obtained on this patient to assess the vascularity of the mass, and to obtain tissue differentiation of the mass from normal tissues (Fig. 59–4). Biopsy is rarely required to differentiate the various tumors that arise in the neck.

Physical and radiographic characteristics of the mass allowed determination that the mass was a lymphangioma. Lymphangioma are uncommon malformations of the lymphatic system. Fifty percent of lymphangiomas are located in the head and neck area. Fifty percent of the lesions are apparent in the neonatal period, while 75% of the cases present within the first year of life.

Lymphangioma are divided into three groups based on their morphology. Cystic hygromas contain discrete dilated spaces that respect tissue planes. Lymphangioma simplex is a mass composed of capillary size lymphatics. Cavernous lymphangioma are composed of large dilated lymphatic spaces. Cavernous lymphangioma contain endothelial buds that extend into surrounding tissues, violating tissue planes and infiltrating into adjacent structures. The invasive growth pattern decreases the potential for complete excision. There is no malignant potential for lymphangioma.

DIAGNOSIS

Cavernous lymphangioma of cervical region.

MEDICAL MANAGEMENT

The neonate must be stabilized after the airway is secured, and thoroughly evaluated for associated anomalies. Only after the child is considered stable should surgical excision of the mass be planned. Pulmonary function must be maximized preoperatively or the resection must be delayed until the neonate's pulmonary function has been optimized.

SURGICAL MANAGEMENT

A large cervicofacial lymphangioma should be excised prior to dismissal of the neonate from the hospital. Lymphangiomas do not spontaneously regress, and they frequently increase in size over time. After the child has been stabilized from a pulmonary standpoint, and all examinations looking for associated anomalies and syndromes have been completed, the resection can be performed. This is generally performed after the first week of life.

The blood volume of the newborn is on the

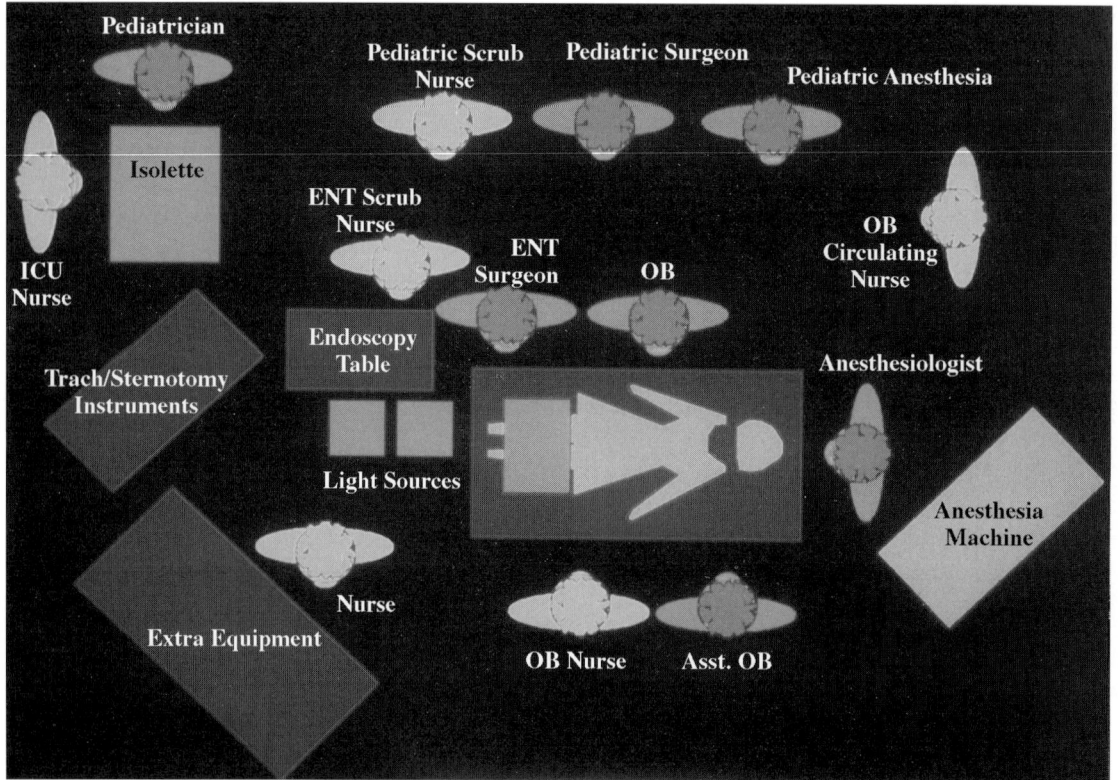

FIGURE 59–2 Diagram of spatial layout of the delivery room. Each team will have access to the patient as the treatment algorithm is followed.

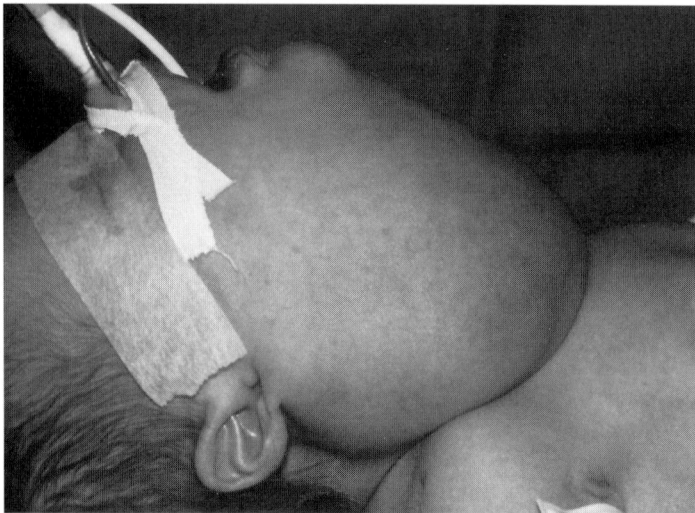

FIGURE 59–3 Newborn with an extensive cervicofacial lymphangioma in the delivery room.

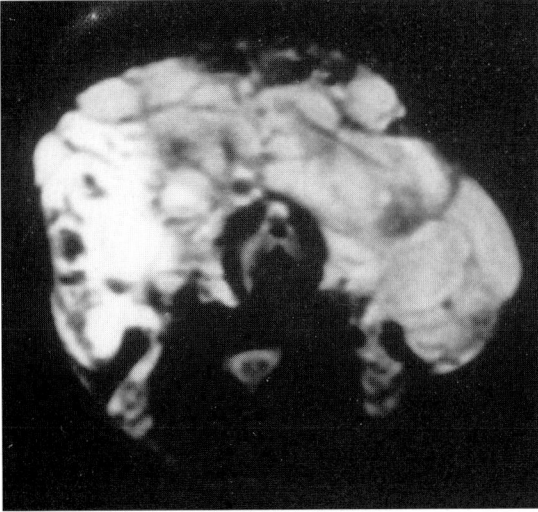

FIGURE 59-4 MRI of the cervicofacial lymphangioma involving bilateral necks, from the skull base to the thorax.

order of 75 cc/kg, making the typical blood volume of a 3-kg neonate approximately 200 cc. Meticulous hemostasis throughout the resection is essential, but despite the best techniques, these neonates will generally require intraoperative transfusions.

The approach to the large cervicofacial lymphangioma is dictated by the extent of the lesion. Unilocular masses can be easily dissected. Infiltrative lesions are resected with the goal of maintaining function. No vital structures should be resected with the mass because lymphangiomas are not malignancies and have no malignant potential. If the lymphangioma is found to be infiltrating into the base of the tongue or lateral pharyngeal wall, the potential for continued growth of the lesion with long-term airway compromise with laryngeal infiltration is high. A tracheotomy may then be required for long-term management of the patient. The airway should always be evaluated, either before or after the resection of a cervicofacial lymphangioma to determine the extent to which the airway is involved with the tumor.

This particular patient was able to breathe spontaneously at birth, but was electively intubated due to the size of the mass and for the potential airway compromise. She underwent excision of the bilateral infiltrating lymphangiomas at 1 week of age. A tracheotomy was performed because of the intense infiltration into the base of tongue, lateral pharyngeal wall, and supraglottic larynx. Residual tumor that causes functional problems will be addressed on a pragmatic basis as she continues to grow (Fig. 59–5).

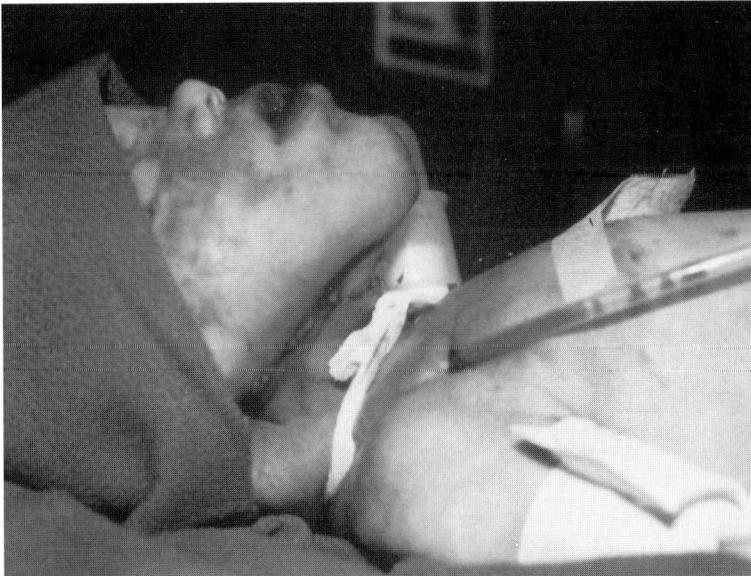

FIGURE 59-5 Postoperative condition of the patient after tracheotomy and resection of the cervicofacial lymphangioma.

REHABILITATION AND FOLLOW-UP

Long-term follow-up of these patients is required. Further resections are based on the location of the persistent disease, the degree to which the recurrent mass becomes symptomatic for the patient, and the degree to which function is impaired. The mere presence of persistent lymphangioma does not necessitate resection.

SUGGESTED READINGS

Barnhart RA, Brown AK Jr. Cystic hygroma of the neck. Report of a case. *Arch Otol.* 1967;86:74–78.

Borecky N, Gudinchet F, Laurini R, et al. Imaging of cervico-thoracic lymphangiomas in children. *Pediatr Radiol.* 1995;25:127–130.

Cohen SR, Thompson JW. Lymphangiomas of the larynx in infants and children. A survey of pediatric lymphangioma. *Ann Otol Rhinol Laryngol.* 1986;127(suppl):1–20.

Filston HC. Hemangiomas, cystic hygromas, and teratomas of the head and neck. *Sem Pediatr Surg.* 1994;3:147–159.

Fonkalsrud EW. Congenital malformations of the lymphatic system. *Sem Pediatr Surg.* 1994;3:62–69.

McCurdy CM, Jr., Seeds JW. Route of delivery of infants with congenital anomalies. *Clin Perinatol.* 1993;20:81–106.

Rothschild MA, Catalano P, Urken M, et al. Evaluation and management of congenital cervical teratoma. Case report and review. *Arch Otolaryngol Head Neck Surg.* 1994;120:444–448.

JUVENILE NASOPHARYNGEAL ANGIOFIBROMA

J. Scott McMurray, M.D.
J. Paul Willging, M.D.

HISTORY

A 14-year-old boy was referred to an otolaryngologist with recurrent self-limiting epistaxis. The epistaxis was spontaneous and usually left sided. He also complained of 6 months of left-sided nasal obstruction. He has had no trauma. He recently had left-sided facial pain and swelling that responded to oral antibiotics. He has had no change in vision or facial sensation. He denied headache.

His medical history was unremarkable. He has no allergies and takes no medication. He has no surgical history.

On physical exam, asymmetry of the left face was noted. His left cheek appeared swollen. It was firm and not tender. His extraocular motion was intact. He had no diplopia. His visual acuity was grossly intact. The other cranial nerves were intact. His oral cavity and oropharynx were unremarkable. He had a fleshy red colored mass in the left nostril, which filled the nasal cavity. The nasal septum was pushed to the right (Fig. 60–1).

DIFFERENTIAL DIAGNOSIS— KEY POINTS

1. The differential diagnosis of a child with a nasal mass includes nasal polyps, nasopharyngeal angiofibroma, hemangiopericytoma, squamous papilloma, inverted papilloma, sinus mucocele, lymphoma, encephalocele, nasal glioma, teratoma, esthesioneuroblastoma, lymphoid hyperplasia, rhabdomyosarcoma, or carcinoma.

2. After benign lymphoid hyperplasia (adenoid hypertrophy), juvenile nasopharyngeal angiofibroma is the most common type of benign nasopharyngeal tumor, accounting for 0.5% of all head and neck tumors. Juvenile nasopharyngeal angiofibroma has a frequency of 1 in 5,000 to 60,000 otolaryngology patients, with the highest occurrence reported in India and Egypt. They most commonly occur in prepubescent boys. Some authors advocate genetic testing if this tumor is found in a phenotypic female.

3. Patients typically present with nasal obstruction and epistaxis. As the tumor progresses, hyponasal speech and cheek and palate deformities may occur. The mass presents as a red, smooth, mucosa-covered compressible mass in the nasal cavity and nasopharynx. Juvenile nasopharyngeal angiofibroma is an aggressive benign vasoformative neoplasm.

4. The embryology of the juvenile nasopharyngeal angiofibroma is still unclear. The most widely accepted theory purports its origin to be from embryonic chondrocartilage during the development of the cranial bones. This explains the site of development of the tumor. The tumor is found at the superior margin of the developing sphenopalatine foramen formed by the trifurcation of the palatine bone, the horizontal ala of the vomer and the root of the pterygoid process. From this location the tumor has easy access to the pterygomaxillary fossa. The tumor may pass into the nasopharynx, the infratemporal fossa or through the skull base intracranially. As the tumor grows, it expands the pterygomaxillary fissure causing anterior bowing of the posterior wall of the maxillary antrum.

TEST INTERPRETATION

The roentgenographic signs thought to be classic for juvenile nasopharyngeal angiofibroma

217

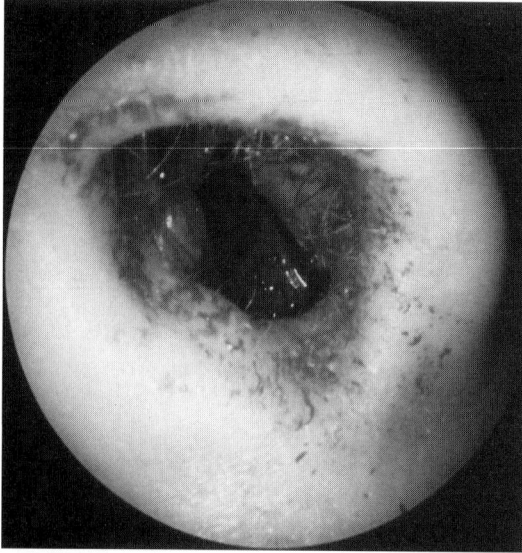

FIGURE 60–1 Clinical photograph of the left nostril of this child at initial presentation. The juvenile nasopharyngeal angiofibroma can be seen at the entrance to the nasal cavity. It is a red, compressible, mucosa-covered mass that fills the nasal cavity.

are (1) a nasopharyngeal mass, (2) anterior bowing of the posterior wall of the maxillary antrum, (3) erosion of the sphenoid bone, (4) erosion of the hard palate, (5) erosion of the medial maxillary sinus, and (6) displacement of the nasal septum. The anterior bowing of the posterior wall of the antrum seen on lateral skull film is known as the Holman–Miller sign and is pathognomonic for juvenile nasopharyngeal angiofibroma.

Computed tomography (CT) with contrast or magnetic resonance imaging (MRI) is helpful for diagnosis and staging. With these imaging studies, the extent of involvement and intracranial extension may be determined. The location and radiographic appearance of the tumor are generally diagnostic.

Biopsy is rarely needed to confirm diagnosis and should be avoided in the office due to the vascular nature of the tumor. The typical histologic appearance is an unencapsulated admixture of vascular tissue and fibrous stroma. The vessel walls lack elastic fibers and have absent or incomplete smooth muscle. This explains the inability of small vessels to contract during injury and the propensity for hemorrhage with minor trauma or biopsy. The cellularity of the

stroma and vessels is benign. There is an abundance of mast cells found in the stroma and a lack of other inflammatory cells (Figs. 60–2A and B).

Several staging systems have been created and modified to describe juvenile nasopharyngeal angiofibroma. Most are based on the extent and location of the tumor. The staging system of Sessions is the most widely used for juvenile angiofibroma. (Table 60–1).

This child's CT scan reveals a massive nasopharyngeal tumor extending from the pterygomaxillary fissure intranasally, causing bowing of the nasal septum and invasion of the infratemporal fossa (Figs. 60–3A and B). This CT scan demonstrates the CT analog of Holman–Miller's sign, expansion of the pterygomaxillary fissure, and anterior bowing of the posterior wall of the antrum. This is pathognomonic for juvenile nasopharyngeal angiofibroma. This tumor extends from the nasal cavity through the pterygomaxillary fissure to the infratemporal fossa. There is also extension into the posterior ethmoid sinuses and the sphenoid sinus. The medial wall of the cavernous sinus has been eroded and the optic nerve and cavernous carotid artery are intimately associated with the tumor. Generally, juvenile nasopharyngeal angiofibroma does not aggressively invade intracranial structures but erodes bone and displaces the meninges. Intracranial extension is important to determine, however, because it greatly affects treatment.

DIAGNOSIS

Juvenile nasopharyngeal angiofibroma, stage IIIA.

MEDICAL MANAGEMENT

Hormonal regulation has been reported in the literature with two case reports using androgen and two case reports using estrogen therapy with marked reduction in tumor size. Receptors for estrogen, progesterone, and androgens are, however, inconsistently found in juvenile nasopharyngeal angiofibroma. The testosterone receptor blocker flutamide reduced stage I and II tumors by an average of 44%. The use of hor-

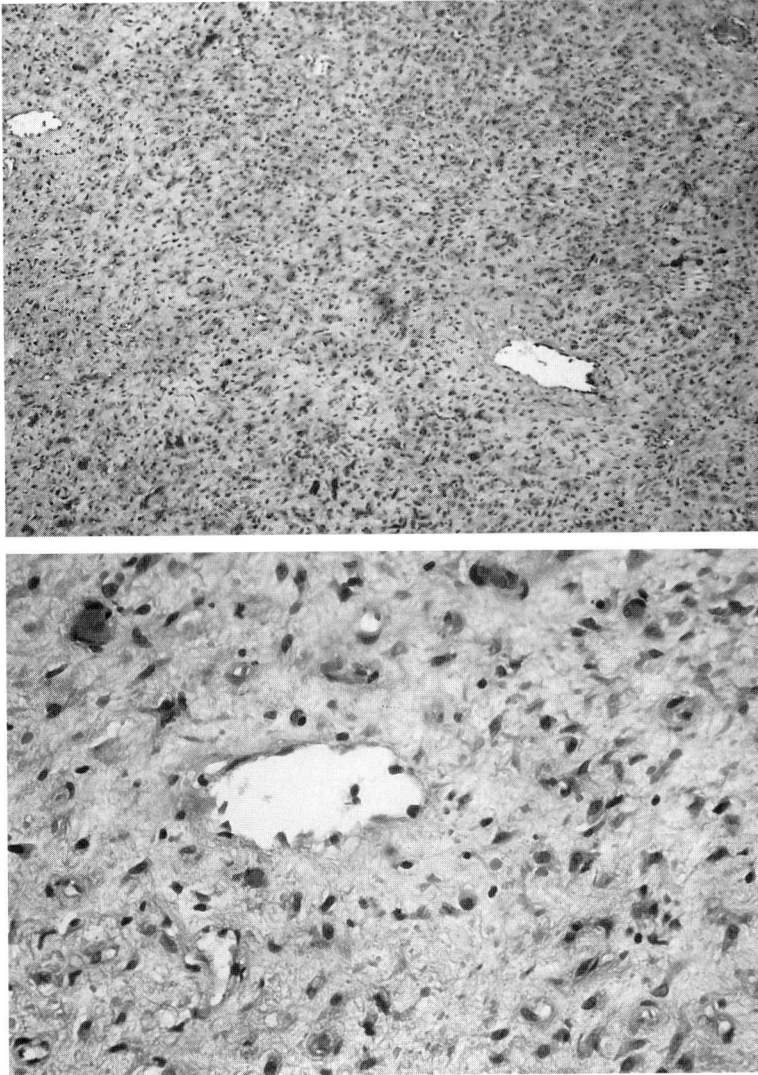

FIGURE 60–2 Photomicrograph of the juvenile nasopharyngeal angiofibroma. (A) An H&E stain at 10×. It shows the mixed stroma and vascular components. The cellularity is benign. The stroma is composed of fibrous tissue with coarse and fine collagen fibers. (B) (H&E; 40×) The thin-walled vascular channel with an absence of smooth muscle. Mast cells are abundant in the myxomatous stroma.

monal therapy has been limited, however, because of hormonal side effects and a variable response to treatment.

Reports of dramatic tumor shrinkage from low-dose external beam radiation have been seen in tumors that are intimately associated with vital structures. The time to maximal effect from radiotherapy can be 12 months to 36 months, however. Some have also proposed that a small asymptomatic nongrowing tumor is adequately controlled. Cummings reported a se-

ries of 55 patients with juvenile nasopharyngeal angiofibroma (stage IIb and greater) of which 42 were treated with primary radiotherapy. Low-dose radiotherapy, 3,000 to 3,500 cGy, achieved tumor control in 44 of these patients (80%), although the exact stage of the irradiated tumors was not reported. A second course of radiotherapy achieved tumor control in 94% of patients. Radiotherapy is not a completely benign treatment, however. Cummings also reported two patients in his series who developed cancer a

TABLE 60–1 Staging of Juvenile Nasopharyngeal Angiofibroma Based on the System Developed by Sessions et al (6)

Stage IA: Tumor limited to the posterior nares and/or nasopharyngeal vault.

Stage IB: Tumor involving the posterior nares and/or nasopharyngeal vault with involvement of at least one paranasal sinus.

Stage IIA: Minimal lateral extension into the pterygomaxillary fossa.

Stage IIB: Full occupation of the pterygomaxillary fossa with or without superior erosion of orbital bones.

Stage IIIA: Erosion of the base of skull (middle cranial fossa/base of pterygoid)—minimal intracranial extension.

Stage IIIB: Extensive intracranial extension with or without extension into the cavernous sinus.

decade after treatment. One patient developed a mixed follicular-papillary carcinoma of the thyroid and another patient developed a basal cell carcinoma of the face. Interestingly, the patient with the basal cell carcinoma of the face also developed hypopituitarism and a cataract. The use of radiotherapy either preoperatively when vital structures are involved to reduce tumor size or postoperatively to help in the management of recurrence is important to consider in large juvenile nasopharyngeal angiofibroma. The risks of radiotherapy must also be considered, however.

SURGICAL MANAGEMENT

The preferred management for juvenile nasopharyngeal angiofibroma is complete surgical extirpation. The morbidity and potential mortality of surgery must be contemplated when planning therapy, however. The surgical approach is tailored to the size and extent of this aggressive benign tumor. Many surgical approaches have been described. These include transnasal, transpalatal, transmandibular, transzygomatic, transantral, combined craniotomy and rhinotomy, and lateral rhinotomy. The lateral rhinotomy incision gives a foundation for excellent exposure. It may be combined with a lip splitting incision and partial maxillectomy for exposure of the infratemporal fossa. Recurrences of

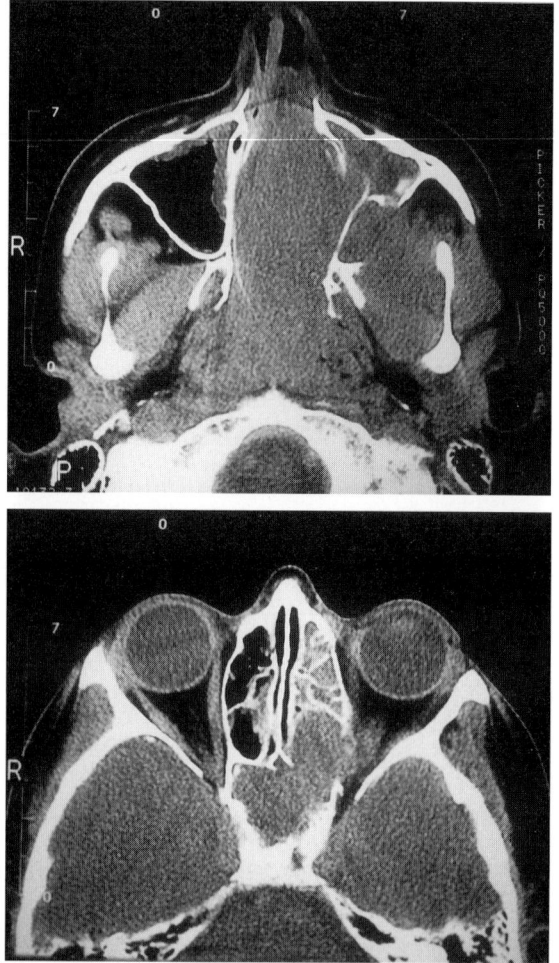

FIGURE 60–3 Axial CT scans. (A) At the level of the pterygomaxillary fissure. The mass can be seen filling the nasal cavity, displacing the nasal septum to the right. The posterior wall of the maxillary sinus has been pushed forward. The pterygomaxillary fissure has been widened dramatically on the left side (CT analogue of the Holman–Miller sign). Not depicted well in the section is the extension into the infratemporal fossa. (B) Erosion of the posterior orbital wall and encroachment on the optic nerve. The posterior ethmoid sinuses and the sphenoid sinus are filled with tumor.

small and medium size tumors treated surgically approach zero.

Angiography is useful to delineate the vascular supply of the tumor and to allow preoperative embolization of the tumor. The main blood supply generally comes from the internal maxillary artery or the ascending pharyngeal artery.

Other likely contributing vessels include the dural, sphenoidal, and ophthalmic branches from the internal carotid artery. Intracranial extension should be seriously considered if the majority of the blood supply is derived from the internal carotid circulation. Contribution from the internal carotid may make embolization impossible. Angiography and embolization should only be undertaken in preparation for extirpative surgery. Other techniques also considered useful in reducing blood loss during surgery include ligation of the internal maxillary artery or the external carotid artery, hypotensive anesthesia, and expedient surgery.

Management of intracranial and skull base invading juvenile nasopharyngeal angiofibroma is more controversial. The recurrence rate after surgical excision increases with the size of the tumor and its association with intracranial structures and skull base suture lines. Erosion of the medial wall of the cavernous sinus has been reported as a poor predictor for complete excision. A recurrence rate of 32% has been found with surgical excision of larger tumors (stage IIIA and B).

REHABILITATION AND FOLLOW-UP

This case illustrates difficult management decisions needed for treatment of a large angiofibroma. Since the medial wall of the cavernous sinus had been eroded, placing the cavernous carotid artery and optic nerve at risk from a combined neurosurgical and otolaryngology craniofacial approach (Fig. 60–3B), radiotherapy with close follow-up and potential surgical salvage was elected. At 3 months the tumor has shown signs of regression (Figs. 60–4A and B). His symptomatology has improved with a cessation of epistaxis and improved nasal airflow. Reevaluation for the need of surgical salvage or further radiotherapy will be made in 18 months.

No studies have accurately evaluated the long-term follow-up for juvenile nasopharyngeal angiofibroma. Some have suggested serial MRI scans starting 2 months after resection and then twice yearly during adolescence. If complete excision has been achieved, the risk of recurrence is low and generally occurs within 2

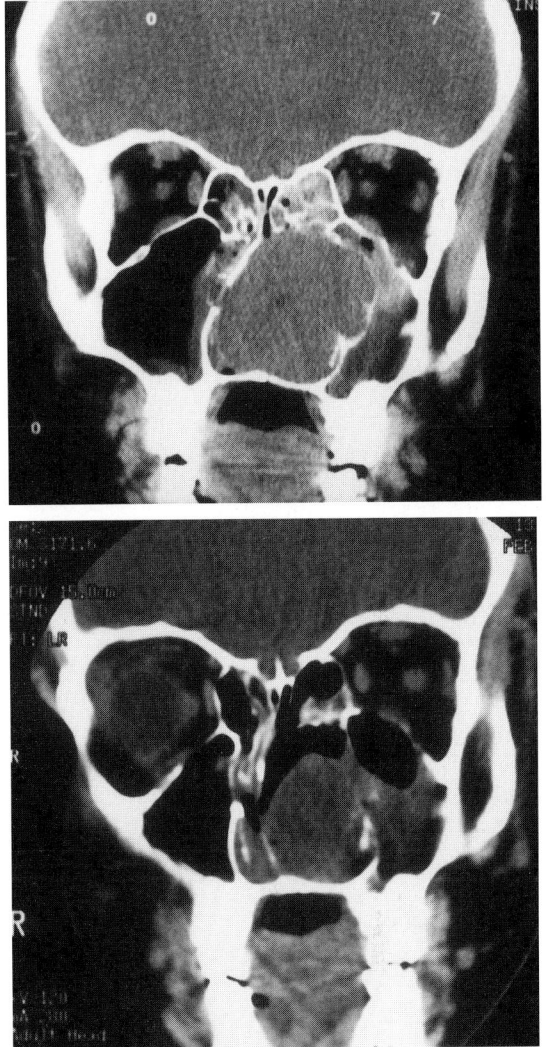

FIGURE 60–4 Coronal CT scans in similar planes of the patient's skull before treatment and 3 months afer radiotherapy. A dramatic decrease in the bulk of the tumor can be seen. Residual tumor persists, however. The complete response to radiotherapy may not be seen for 12 to 36 months.

years. Recurrence rates increase with size and intracranial extension. Rare reports of spontaneous regression have been made but also reported are rare cases of malignant transformation. Although very rare, sarcomatous changes have been seen usually in irradiated nasopharyngeal angiofibroma. Reexcision or adjuvant radiotherapy should be considered for recurrences.

SUGGESTED READINGS

BATSAKIS JG. *Tumors of the Head and Neck: Clinical and Pathological Considerations.* 2nd ed. Baltimore, MD: Williams & Wilkins; 1979.

BREMER JW, NEEL HB, DESANTO LW, JONES GC. Angiofibroma: treatment trends in 150 patients during 40 years. *Laryngoscope.* 1986;96:1321–1329.

CUMMINGS BJ, BLEND R, KEANE T, et al. Primary radiation therapy for juvenile nasopharyngeal angiofibroma. *Laryngoscope.* 1984;94(12 part 1):1599–1605.

DUVAL AJ, MOREANO AE. Juvenile nasopharyngeal angiofibroma: diagnosis and treatment. *Head Neck Surg.* 1987;97:537.

FITZPATRICK PJ, BRIANT TDR, BERMAN JM. The nasopharyngeal angiofibroma. *Arch Otol.* 1980;106:234–236.

GATES GA, RICE DH, KOOPMANN CF JR, SCHULLER DE. Flutamide-induced regression of angiofibroma. *Laryngoscope.* 1992;102(6):641–644.

HOLMAN CB, MILLER WE. Juvenile nasopharyngeal fibroma: roentgenologic characteristics. *Am J Roentgenol.* 1965;94:292–298.

RADKOWSKI D, McGILL T, HEALY GB, OHLMS L, JONES DT. Angiofibroma: changes in staging and treatment. *Arch Otolaryngol Head Neck Surg.* 1996;122(2):122–129.

SCHIFF M. Juvenile nasopharyngeal angiofibroma: a theory of pathogenesis. *Laryngoscope.* 1959;69:981–1016.

SESSIONS RB, BRYAN RN, NACLERIO RM, ALFORD BR. Radiographic staging of juvenile angiofibroma. *Head Neck Surg.* 1981;3:279–283.

WENIG BM. Neoplasms of the oral cavity, nasopharynx, tonsils, and neck. In: *Atlas of Head and Neck Pathology.* Philadelphia, PA: WB Saunders; 1993:143–201.

WIATRAK BJ, KOOPMANN CF, TURRISI AT. Radiation therapy as an alternative to surgery in the management of intracranial juvenile nasopharyngeal angiofibroma. *Int J Pediatr Otorhinolaryngol.* 1993;28(1):51–61.

POST-TONSILLECTOMY BLEEDING

Yoram Stern, M.D.
Charles M. Myer, III, M.D.

HISTORY

A 4-year-old white male presented to the emergency room because of oral bleeding 20 hours after a tonsillectomy. The procedure was done by means of electrocautery, and hemostasis was obtained with electrocautery and suture ligatures. The physical examination revealed an alert child with a pulse of 110/minute and a blood pressure of 110/70. Examination of the oropharynx revealed no active bleeding or clot in the tonsillar fossa. Complete blood count (CBC), prothrombin time (PT), activated partial thromboplastin time (PTT), and bleeding time (BT) were within normal limits. The child was admitted to the hospital for observation and discharged after 24 hours with no bleeding. Three days later (5th postoperative day), the child was admitted to the hospital again due to oral bleeding. Examination at the time of admission revealed no active bleeding or clot. CBC and coagulation tests were repeated and were normal again except for a hematocrit of 21.3 grams %. A blood transfusion was required due to orthostatic changes. The child remained in the hospital for observation and 7 days later (12th postoperative day) had oral bleeding again, which could not be controlled at the bedside. The child underwent exploration of the tonsillar fosse under general anesthesia in the operating room where a blood clot in the right tonsillar fossa was removed and hemostasis was achieved with the electrocautery. Three days later (15th postoperative day), the child again had bleeding, which was controlled with local measures. Due to a low hematocrit (19.4 grams %), another blood transfusion was required. At this point, a carotid arteriogram was ordered. Based on the history and the radiographic studies demonstrating an aneurysm arising from the right facial artery, the patient underwent right neck exploration with ligation of the right facial artery. No further bleeding was noted and the child was discharged from the hospital 2 days later.

DIFFERENTIAL DIAGNOSIS— KEY POINTS

1. This patient presented initially with post-tonsillectomy bleeding within the first 24 hours after adenotonsillectomy. This is considered primary hemorrhage and is usually due to improper hemostasis during the primary surgery. Secondary post-tonsillectomy hemorrhage is defined as any bleeding after the first 24 postoperative hours. Such bleeding usually occurs between the 5th and 10th postoperative day and commonly is associated with premature separation of the granulation membrane that forms over the pharyngeal surface after tonsillectomy. The rate of primary hemorrhage generally ranges from 0.2 to 2.2% and of secondary hemorrhage from 0.1 to 3%.

2. Repeated postoperative bleeding should raise the possibility of a coagulation disorder. A thorough preoperative medical history regarding the patient and immediate family members should be obtained. Points that need to be addressed are history of easy bruising, epistaxis, oral bleeding, post-traumatic hemorrhage, excessive circumcision bleeding, postoperative or dental hemorrhage, hemarthrosis, perinatal bleeding and recent usage of any medication, especially nonsteroidal anti-inflammatory and anticoagulant medications. Systemic disorders that might result in excessive bleeding, such as liver disease, renal disease, or hematologic disease, should be addressed as well.

   The preoperative physical examination may help one detect possible coagulopathies and provides additional information. The presence of petechiae might suggest vascular or platelet disorders. Mucosal and gastrointestinal hemorrhage may be associated with vascular abnormalities such as bleeding into an elbow or knee joint, which is characteristic of hemophilia A (factor VIII deficiency) or factor IX deficiency. The presence of hepatosplenomegaly may indicate a liver disorder or hemolytic neoplasm.

3. In cases of recurrent bleeding with normal coagulation studies, vascular abnormalities would be expected and evaluation by angiography should be done.

TEST INTERPRETATION

Platelet count, activated PTT, PT, and BT are useful in the detection of inherited and acquired coagulation disorders. These tests should always be obtained preoperatively if the history or medical examination suggests a coagulation disorder. If the patient's clinical history raises the definite possibility of a specific coagulation disorder, specific tests should be performed. For example, if the patient has a history of spontaneous bruising or if the BT is prolonged and the platelet count is normal, additional laboratory tests should be focused on the possibility of von Willebrand's disease (VW) or a primary platelet disorder. Actual preoperative detection of a coagulation defect allows for vital preoperative management that improves patient care by reducing perioperative complications and may prevent a disastrous surgical outcome. The use of routine preoperative laboratory screening tests is questionable since these tests are regarded to have low positive predictive value due to poor sensitivity. Coagulation testing should be obtained following a bleeding episode and, if abnormal, hematology consultation and additional coagulation testing should be obtained. A CBC also should be obtained in order to assess the degree of hemorrhage and as a baseline in case further bleeding develops. In this case, laboratory analysis revealed a platelet count of 300,000/nm^3 (normal range, 150,000 to 400,000/nm^3), PT 12.9 seconds (normal range, 11.5 to 13.5 seconds), a PTT 29 seconds (normal

range, 21 to 30.2 seconds), and bleeding time of 6 minutes (normal range, 2 to 9 minutes) after the initial bleeding episode. Hematocrit was initially 35 grams % but dropped to 21.3 and 19.4 grams % after the second and fourth bleeding episodes, respectively. The combination of multiple bleeding episodes with normal coagulation tests should raise the suspicion of a vascular abnormality and this needs to be evaluated by angiography. Arteriography has a low but significant risk of morbidity and mortality. Yet, in cases of repeated postoperative bleeding, this study is essential in order to detect possible vascular abnormalities that might cause the repeated episodes of bleeding. In this case, the carotid arteriogram revealed an aneurysm of the proximal facial artery on the right side (Fig. 61–1).

DIAGNOSIS

Aneurysm of the right facial artery.

MEDICAL MANAGEMENT

Any coagulation disorder detected preoperatively or postoperatively should be addressed and treated as necessary. Two of the most common coagulation defects encountered are platelet dysfunction and VW. More than 20 subtypes of VW have been recognized to date. Some of these subtypes respond to desmopressin acetate

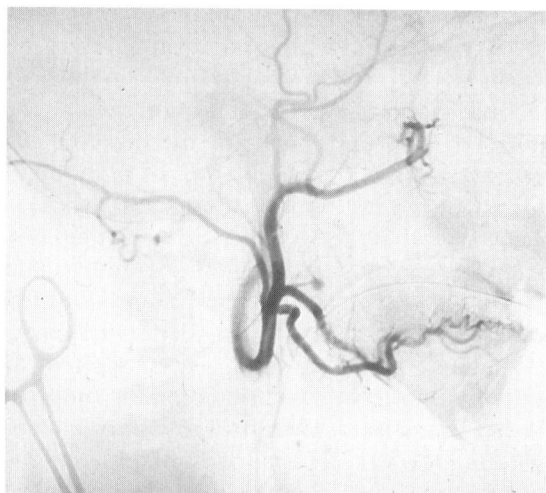

FIGURE 61–1 Aneurysm of the right facial artery.

(DDAVP) treatment. This should be evaluated by a challenge test with this drug 1 or 2 weeks prior to surgery. If DDAVP is to be used, treatment should be given about 1 hour before surgery at a dose of 0.3 mg/kg of body weight during a 30-minute infusion and once daily thereafter until wound healing is complete. Cryoprecipitate or factor VIII concentrates, which contain VW multimers, should be available in the event that the DDAVP fails to control hemorrhage. Other subtypes of VW are treated with exogenous VW factor replacement in the form of cryoprecipitate or factor VIII concentrate. Drugs are the most common causes of platelet dysfunction and aspirin is probably the most commonly used drug known to affect platelet function. When a hemostatically normal patient who is taking aspirin requires a surgical procedure, aspirin should be discontinued for at least 2 weeks. If severe hemorrhage due to deficient platelet function is suspected, either a random donor platelet transfusion or DDAVP would be rapidly effective.

Patients with post-tonsillectomy bleeding usually are admitted for observation and blood tests. An exception to this rule may be a delayed bleeding episode without signs of clot or active bleeding. This patient can be kept in an observation unit for about 4 hours while being hydrated before discharge. If the blood loss is excessive and the patient is symptomatic, blood transfusion should be considered.

SURGICAL MANAGEMENT

The most important factor in management of postoperative tonsillectomy bleeding is prevention. The actual method of removal of tonsils, either by dissection or electrocautery, is probably not as important as attention to the detail of staying in the proper plane between the tonsillar capsule and its surrounding fossa. Hemostasis generally is obtained with either a suture tie or electrocautery. The operating surgeon must not terminate the procedure until she or he is absolutely confident of hemostasis. If any bleeding is noted in the mouth during emergence from anesthesia, the surgeon should not be reluctant to have the anesthesiologist deepen the plane of anesthesia so that the

pharynx can be reexamined and any bleeding stopped. While a small amount of blood-tinged saliva is acceptable in the recovery room and for the first 24 hours, any amount of bright red blood coming from the mouth or nose should alert the surgeon to the possibility of postoperative bleeding and initiate a complete examination of the oropharynx and the possibility of exploration of the area in the operating room. Frequent swallowing and tachycardia also have been reported as indirect evidence of possible postoperative bleeding. In addition, if the child has continued emesis with coffee ground material, suspicion should be aroused that there may be active pharyngeal bleeding and appropriate investigation and treatment should take place. If a clot is revealed in the tonsillar fossa during the physical examination, this should be removed because it can prevent normal tissue retraction and subsequent healing. The age and cooperativeness of the child are important in the decision-making process. In the cooperative patient, local or topical anesthesia may be sufficient to allow direct examination and removal of the clot. If this fails or if the patient is unable to tolerate care in an awake state, general anesthesia will be required to control the airway and allow the surgeon to work without distraction. The initial step in hemostasis is suctioning off any fresh clot from the tonsillar fossa. Identified bleeding sites are controlled with electrocautery or a suture tie. If these measures are not successful, suture ligature may be required to stop the bleeding. However, this must be done with extreme care. The tissue in the postoperative tonsillar fossa is very fragile. Placement of sutures is often difficult because the suture tends to tear through the tissue and pull out. The surgeon then may attempt to place the suture deeper to hold more securely and may inadvertently lacerate a major vessel deep to the fossa, possibly leading to aneurysm formation. If the measures mentioned are not successful in stopping the bleeding, consideration must be given to exploration of the neck and ligation of the external carotid artery or its small distal branches. If possible, preoperative angiography may be helpful and embolization might be considered as a surgical alternative or adjunct.

REHABILITATION AND FOLLOW-UP

If any coagulation disorder is discovered during the preoperative or postoperative period, this should be properly addressed and treated. The patient and his parents should receive a complete hematologic consultation and should be followed periodically as necessary.

SUGGESTED READINGS

Bolger WE, Parsons DS, Potempa L. Preoperative hemostatic assessment of the adenotonsillectomy patient. *Otolaryngol Head Neck Surg.* 1990;103:396–405.

Burk CD, Miller L, Handler SD, Cohen AL. Preoperative history and coagulation screening in children undergoing tonsillectomy. *Pediatrics.* 1993;89:691–695.

Franco KL, Wallace RB. Management of postoperative bleeding after tonsillectomy. *Otonlaryngol Clin North Am.* 1987;20:291–297.

Handler SD, Miller L, Richmond KH, Baranak CC. Post-tonsillectomy hemorrhage; incidence, prevention and management. *Laryngoscope.* 1986;96:1243–1247.

Tami TA, Parker GS, Taylor RE. Post-tonsillectomy bleeding: an evaluation of risk factors. *Laryngoscope.* 1987;97:1307–1311.

STRIDOROUS CHILD

Yoram Stern, M.D.
Charles M. Myer, III, M.D.

HISTORY

A 4-month-old full-term female infant presents with "noisy breathing." The parents indicate that the "noise" becomes worse when the child is agitated or excited but is not influenced by position. No change in cry is reported. The child has had no apneic or cyanotic episodes and weight gain has been appropriate. On physical examination, no increase in respiratory rate, retraction, or flaring of the nostrils is noted. Auscultation reveals biphasic stridor. A small cutaneous posterior cervical hemangioma is observed. Flexible nasolaryngoscopy demonstrates normal vocal cord mobility with no supraglottic abnormalities. Airway radiographs, including views of the chest and neck, demonstrate asymmetric subglottic narrowing. Based on the history, physical examination and radiographic evaluation, microlaryngoscopy and bronchoscopy are performed.

DIFFERENTIAL DIAGNOSIS— KEY POINTS

1. This patient's primary symptom is biphasic stridor, which developed gradually in the first few months of life.

2. Lack of acute onset of the stridor and absence of any signs of acute inflammation such as fever usually rule out inflammatory causes of upper airway obstruction, including croup, epiglottitis, or bacterial tracheitis.

3. The stridor did not present immediately after birth. Therefore, causes for immediate respiratory distress such as laryngeal atresia or congenital bilateral vocal cord paralysis can be excluded.

4. No history of intubation or other laryngotracheal trauma was obtained. Therefore, the diagnosis of acquired subglottic stenosis is un-

likely although congenital subglottic stenosis cannot be ruled out.

5. Normal flexible laryngoscopy usually excludes the diagnosis of laryngomalacia and impaired vocal cord mobility, which are two of the most common causes of stridor in infants. In addition, these patients usually present at an earlier age.

6. The possibility of foreign body aspiration should always be considered. This should be discussed carefully with the parents. However, airway difficulties due to a foreign body usually have a rapid course and the aspiration events usually occur between 1 and 3 years of age.

7. Normal flexible laryngoscopy and biphasic stridor may suggest the possibility of a subglottic or tracheal lesion. Direct endoscopy under general anesthesia is required in order to evaluate properly this region as well as the rest of the tracheobronchial tree.

TEST INTERPRETATION

Anteroposterior and lateral high-kilovoltage radiographs that are tightly coned to the trachea will allow visualization of subglottic space. Normally, the airway appears slightly narrowed between the vocal cords, and the subglottic space is convex or shouldered.

An anteroposterior neck film demonstrated asymmetric narrowing in the subglottic region (Fig. 62–1), and a lateral radiograph demonstrated a possible posterior subglottic mass in the patient presented. Direct endoscopy of the upper airway revealed a normal supraglottis and glottis. In the immediate subglottis, a pink submucosal mass was noted in the left posterior/lateral quadrant (Fig. 62–2). The mass occupied about 40% of the subglottic lumen and could be compressed by the endo-

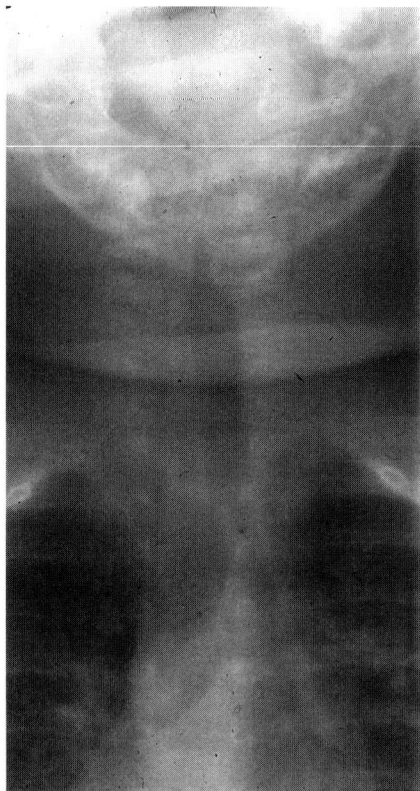

FIGURE 62–1 Anteroposterior high-kilovoltage plain film demonstrating asymmetric narrowing of the subglottis.

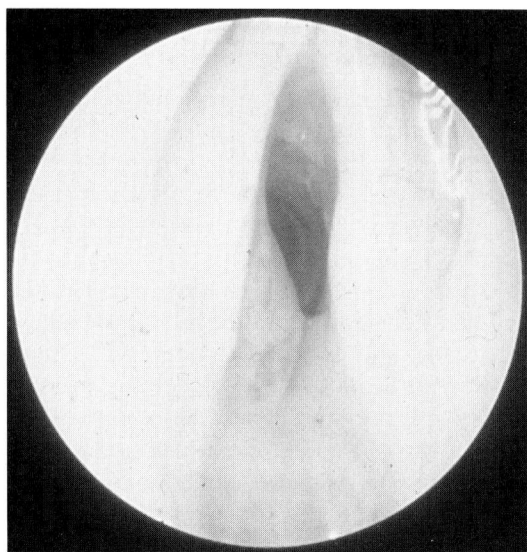

FIGURE 62–2 Smooth submucosal mass arising from posterior/lateral portion of the subglottis.

scope. The rest of the tracheobronchial tree was normal.

DIAGNOSIS

Subglottic hemangioma.

MEDICAL MANAGEMENT

Systemic steroid therapy has been attempted frequently in the treatment of subglottic hemangiomas with mixed results. The mechanism of the steroid effect on hemangioma is not clear. The use of steroids is not without potential long-term complications such as growth suppression and the development of cushingoid features. Therefore, when steroid use is considered, a maximal initial dose should be used to obtain the greatest effect on the hemangioma (dexamethasone sodium phosphate 1 mg/kg/day). The dose should be reduced rapidly to avoid long-term complications. Rebound growth of the hemangioma may occur after the completion of steroid treatment. A reasonable treatment plan would be the use of prednisone 2 to 3 mg/kg/day every other day. Interferon alpha also has been used for the treatment of a subglottic hemangioma with good results.

SURGICAL MANAGEMENT

When a large obstructive hemangioma is present, a tracheostomy usually is required. This will bypass the obstruction until another mode of therapy can be used or the lesion spontaneously regresses. When the lesion is somewhat smaller, it can be treated endoscopically alone or in combination with systemic steroids. The carbon dioxide (CO_2) laser has the ability to decrease the size of the lesion with minimal resultant edema or adjacent tissue injury. When the hemangioma is treated by the CO_2 laser, care is taken not to create a circumferential defect and to avoid injury to the cricoid perichondrium. The patient usually is intubated postoperatively for several days. Repeat laser treatment is then performed as needed. Open surgical excision, which is generally thought to be associated with higher morbidity, has gained some recent support, especially for isolated lesions. Other modes of therapy that have not gained much popularity are cryotherapy, electrocautery, embolization, and radiation.

REHABILITATION AND FOLLOW-UP

The natural history of this lesion can be unpredictable but most have a favorable natural history and usually resolve spontaneously after 12 to 18 months. Therefore, any type of surgical intervention should be limited unless there is significant airway obstruction. Surgical intervention may result in severe complications of the larynx, including subglottic stenosis, and any therapeutic maneuver that has significant long-term sequelae should be avoided. Repeated endoscopies are necessary to follow the lesion's response to therapy and possible spontaneous regression.

SUGGESTED READINGS

CHOA DI, SMITH MCF, EVANS JNG, BAILEY CM. Subglottic hemangioma in children. *J Laryngol Otol.* 1986;100:447–457.

GREGG CM, WIATRAK BJ, KOOPMAN CF JR. Management of options for infantile subglottic hemangioma. *Am J Otolaryngol.* 1995;16:409–414.

RIDING K. Subglottic hemangioma: a practical approach. *J Otolaryngol.* 1992;21:419–421.

SEIKALY H, CUYLER JP. Infantile subglottic hemangioma. *J Otolaryngol.* 1994;23:135–137.

SHIKHANO AH, JONES MM, MORSH BR, et al. Infantile subglottic hemangioma: an update. *Ann Otol Rhinol Laryngol.* 1986;95:336–347.

SIE KC, MCGILL T, HEALY GB. Subglottic hemangioma: ten year's experience with carbon dioxide laser. *Ann Otol Rhinol Laryngol.* 1994;103:167–172.

WANER M, SUEN JY, DINEHART S. Treatment of hemangiomas of the head and neck. *Laryngoscope.* 1992; 102:1123–1132.

Case 63

CYSTIC FIBROSIS

Sally R. Shott, M.D.

HISTORY

C.C. is an 8-year-old female with a history of cystic fibrosis (CF), asthma, sinusitis, allergies, and recurrent gastrointestinal problems. She presents to the office complaining of chronic headaches. She has had multiple admissions to the hospital for CF exacerbations, but has never required endotracheal intubation for these. She has been on multiple courses of oral antibiotics and most recently has had a precutaneous intravenous catheter (PIC) line for home intravenous antibiotics. She reports that the antibiotics, given specifically for her lung infections, seem to ease the headaches but they never totally resolve.

Medical history includes an adenotonsillectomy at age 5 years.

Physical exam revealed a thin, but active young lady in no acute distress. Examination of her nose revealed erythematous and boggy nasal turbinates and nasal polyps. Palpation of the face was positive for mild tenderness over the maxillary sinuses.

DIFFERENTIAL DIAGNOSIS— KEY POINTS

1. Cystic fibrosis is an inherited, autosomal recessive disorder that results in abnormal function of the exocrine glands. Exocrine glands and ducts are obstructed throughout the body, resulting in the most common clinical manifestations of chronic obstructive pulmonary disease and gastrointestinal malabsorption secondary to pancreatic insufficiency.

2. Sinusitis is also common, if not universal, in patients with CF. Identified as a component of CF in the 1950s, Lurie first described the association of nasal polyposis and CF in 1957. The incidence of nasal polyps has been reported to be almost 50%. The most common symptoms include nasal obstruction, rhinorrhea, and headache.

3. Sinus radiographs are usually abnormal in children with CF. Computed tomography (CT) scans have been reported to be abnormal in 100% of those evaluated.

4. The most likely diagnosis in this patient is chronic sinusitis with nasal polyposis. Further evaluation is needed to determine the extent of the disease and specifically to determine if there is evidence of bony erosion from the chronic disease process.

TEST INTERPRETATION

A CT scan of the paranasal sinuses was performed on this patient. As seen in Figure 63–1, there is erosion of the medial wall of the maxillary sinus bilaterally and soft tissue extruding into the nasal cavity from the maxillary sinus consistent with polyps.

DIAGNOSIS

Chronic sinusitis with evidence of bone erosion, in a patient with cystic fibrosis.

MEDICAL MANAGEMENT

The effectiveness of medical management of sinusitis and nasal polyps in children with CF has been extremely disappointing. Studies evaluating the bacteriology of sinusitis in children with CF commonly identify *Pseudomonas aeruginosa*, *Staphylococcus aureus*, and *Haemophilus influenzae* as well as anaerobes. Prolonged courses of antibiotics and steroids, both intranasal and systemic, decongestants, and antihistamines are the mainstay of medical management. Although only partially successful in controlling disease, it is thought the use of antibiotics may contribute to the lower incidence of complications of sinusitis in this patient population including orbital cellulitis and osteomyelitis. Unfortunately, however, these therapies have not been shown to affect the initial development of nasal polyps

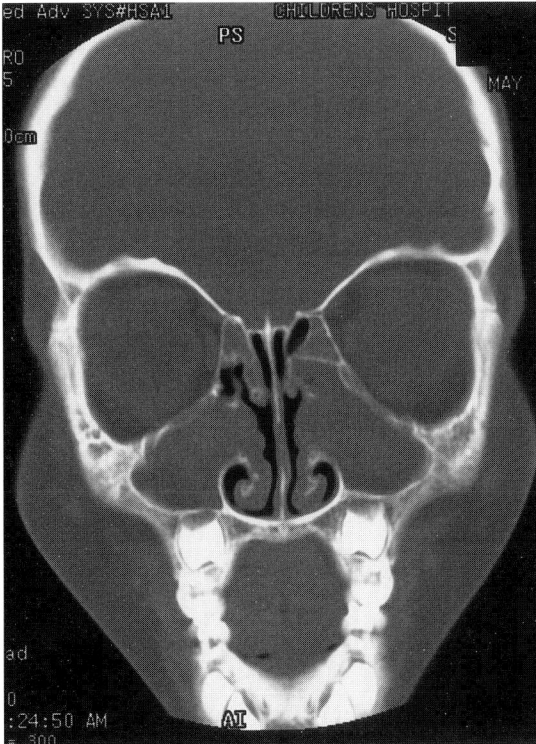

FIGURE 63–1 CT of the paranasal sinuses in this patient with cystic fibrosis shows erosion of the medial wall of the maxillary sinus bilaterally and soft tissue, consistent with nasal polyps, extruding from the maxillary sinuses into the nose.

or to decrease the incidence of recurrence of the sinusitis and polyps.

Because of the high incidence of nasal polyps, the role of allergy has been studied. However, the incidence of allergy in children with CF is no different from the general population. Other studies have shown that the pathologic nature of the nasal polyps due to CF is different from allergic polyps.

Hypertonic saline irrigations can be helpful. This solution, made up of water or saline, pickling salt, and baking soda helps to mobilize the thick, tenacious nasal and sinus secretions seen in children with CF.

SURGICAL MANAGEMENT

Although surgical intervention has been shown to provide symptomatic relief especially in terms of controlling the congestion and head-

aches associated with sinusitis and nasal polyps, the long-term effectiveness of surgery can also be disappointing. Studies evaluating the effectiveness of different surgical procedures discuss results in terms of "fewer recurrences" and "longer symptom-free" periods, but not in terms of cure rates.

However, some improvement in this regard has been made. Simple nasal polypectomy in a child with CF and nasal polyps is usually not effective. More aggressive sinus surgery has been shown to decrease the frequency of recurrences and provide longer symptom-free intervals, but is rarely curative. Functional endoscopic sinus surgery with intranasal ethmoidectomies and maxillary antrostomies with removal of polyps from the maxillary sinuses are usually required. Moss and King reported a further increase in the symptom-free period by the addition of serial antimicrobial lavage in addition to the endoscopic surgery. Placing catheters into the maxillary sinuses via the antrostomy at the time of surgery, they then treated their patients with tobramycin irrigations for 7 to 10 days postoperatively. They reported an increase in the symptom-free interval to at least 2 years.

The improvement seen with the postoperative antimicrobial irrigations stresses the need for continued medical management following surgical intervention in this ongoing, relentless disease. Hypertonic saline nasal irrigations are also quite helpful in mobilizing the tenacious secretions out of the opened sinus cavities.

Because of the chronic nature of this disease process, the need for revision surgery should be expected and these expectations need to be openly discussed with the patient and their family. The timing of such revision surgery depends on the severity of the symptoms of nasal obstruction, headache, and facial pain and the possible effects of the purulent postnasal drainage on the pulmonary status of the patient. Exacerbations of the patient's lung disease may be linked to exacerbations of the sinusitis. At revision surgery one may find that all that is required is suctioning of the thick, paste-like secretions from the sinuses. It is also possible, however, that one will find recurrence of the extensive polyposis seen at the original surgery.

Because of the underlying pulmonary disease, special considerations need to be taken with regard to general anesthesia and surgery. Because of the effects of CF on the child's cardiopulmonary systems, a full medical evaluation should be done by the child's pulmonologist and by the anesthesiologist prior to surgery. Maximization of the patient's pulmonary status prior to surgery is required with possible inhouse preoperative antibiotics and pulmonary physiotherapy. Hydration prior to surgery is also important. All of the potential medical problems associated with CF including pancreatic dysfunction and diabetes and coagulation abnormalities should be considered. Communication between the surgeon, the anesthesiologist, the primary care physician, and the various specialists participating in the patient's care is imperative.

REHABILITATION AND FOLLOW-UP

Due to the chronic nature of sinusitis in children with cystic fibrosis it is wise to encourage open communication not only with the patient and his or her family but also with the patient's pulmonologist, the most likely primary manager of the patient's care. This will provide better decision making in terms of timing of revision surgery and will keep you informed as to the pulmonary status of the patient, especially if a general anesthetic is being considered.

SUGGESTED READINGS

COLE RR, COTTON RT. Preventing postoperative complications in the adult cystic fibrosis patient. *Int J Pediatr Otorhinolaryngol.* 1990;18:263–269.

CROCKETT DM, MCGILL TJ, HEALY GB, et al. Nasal and paranasal sinus surgery in children with cystic fibrosis. *Ann Otol Laryngol.* 1987;96:367–372.

CUYLER JP, MONAGHAN AJ. Cystic fibrosis and sinusitis. *J Otolaryngol.* 1989;18:173–175.

DRAKE-LEE AB, MORGAN DW. Nasal polyps and sinusitis in children with cystic fibrosis. *J Laryngol Otol.* 1989;103:753–755.

MOSS RB, KING VV. Management of sinusitis in cystic fibrosis by endoscopic surgery and serial antimicrobial lavage. *Arch Otolaryngol Head Neck Surg.* 1995; 121:566–572.

Case 64

DOWN SYNDROME

Sally R. Shott, M.D.

HISTORY

A 12-year-old with Down syndrome presents to the emergency room with a 2-day history of sore throat, increasing difficulty swallowing, poor oral intake, and inability to handle his secretions. His mother reports that he has had a long history of trouble breathing at night, preferring to sleep in the sitting position. She had not been particularly concerned about this because she just assumed that this was normal for children with Down syndrome. Since the sore throat started, however, the breathing had become more labored and he seemed to be holding his breath when he was sleeping.

The patient's history was significant for recurrent episodes of croup. The mother denied any history of cardiac or pulmonary problems. She did note, however, that her son's gait had become somewhat unsteady, particularly after he was playing in the yard, rolling on the ground, and seemed to lose his balance more easily.

Physical exam revealed a mildly obese 12-year-old with trismus and physical exam consistent with a right peritonsillar abscess. He was drooling and had mild retraction and significant upper airway congestion.

DIFFERENTIAL DIAGNOSIS— KEY POINTS

Several key points in this history point to potential problems in the care of this child:

1. The patient has a history consistent with sleep apnea that has now been exacerbated by his current acute infection. Unfortunately, because a large percentage of children with Down syndrome have airway obstruction during sleep and sleep apnea, starting at a very young age, parents frequently assume that this is "normal" for their child. Although the acute situation of a peritonsillar abscess

has caused an acute exacerbation to his underlying upper airway obstruction, airway obstruction in children with Down syndrome can be caused by medially displaced tonsils in the face of midface hypoplasia and a contracted oropharynx, hypotonia with oropharyngeal and hypopharyngeal collapse during sleep, and macroglossia with its associated airway obstruction. In addition, central apnea can be seen.

2. This child presents with a history of recurrent croup. Children with Down syndrome are known to have smaller subglottic airways than the normal population and are prone to recurrent episodes of croup. This is important from an anesthetic standpoint when intubation is being considered. It is important to use the appropriate size endotracheal tube in this child's airway.

3. The patient's history of recently noted abnormal gait, particularly after active play and rolling on the ground may be due to some coordination problems but could also be due to atlantoaxial instability and resultant compression of the spinal cord. This is of particular importance if contemplating a surgical procedure where the patient's neck will be manipulated.

INTERPRETATION

1. *Cervical spine films.* Prior to any surgical procedure where manipulation of the neck is done, and particularly in view of the patient's history of change in gait, cervical spine films should be done. Cervical spine abnormalities seen in Down syndrome include atlantoaxial instability, abnormal congenital fusion of the vertebral bodies, degenerative changes in the C2-3 and C3-4 cervical interspaces, and spinal cord compression. Hyperextension, in the presence of atlantoaxial instability, can cause compression of the spinal cord. Lateral neck

x-rays in the extension, flexion, and neutral position should be performed. If there is any question of abnormality as in this patient's case, a CAT scan evaluation is also helpful. Figure 64–1, although not the patient described in this case, shows an example of some of the cervical spine abnormalities seen in children with Down syndrome. The cervical spine film of the patient described in this case was normal.

2. *Polysomnogram.* Although a polysomnogram would not be indicated at this point for this patient's treatment course, this should be considered postoperatively. Because of the multiple potential sources of airway obstruction, although this patient may improve after a tonsillectomy, airway obstruction and sleep apnea may continue. In addition, a sleep study would rule out central apnea. The need for further airway support such as continuous positive airway pressure (CPAP) or oxygen supplementation could then be determined.

3. *Airway films.* With this patient's history of recurrent croup, airway films may suggest some subglottic narrowing but in the face of this patient's peritonsillar abscess and resultant inflammation it should be assumed that this is present until proven otherwise. Special precautions, particularly in terms of the size of endotracheal tubes used and documentation of an air leak around the endotracheal tube, should be taken at the time of surgery.

4. *Laboratory tests.* A complete blood count is helpful in these situations, not only in terms of the acute infection but also because children with Down syndrome have a higher incidence of leukemia than the general population. This patient's complete blood count was consistent with an acute infection.

5. *Chest x-ray.* With this patient's long history of upper airway obstruction, a chest x-ray would be helpful to rule out signs of cor pulmonale secondary to the chronic upper airway obstruction. His x-ray was normal.

6. *Metabolic studies.* Patient's with Down syndrome have a higher incidence of hypothyroidism. Again, this would be an important piece of information to know if general anesthesia is considered. If not done previously, these laboratory studies should be done.

DIAGNOSIS

Right peritonsillar abscess in a 12-year-old with Down syndrome.

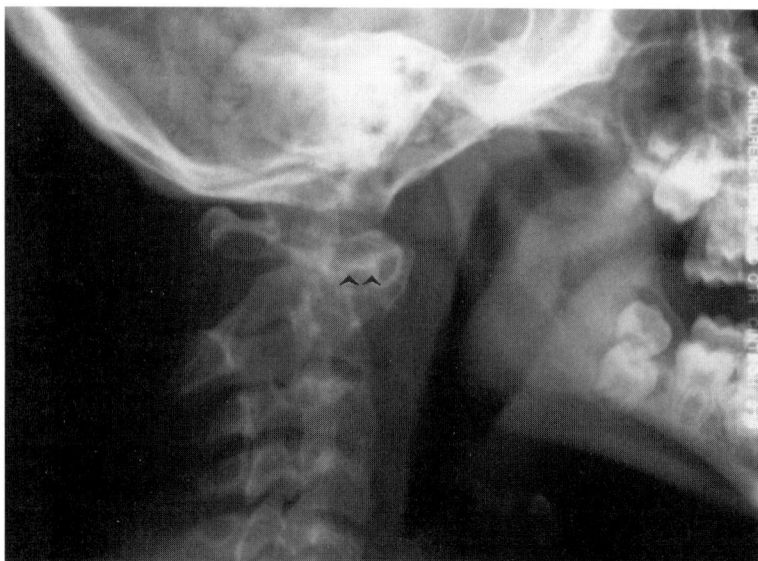

FIGURE 64–1 Cervical spine film in the lateral flexion view of an 8-year-old male with Down syndrome. The first cervical vertebrae is hypoplastic. The space anterior to the dens is increased (arrowheads), whereas the space posterior to the dens is markedly decreased (dots).

MEDICAL MANAGEMENT

The medical management of peritonsillar abscess is no different in a child with Down syndrome. IV fluids and parental antibiotics are used. If it is unclear whether the infection represents an abscess or a cellulitis, the patient may benefit from IV hydration and antibiotics for 24 hours prior to surgical consideration. If the infection is limited to cellulitis, there will most likely be improvement and medical management may be all that is necessary. However, in this patient's case, the history of upper airway obstruction prior to this acute event must not be forgotten. Follow-up management must include evaluation to determine the degree and severity of obstruction during sleep.

SURGICAL MANAGEMENT

In this patient's case, surgical management of a peritonsillar abscess is no different than that for a child without Down syndrome. However, special precautions must be taken during the surgical procedure. Because this is an emergency procedure, full evaluation of the patient's complaints of changing gait and potential cervical spine abnormalities may not have occurred. Because of the hyperextension used during tonsillectomy, the technique must be altered. The surgery is performed with the patient in the neutral position. No shoulder rolls are used and the head is kept in as horizontal of a position as is possible.

With this patient's history of recurrent croup, at the time of intubation, a smaller tube than would be expected for the patient's age and size should be used. The appropriateness of the tube chosen should be confirmed with the presence of an air leak around the endotracheal tube.

Postoperatively, patients may have a higher rate of complications than in children without Down syndrome. Because of the other potential sources of airway obstruction, that is, hypotonia, macroglossia, and central apnea, there is a higher incidence of postoperative airway obstruction that will need to be monitored closely.

REHABILITATION AND FOLLOW-UP

Following this patient's treatment for the peritonsillar abscess by a tonsillectomy, this patient should undergo a polysomnogram to better document the degree of airway obstruction during sleep. Other potential treatment includes CPAP, supplemental oxygen, and even tracheotomy if the obstruction is severe. The patient should be further followed in the future to rule out the development of cardiac disease such as cor pulmonale or pulmonary hypertension from long-standing airway obstruction.

SUGGESTED READINGS

BALKANY TJ, DOWNS MP, JAFEK BW, KRAJICEK MJ. Hearing loss in Down syndrome. *Clin Pediatr.* 1979;18:116–118.

DAHLE AJ, MCCOLLISTER FP. Hearing and otologic disorders in children with Down syndrome. *Am J Ment Defic.* 1986;90:636–642.

HARLEY EH, COLLINS MD. Neurologic sequelae secondary to atlantoaxial instability in Down syndrome: implications in otolaryngologic surgery. *Arch Head Neck Surg.* 1994;120:159–165.

LEVINE OR, SIMPSER M. Alveolar hypoventilation and cor pulmonale associated with chronic airway obstruction in infants with Down syndrome. *Clin Pediatr.* 1982;21:25–29.

MARCUS CL, KEENS TG, BAUTISTA DB, et al. Obstructive sleep apnea in children with Down syndrome. *Pediatrics.* 1991;88:132–139.

MILLER R, GRAY SD, COTTON RT, MYER CM III. Subglottic stenosis and Down syndrome. *Am J Otol.* 1990;11:274–277.

PUESCHEL SM, SCOLA FH. Atlantoaxial instability in individuals with Down syndrome: epidemiologic, radiologic, and clinical studies. *Pediatrics.* 1987;80:555–560.

STROME M. Down's syndrome—A modern otorhinolaryngological perspective. *Laryngoscope.* 1981;41:1581–1594.

LARYNGEAL PAPILLOMA

Yoram Stern, M.D.
Sally R. Shott, M.D.

HISTORY

A 4-year-old boy presented to the otolaryngology clinic with a history of hoarseness, which has progressed relentlessly for the previous 5 months. The parents denied any history of respiratory difficulties or dysphagia. His primary care physician had treated him with antibiotics. However, his symptoms continued to worsen. The patient was the firstborn child of young parents and his medical history was unremarkable.

Physical examination revealed a child with no respiratory distress. Examination of the ears, oropharynx, nose, and neck was unremarkable. Flexible nasopharyngoscopy revealed a mass involving the right vocal cord. Vocal cord mobility was normal.

Based on the history and physical examination, direct laryngoscopy and bronchoscopy with biopsy were performed.

DIFFERENTIAL DIAGNOSIS— KEY POINTS

1. The patient's main symptom, hoarseness, tends to be overlooked in children until it reaches a certain level of severity.

2. Short-term hoarseness is usually related to laryngeal inflammation. This is usually accompanied by other airway complaints or dysphagia, and systemic manifestations.

3. Progressive hoarseness is usually due to vocal cord lesions. The most common lesion in the pediatric age group is the simple laryngeal nodules, polyps, or keratosis of the vocal cord caused by vocal abuse. In addition to progression of hoarseness, there is fluctuation in the severity of symptoms.

4. Acquired recurrent laryngeal nerve involvement causing hoarseness may be seen as part of a host of peripheral neuropathies (including metal poisoning, deficiency states, diabetic and postinfectious polyneuropathy). Impaired vocal cord mobility can also be due to cricotracheal joint dislocation due to traumatic intubation or neck trauma. Flexible nasopharyngoscopy can usually rule out vocal cord mobility problems even in uncooperative patients.

5. Relentlessly progressive hoarseness should suggest neoplasms of which juvenile laryngeal papillomas are the most common lesion. Other possible lesions are laryngeal hemangiomas, although these tend to occur before 6 months of age. Rare neoplasms include neurogenic tumor, benign and malignant mesenchymal tumors, and squamous cell carcinoma. Final diagnosis needs to be made by biopsy.

INTERPRETATION

In any infant or young child with symptoms of hoarseness or voice change, flexible nasopharyngoscopy should be performed. If this reveals a mass involving the larynx, direct laryngoscopy with biopsy is indicated for definitive diagnosis.

Direct laryngoscopy revealed an irregular subglottic mass involving the right vocal cord (Fig. 65–1). The mass was excised and sent for biopsy. Histologic evaluation of the biopsied tissue revealed projections of connective tissue cores covered by stratified squamous epithelium (Fig. 65–2).

Malignant degeneration is rare but possible. Therefore, the biopsy should be repeated in cases of rapid growth or grossly suspected lesions.

DIAGNOSIS

Respiratory papillomatosis.

MEDICAL MANAGEMENT

The variety of medical control options for this disease reflects the difficulty in defining a definitive corrective therapy. Variable response was reported in several prospective studies using interferon treatment. Interferon is usually given for at least 6 months and exacerbation is possible after discontinuation of treatment (rebound phenomenon). Other treatment modalities include retinoids (vitamin A analogues), acyclovir, antimetabolites, and photodynamic therapy. None are of proven value.

SURGICAL MANAGEMENT

Currently the procedure of choice for recurrent respiratory papillomas is microsuspension laryngoscopy with CO_2 laser removal of the papillomas. The laser allows vaporization of the papilloma while preserving normal tissue around it. Anesthetic options during the procedure include laser-safe endotracheal tube, jet ventilation, apneic technique, and spontaneous ventilation. Although a better knowledge of laser application has resulted in fewer intraoperative complications, there have been reports of delayed local tissue damages in up to 35% of the patients. In some patients rapid and extensive growth of the papilloma may result in life-threatening airway obstruction. In these cases

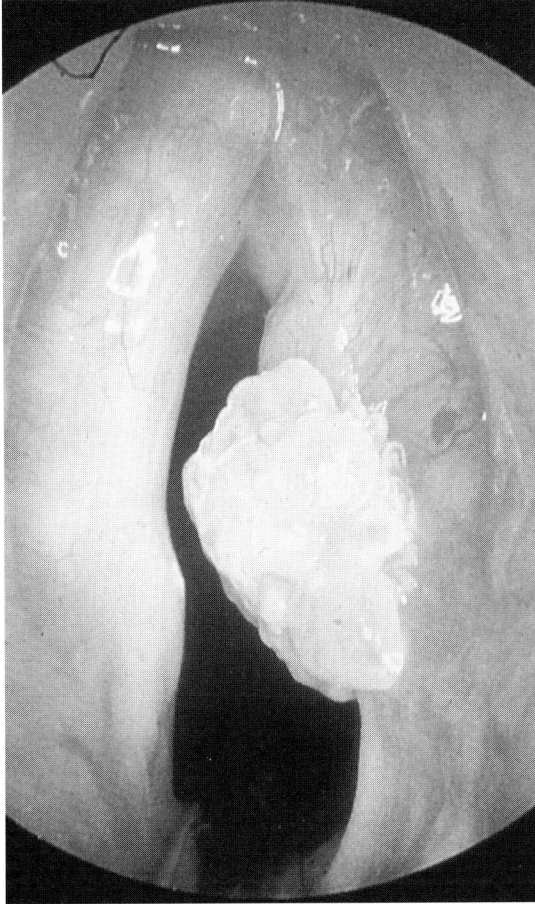

FIGURE 65-1 Laryngoscopy reveals an irregular subglottic mass involving the right vocal cord.

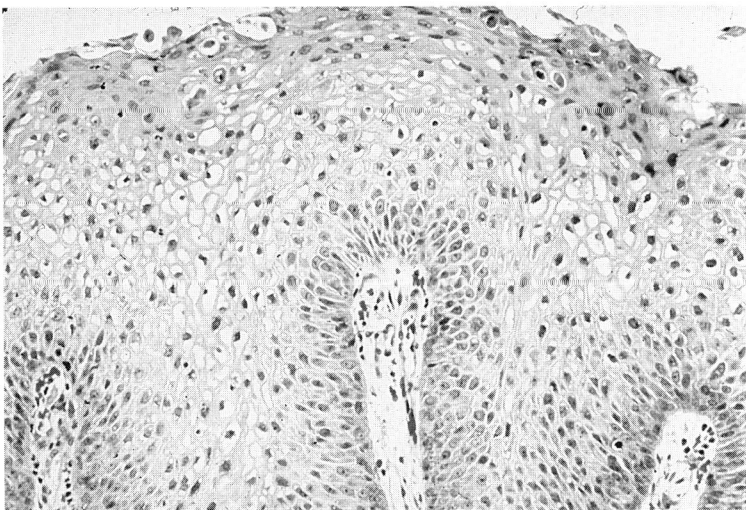

FIGURE 65-2 Histologic evaluation of the biopsied tissue demonstrates projections of connective tissue cores covered by stratified squamous epithelium.

tracheotomy may be required to provide a safe airway. However, association between tracheostomy and distal spread of the papillomas has been noted.

The natural course of the disease often results in spontaneous regression over the years, and complete removal of the papillomas is unrealistic and unnecessary. Therefore, inappropriately aggressive treatment should be avoided.

REHABILITATION AND FOLLOW-UP

Characteristically, the clinical course of the disease is unpredictable. The papilloma may respond to a single treatment or recur chronically, arising from multiple sites and spreading to the distal tracheobronchial tree. The papillomas may regress spontaneously during puberty but some progress into adulthood. Malignant transformation has been described. Therefore, periodic biopsies should be done. Chest x-ray should be performed annually. When distal spread is suspected, chest CT should be obtained. Because of the morbidity and the emotional strain associated with this disease, moral support to the patient and the family is of great importance.

SUGGESTED READINGS

ABRAMSON AL, SHIKOWITZ MJ, MULLOOLY VM, et al. Clinical effects of photodynamic therapy on recurrent laryngeal papillomas. *Arch Otolaryngol Head Neck Surg.* 1992;188:25–29.

AVIDANO MA, SINGLETON GT. Adjuvant drug strategies in the treatment of recurrent respiratory papillomatosis. *Otolaryngol Head Neck Surg.* 1995;112:197–202.

COLE RR, MYER CM, COTTON RT. Tracheostomy in children with recurrent respiratory papillomatosis. *Head Neck.* 1989;11:226–230.

CROCKETT DM, MCCABE BF, SHIVE CJ. Complication of laser surgery for recurrent respiratory papillomatosis. *Ann Otol Rhinol Laryngol.* 1987;96:639–644.

HEALY GB, GELBER RD, TROWBRIDGE AL, et al. Treatment of recurrent respiratory papillomatosis with human leukocyte interferon. *N Engl J Med.* 1980;314:401–407.

LEVENTHAL BG, KASHIMD HK, MOUNTS P, et al. Long-term response of recurrent respiratory papillomatosis to treatment with lymphoblastoid interferon ALFA-n1. *N Engl J Med.* 1991;325:613–617.

SCHNADIG VJ, CLARK WD, CLEGG TJ, YAO CS. Invasive papillomatosis and squamous carcinoma complicating juvenile laryngeal papillomatosis. *Arch Otolaryngol Head Neck Surg.* 1986;112:966–971.

PLASTIC AND RECONSTRUCTION

MANDIBULAR DEFECT
Lyon L. Gleich, M.D.

HISTORY

The patient is a 62-year-old male who presented with a T4N2cM0 squamous cell carcinoma of the floor of the mouth. The tumor involved the entire anterior oral tongue and invaded the mandible widely in its anterior segment. The palpable adenopathy consists of two 2-cm mid-jugular nodes on the left and one 1.5-cm mid-jugular node on the right. He has a 80 pack/year smoking history and drinks 20 beers per week. He has mild chronic obstructive pulmonary disease. He lost 10 pounds in the past 6 months.

After thorough consultation, the patient opted for surgical treatment with planned post-operative radiation. The surgery was begun and consisted of a left radical neck dissection and right modified neck dissection preserving the internal jugular vein. The primary tumor resection was accomplished by performing mandibulotomies just posterior to the mandibular angle on the left and just anterior to the angle on the right and resecting nearly the entire tongue. The necks and primaries were removed en bloc. The resected specimen is shown in Figure 66–1 and the defect is shown in Figure 66–2. (Arrows on both figures point to mandibular osteotomy sites.)

DIFFERENTIAL DIAGNOSIS—
KEY POINTS

1. Mandibular reconstruction aims to restore the continuity and function of the mandible. For lateral segmental mandibular defects this is often easier than for anterior defects. For lateral defects osseous reconstruction is not essential. The soft tissues can be reconstructed with appropriate flaps and the patient will have adequate function and cosmesis. Restoration of mandibular continuity with a plate or osseous reconstruction can be performed for lateral defects, but the functional and cosmetic benefits are not as great as for anterior defects.

2. Anterior mandibular defects require osseous reconstruction to prevent the "Andy Gump" deformity. The reconstruction is complicated and adds additional hours to the surgery. The anterior bone should therefore only be sacrificed when it is clearly at risk of invasion. If the risk of mandibular invasion by the cancer is not high, either a stripping of the mandibular periosteum or a marginal mandibulectomy may prevent the need for a complex reconstruction. The relationship of the cancer to the mandible can best be assessed on clinical exam. Firm fixation of the tumor to the bone, loose teeth adjacent to the tumor, or decreased sensation in the region of the mental nerve all are highly suggestive of mandibular invasion. Scans and panorex films are helpful as supplements to a thorough exam.

3. This patient has a significant osseous and soft tissue defect as a result of the necessary surgery to adequately resect his tumor. The bony defect is sizable, measuring in excess of 12 cm. Additionally, the soft tissue reconstruction needs to replace the floor of the mouth to permit oral alimentation without aspiration. In this patient a significant portion of the tongue base was not resected and would

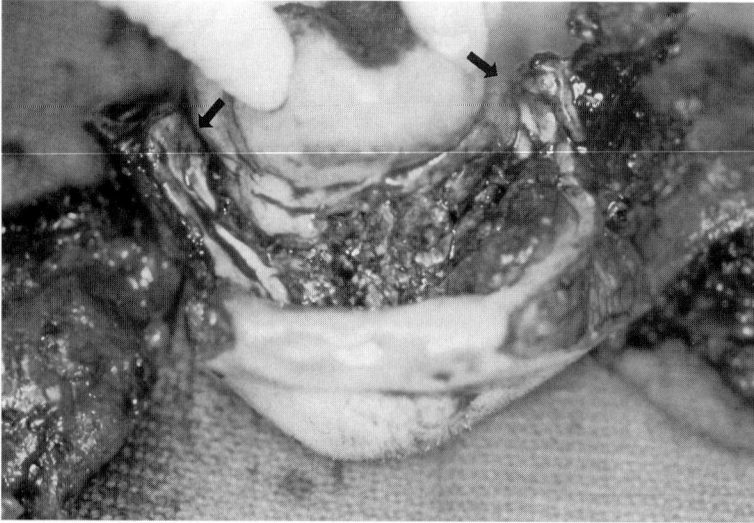

FIGURE 66–1 Resected specimen.

provide sufficient protection of the larynx. If this patient's tumor resection required a complete glossectomy or the patient was debilitated, consideration should be given to also resecting the larynx to prevent severe aspiration.

TEST INTERPRETATION

1. Preoperative computed tomography (CT) scan and panorex film confirmed invasion of the mandible, thus necessitating complete mandibulectomy.

2. Intraoperative frozen sections confirmed clear margins prior to attempting this major reconstructive procedure.

DIAGNOSIS

Anterior postsurgical mandibular defect.

MEDICAL MANAGEMENT

A large osseous defect such as this requires surgical correction to permit function and prevent the "Andy Gump" deformity. Intraoperatively intensive medical management of fluids and electrolytes is necessary to keep the patient stable for the long surgical procedure. Postoperatively the medical management will require intensive pulmonary toilet and nutritional supplementation to permit healing.

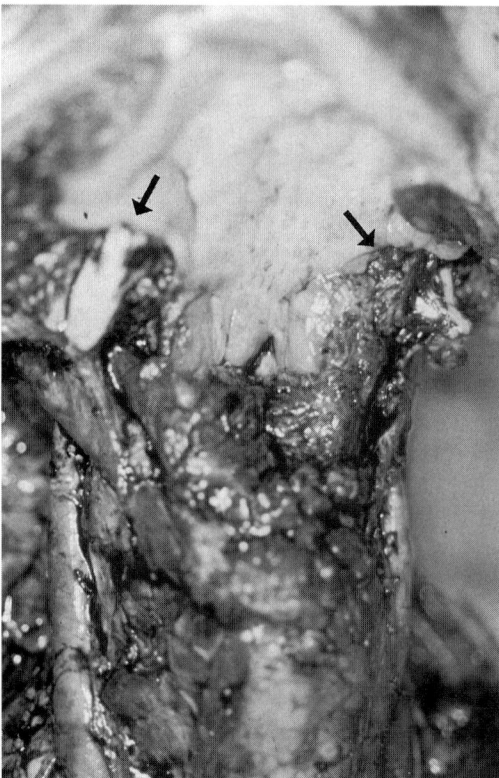

FIGURE 66–2 Surgical defect of mandible.

SURGICAL MANAGEMENT

In the past alloplasts, plates, and trays were the best options for mandibular reconstruction. Vascularized osteocutaneous flaps are now the accepted standard for reconstructing anterior mandibular defects. Potential donor sites for the osteocutaneous flaps include iliac crest, fibula, and scapula. Radial forearm has been used for mandibular reconstruction, but the donor site morbidity is great from harvesting radius and the amount of bone available is often insufficient.

The iliac crest osteocutaneous flap is supplied by the deep circumflex iliac vessels and is harvested with the overlying skin and internal oblique muscle. The iliac crest curvature resembles the mandible and can be used to reconstruct defects up to 16 cm in size. The internal oblique muscle has an axial blood supply and can be positioned relatively freely to aid in the oral reconstruction. The skin paddle, however, has a fixed relationship to the ilium due to multiple perforating vessels, limiting its reconstructive ability. If the soft tissues are insufficient for reconstruction additional flaps can be combined with the iliac crest flap. The harvesting of the iliac crest flap can result in significant morbidity, especially hip pain. Additionally, harvesting of the oblique muscles can result in abdominal herniation. The iliac crest bone can support osteointegrated implants for dental restoration.

The scapular osteocutaneous flap is supplied by the circumflex scapular vessels, which are large-caliber long vessels. Up to 10 to 14 cm of bone can be harvested and osteotomies can be made in the bone to achieve an appropriate shape. The soft tissue paddle is supplied by descending branches of the circumflex scapular vessel and is a fasciocutaneous flap, referred to as the parascapular flap, which can be separated significantly from the bone and rotated to aid in reconstruction. Extensive skin paddles can be transferred based on these vessels. Harvesting the scapular flap can result in injury to the brachial plexus, shoulder joint, and axillary muscles. In particular, teres major is often injured. If extensive skin is harvested, closure of the donor site may be difficult. A significant limitation of this flap is that the harvesting must wait until after the resection is completed since the patient needs to be repositioned. Finally, the bone is of insufficient thickness to support osteointegrated implants.

The fibula osteocutaneous flap is supplied by the peroneal vessels, and greater than 20 cm of bone can be harvested. This is therefore the ideal flap for reconstructing a defect such as in this patient since so much bone is needed. Multiple wedge-shaped osteotomies, without injuring the peroneal vessels that run the length of the bone, are necessary to convert the straight fibula into an appropriate shape for mandibular reconstruction. The overlying skin flap is supplied by perforators from the peroneal vessels of varying reliability. If the perforators are not seen the skin flap is less viable. Harvesting the lateral sural cutaneous nerve and anastomosing this to a sensory nerve may increase oral sensation after reconstruction. As with the other flaps, the fibular flap has its limitations. Anatomic variations may result in an absent or malformed fibula. The peroneal artery contributes a significant portion of the blood supply to the foot in 10 to 20% of people, and harvesting can result in ischemia in these cases. Preoperative assessment of pedal pulses can help prevent this. Harvesting can result in injury to the peroneal nerve as well as muscle weakness, edema, and cold intolerance. Skin grafts are often needed to close the skin donor site. Closing the donor site tightly can result in compartment syndrome. The skin flap fails in 5 to 10% of cases and a second flap for soft tissue reconstruction should be considered at the time of surgery. The fibular flap can accept osteointegrated implants; however, the implant must be shorter than that which would be placed in an iliac crest graft.

For this patient a fibula flap was used in conjunction with a radial forearm flap for additional soft tissue. The fibula permitted reconstruction of this extensive bony defect and the radial forearm was used to line the soft tissue of the floor of the mouth. A gastrostomy was placed as well as a tracheostomy.

REHABILITATION AND FOLLOW-UP

One week after surgery the patient was begun on a course of ambulation with assistance from physical therapy. Decannulation is usually possible by 14 days after surgery. A limited oral diet is usually tolerated by 2 months after surgery, permitting gastrostomy tube removal. External beam radiation can usually be started by 6 weeks following surgery.

In patients who undergo extensive surgery, intensive pulmonary care must be given to prevent pneumonia. In particular, this should include frequent tracheal suctioning and early mobilization.

A gastrostomy tube should be used to maintain adequate nutrition for wound healing. Swallowing can be aided by a therapist. A supraglottic-type diet, which consists of soft foods, but not liquids is usually preferred. Liquids, while easiest to move to the oropharynx, are also the easiest material to aspirate. The therapist utilizes a variety of head positions to aid swallowing therapy, in particular, bending of the neck at the pharyngeal phase to open the hypopharynx. The patient is instructed to cough after each swallow to expunge aspirated material. With this regimen most patients can slowly expand their oral diet.

The fibula flap can usually accept osteointegrated implants. Implants can aid in dental restoration, further improving cosmesis and function. However, these patients have already been through extensive therapy and rehabilitation, and often do not wish to undergo any further elective treatment.

SUGGESTED READINGS

HIDALGO DA, REKOW A. A review of 60 consecutive fibula free flap mandible reconstructions. *Plast Reconstr Surg.* 1995;96:585–596.

KOMISAR A. The functional result of mandibular reconstruction. *Laryngoscope.* 1990;100:364–374.

URKEN ML. Composite free flaps in oromandibular reconstruction. Review of the literature. *Arch Otolaryngol Head Neck Surg.* 1991;117:724–732.

HYPOPHARYNGEAL RECONSTRUCTION

Lyon L. Gleich, M.D.

HISTORY

A 65-year-old male had undergone a total laryngectomy and partial pharyngectomy with a left radical neck dissection, right neck dissection preserving the internal jugular vein and cranial nerve XI, and reconstruction with a pectoralis flap for a T3N1M0 squamous cell carcinoma of the left pyriform sinus. He did well in the initial postoperative period; however, on the fifth postoperative day saliva was noted superior to the stoma. The right side of the wound was opened to permit drainage. Wound care with wet to dry dressings was then attempted, but there was no evidence of healing over a 2-week period. During this period a gastrostomy was performed and the nasogastric feeding tube removed.

DIFFERENTIAL DIAGNOSIS— KEY POINTS

1. Fistulas following major head and neck surgery with myocutaneous flap reconstructions are common, occurring in nearly 25% of cases. In this instance a pectoralis flap was used for reconstruction of a hypopharyngeal defect. The pectoralis flap is advantageous in that it has an excellent blood supply, easily reaches the hypopharynx, is familiar to otolaryngologists, and does not require microscopic techniques. In reconstructing the hypopharynx, though, the pectoralis flap needs to be partially curved and has a tendency to unfurl. This may result in fistula formation.

2. The initial treatment of any fistula of the head and neck is to establish appropriate drainage. Most fistula will heal thereafter with basic wound care. When healing does not occur it is important to reassess the situation. Many factors may delay wound healing, but the most significant in this situation would be (1) persistent cancer, (2) nutritional depletion, or (3) inadequate or poorly vascularized tissues.

3. The pathology should be carefully examined to determine if the surgical margins were negative. If the margins were not clear, an attempt should be made to determine where the positive margin was and to resect the persistent tumor if possible. If the margins were clear the patient should be assessed for nutritional factors that may influence wound healing. The patient may be receiving insufficient enteral nutrition, and malnourishment can result in a nonhealing wound. If the enteral intake is sufficient laboratory values related to wound healing should be checked. In particular, albumin level can be used to determine the degree of malnourishment. Additionally, poor thyroid function can impair wound healing, so thyroid hormone levels should be assessed. Electrolyte insufficiencies, particularly for magnesium can impair healing and should also be checked and replaced if necessary.

4. While these nutritional factors are being managed wound care should be continued. If there is still impaired healing then the problem is related to insufficient or poorly vascularized tissue. Prior radiation therapy is a frequent cause of wound breakdown; however, in this case the patient has not been irradiated. Diabetes and other systemic diseases, such as liver failure can also impair wound healing. However, most often in head and neck cancer patients poor healing occurs due to marginal nutritional status compounded by the effects of tobacco smoking.

TEST INTERPRETATION

In this patient the surgical margins were negative for malignancy. There were two positive nodes in the left neck. The patient has been tolerating adequate nutritional supplementation. The albumin level is at the lower limits of normal. The magnesium level was low, but normalized after replacement. No other electrolyte abnormalities were detected. The hematocrit is 32. The thyroid hormone level was low and was replaced with levothyroxine sodium. Despite this the fistula persisted and the patient is now at 1 month after surgery (Fig. 67–1).

DIAGNOSIS

Fistula following reconstruction of a hypopharyngeal defect.

MEDICAL MANAGEMENT

A persistent fistula is a difficult complication to manage. This patient has now been medically optimized for healing, with appropriate nutrition, thyroid hormone, electrolyte replacement, and smoking cessation.

SURGICAL MANAGEMENT

The next concern is to formulate a plan to recreate a pharynx without additional untoward effects. Additionally, this patient needs to be irradiated, and this should begin within 6 weeks of his surgery. Further surgery will most likely delay the irradiation, and while radiation can be given to open wounds, it does complicate the final reconstruction.

In this patient the wound was explored and the edges trimmed. The resultant defect is shown in Figure 67–2. The pectoralis flap had indeed unfurled, and the remaining posterior mucosa had become scarified. There was insufficient tissue to close the wound directly. The options for reconstructing this hypopharyngeal defect would include (1) another myocutaneous flap, (2) a free flap, or (3) a gastric pull-up. Other procedures, such as the Bakamjian deltopectoral flap for reconstruction, are now rarely utilized due to the need for multiple procedures. While another myocutaneous flap, such as the opposite pectoralis flap, could be used to close this defect, sewing two myocutaneous flaps together would have a high risk of further complications and was not done. The gastric pull-up, while a viable option for hypopharyngeal reconstruction, is highly morbid due to the need to traumatize both the chest and abdomen. Free vascularized flaps were therefore the best option in this patient.

The hypopharynx can be reconstructed using either jejunal free flaps or tubed radial forearm flaps. The radial forearm flap reduces the need for a laparotomy, but an additional suture line is necessary to tube this flap. The jejunal flap requires suturing only superiorly and inferiorly

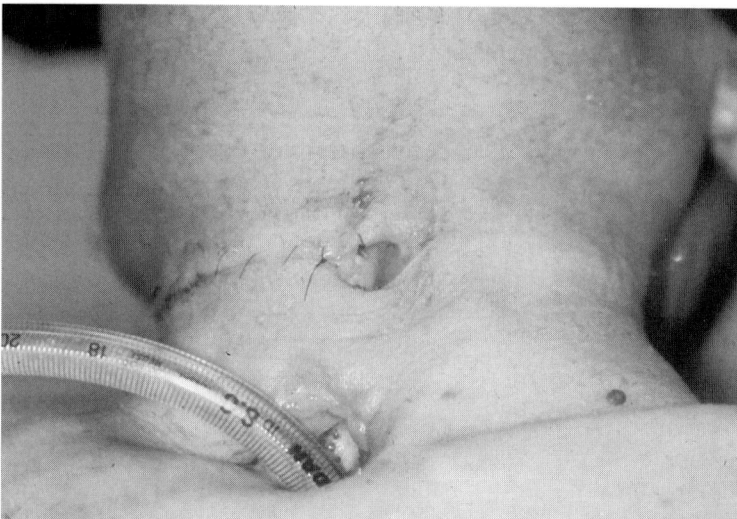

FIGURE 67–1 Fistula resulting from reconstruction of a hypopharyngeal defect.

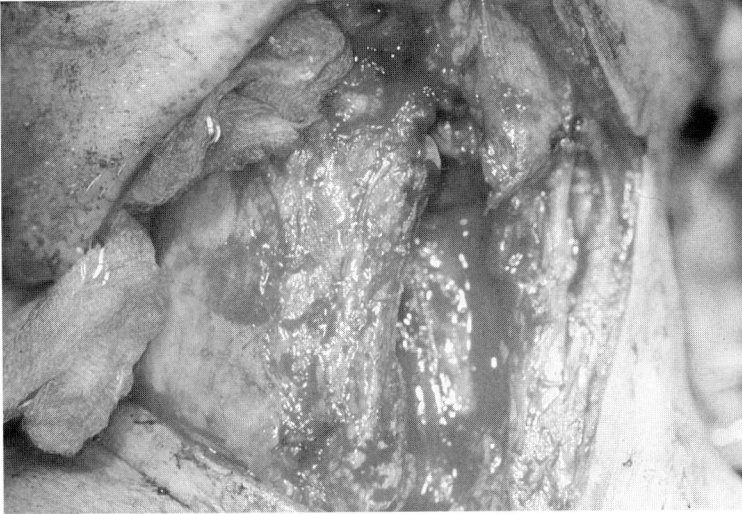

FIGURE 67-2 Note that the pectoralis flap has unfurled and the remaining posterior mucosa is scarified.

and has proven efficacy in reconstructing complex hypopharyngeal defects. The jejunum was therefore utilized to reconstruct this patient's hypopharynx (Fig. 67-3). The remaining posterior pharyngeal wall mucosa was removed and the pectoralis flap was permitted to remain in the neck. There was a persistent significant skin defect by the stoma, which was closed with a deltopectoral flap. The patient healed well and was able to tolerate a diet on postoperative day 10. Radiation began 7 weeks after the initial surgery.

REHABILITATION AND FOLLOW-UP

The patient's swallowing did become partially impaired during the radiation therapy, and he resumed using his gastrostomy tube. One month following radiation the patient tolerated all of his feeding orally and the tube was removed. Speech was rehabilitated with an electrolarynx. It is possible to develop either tracheoesophageal puncture (TEP) or esophageal speech after jejunal reconstruction, but the results are inferior to those obtained in other patients. This patient was satisfied with electrolarynx speech and did not wish to try other techniques. The patient was seen for routine follow-up visits. The thyroid levels were monitored and replacement continued. Annual chest x-rays and laboratory evaluation were performed.

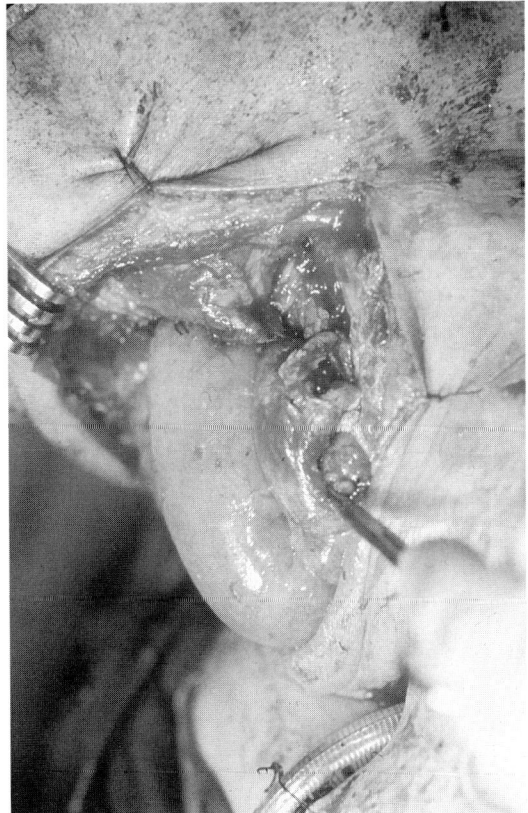

FIGURE 67-3 Reconstruction of the hypopharynx using the jejunum.

SUGGESTED READINGS

Ariyan S. The pectoralis major myocutaneous flap: a versatile flap for reconstruction in the head and neck. *Plast Reconstr Surg.* 1979;63:73–81.

Fabian RL. Reconstruction of the laryngopharynx and cervical esophagus. *Laryngoscope.* 1984;94:1334–1350.

Gluckman JL, McDonough J, Donegan JO, et al. The free jejunal graft in head and neck reconstruction. *Laryngoscope.* 1981;91:1887–1895.

NASAL RECONSTRUCTION OF A MOH'S SURGICAL DEFECT

James Clemens, M.D.
Kevin A. Shumrick, M.D.

HISTORY

A 75-year-old white male presents for surgical repair after Moh's excision of a cutaneous malignancy of the nose. The defect is 2.1 cm and involves the majority of the nasal tip (Fig. 68–1). The lower lateral cartilage is exposed, but intact. There is no communication to the intranasal cavity.

DIFFERENTIAL DIAGNOSIS— KEY POINTS

1. Mohs' micrographic surgery was developed by Dr. Frederick E. Mohs in 1936. The basic principle of this technique is complete evaluation of the margin of the resection, and serial excisions of residual tumor-positive areas only. After removing the bulk of the lesion with a small rim of normal appearing skin, the specimen is flattened with releasing incisions, so that the cut surface is in one plane. Frozen sections are then taken and evaluated for residual tumor. The stained borders orient the specimen and direct the surgeon to areas of residual tumor, which are excised. The entire process is repeated until all margins are negative for tumor.

2. Basal cell carcinoma (BCCA) commonly occurs on the nose and is the most common form of malignant skin neoplasm, accounting for 77% of all cases. Originating at the basal layer of the skin, its histologic borders are often wider than they appear clinically. Sun exposure is the major risk factor for this tumor, with 90% of BCCA occurring on the head and neck. BCCA rarely metastasizes.

3. Squamous cell carcinoma (SCCA) accounts for 20% of cutaneous malignancies. While SCCA may metastasize, it is uncommon except in cases where the primary is extremely large or deeply invasive. Regional nodal groups deserve close clinical evaluation and follow-up.

4. Melanoma accounts for less than 10% of skin cancers; however, 20% of these arise on the head and neck. The most common locations in decreasing frequency are the cheek, scalp, ear, and neck. Sun exposure and congenital nevi are primary risk factors.

5. When planning closure of any surgical defect it is important to consider host factors that may reduce the success of the closure. Tobacco usage, diabetes, and poor nutritional status can all adversely affect the ability of skin grafts to take and pedicled flaps to survive. In these patients delaying a flap may be a consideration.

TEST INTERPRETATION

Lesions of the skin can be treated under local anesthesia in most cases. Unless intravenous sedation or general anesthesia is planned, minimal preoperative laboratory testing is indicated.

If this lesion had not been excised by a Moh's surgeon, a tissue diagnosis would be necessary. Biopsy options include excisional biopsy, punch biopsy, incisional biopsy, or shave biopsy. In general, shave biopsies should be avoided because if melanoma is diagnosed tumor thickness can not be assessed on a shave biopsy specimen.

Further workup such as computed tomography scans are rarely indicated unless the malignancy is quite large with obvious deep invasion, cranial nerve involvement, or possibly evidence of metastasis.

DIAGNOSIS

Moh's defect following excision of a basal cell carcinoma of the nose.

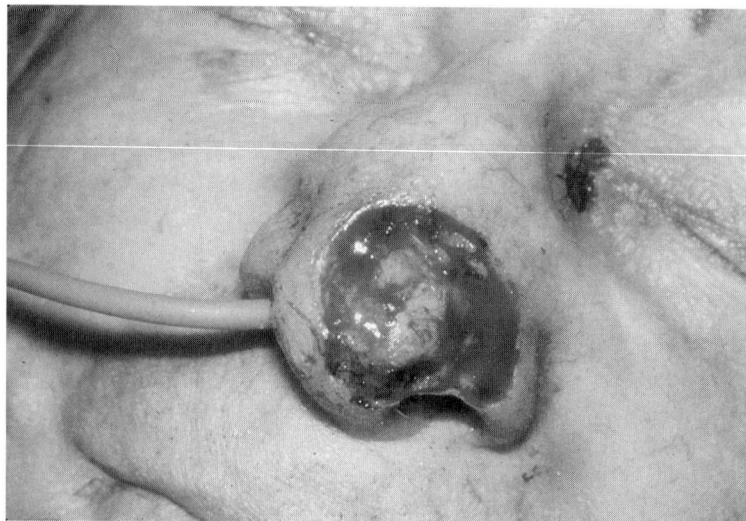

FIGURE 68–1 Moh's excision of a cutaneous malignancy of the nose. The lower lateral cartilage is exposed but intact and there is no communication to the intranasal cavity.

MEDICAL MANAGEMENT

There is little role for medical treatment of malignancies of the skin. Topical 5-fluorouracil has been applied to actinic keratoses but is not suggested for malignancies. At present no effective chemotherapy or immunotherapy exists.

Medical management should instead be directed at prevention. Patients should be educated about the harmful effects of ultraviolet (UV) exposure, tanning booths, and sun bathing. The use of sun blocks, brimmed hats, and clothing to limit the amount of UV exposure should be encouraged. In addition, education should be directed toward early diagnosis. Parents should be encouraged to provide children with adequate sun protection during outdoor activities.

SURGICAL MANAGEMENT

This type of a nasal defect can be reliably managed with a paramedian forehead flap (Fig. 68–2). Other flaps to consider include nasolabial, inner canthal, bilobe, and glabellar flaps. The paramedian forehead flap is based on the supratrochlear vessels. These vessels are terminal branches of the ophthalmic artery and exit the orbit medially traveling between the corrugator and orbicularis. At approximately the level of the medial aspect of the eyebrow they pierce the frontalis muscle and travel in the subcutaneous tissue toward the scalp. In planning this flap, the level of the medial brow (or slightly lower) is used as the point of rotation. A template of the defect and proposed stalk of the flap is made using the metal packaging from a suture pack or Vaseline gauze. The template is rotated onto the forehead over the course of the supratrochlear vessels. If needed a doppler may be used to confirm the position of these vessels. If necessary, hair-bearing scalp may be taken on the pedicle since this is easily shaved or can be treated using electrolysis. The flap is elevated in a plane under the frontalis muscle which serves to protect these vessels. The muscle is then removed under direct visualization to thin the flap. After the flap is sewn into position, the stalk is wrapped in Vaseline gauze for protection. The pedicle is divided and the remainder of the flap inset in 2 to 3 weeks (Fig. 68–3).

Full thickness or split thickness skin grafts could be employed as alternative techniques. These have the advantages of being easy to obtain with minimal donor site morbidity and they provide a thin covering of the defect, which will readily demonstrate tumor recurrence. Some advocate allowing the wound to granulate until the defect is near level to the epidermis with granulation tissue. A skin graft is then applied to the rich vascular bed of granulation tissue,

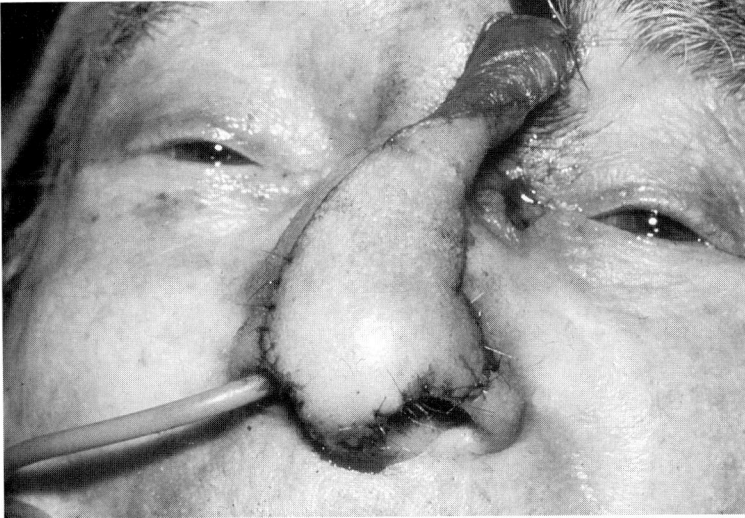

FIGURE 68-2 Paramedian forehead flap.

resulting in less of a sunken appearance over the defect.

Finally, this defect could heal by secondary intention as long as the exposed cartilage was

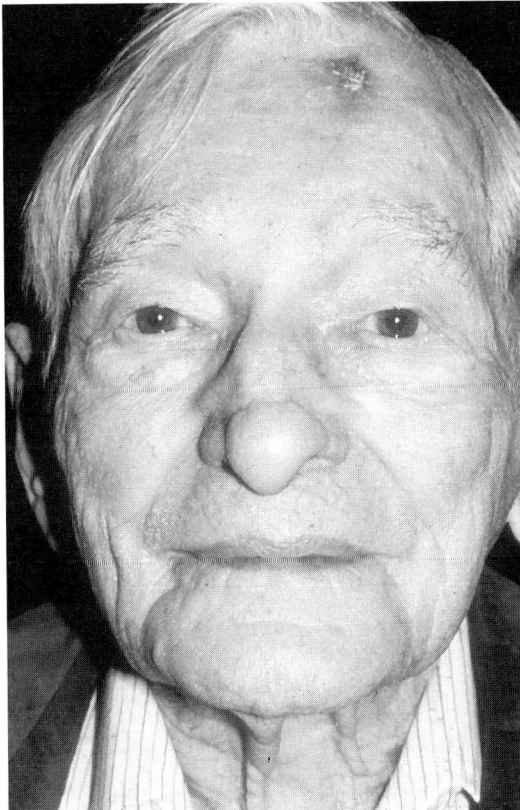

FIGURE 68-3 Postoperative result following division of pedicle.

kept covered. Disadvantages to this approach include scarring with alar retraction following a prolonged coarse of open wound care.

If the defect was through and through to the nasal cavity, a lining would be necessary. Options (depending on the size) include a septal flap, an epithelial turn-in flap, and a radial forearm free flap. A nasal lining is crucial to avoid unpredictable scarring resulting in alar retraction and/or nasal stenosis.

If cartilage is missing, it should be replaced to prevent retraction of the flap margins during healing. Conchal or septal cartilage are reliable sources for cartilage.

Consider excising complete nasal subunits before the contouring flap, especially if greater than 50% of the subunit has been removed. This generally results in improved osmesis. Avoid placing plugs which cross the alar or nostril margins if possible. Send all excised skin for pathologic exam to rule out persistent tumor.

REHABILITATION AND FOLLOW-UP

Depending on the suture material, stitches are generally removed within 1 week. If forehead flap has been used, the pedicle division takes place between 2 and 3 weeks. Some flaps may require defatting at the time of pedicle division or at a subsequent sitting if unsatisfactory. Wounds generally heal rapidly with minimal morbidity. The patient requires follow-up for the development of new or recurrent skin lesions on an annual basis by either a Moh's or a head and neck surgeon. All patients should be encouraged to use sunscreens to avoid additional actinic damage.

SUGGESTED READINGS

Baker SR, Swanson NA. *Local Flaps in Facial Reconstruction.* St. Louis, MO: Mosby–Year Book; 1995.

Burget GC, Menick FJ. *Aesthetic Reconstruction of the Nose.* St. Louis, MO: Mosby–Year Book, 1994.

Fleming ID et al. Principles of management of basal and squamous cell carcinoma of the skin, *Cancer.* 1995;75(2, suppl):699–704.

Morrison WA et al. Island inner canthal and glabellar flaps for nasal tip reconstruction. *Br J Plast Surg.* 1995;48:236–270.

Park SS et al. The epithelial turn in flap in nasal reconstruction. *Arch Otolaryngol Head Neck Surg.* 1995;121:1122–1127.

Shumrick KA. Nasal reconstruction, excluding the TIP. *Curr Opin Otolaryngol Head Neck Surg.* 1995;3: 286–292.

Shumrick KA. The anatomic basis for the design of forehead flaps in nasal reconstruction. *Arch Otolaryngol Head Neck Surg.* 1992;118:373–379.

Case 69

CONGENITAL NASAL MASS

Yoram Stern, M.D.
Charles M. Myer, III, M.D.

HISTORY

A 8-year-old girl presented with a long history of nasal obstruction and snoring. No rhinorrhea or epistaxis was reported. Physical examination revealed a pulsatile, bluish compressive mass in the right nasal cavity. Enlargement of the mass was noted with compression of the jugular vein (positive Furstenberg sign). No external deformity of the nose was noted. Examination of the nasopharynx and oropharynx was unremarkable as was the remainder of the head and neck examination. A computed tomography (CT) scan and magnetic resonance image (MRI) of the cranial fossa, orbits, paranasal sinuses, and nasopharynx were ordered.

DIFFERENTIAL DIAGNOSIS— KEY POINTS

1. This child presents with a prolonged history of nasal obstruction. The most common etiologies for nasal obstruction in children are chronic rhinosinusitis or adenoid hypertrophy. These potential causes can be identified generally while taking the history and performing the physical examination. An imaging study of the nasopharynx (lateral neck film) and a paranasal sinus CT scan can help in making the diagnosis.

2. Given the age of the patient, an acquired disorder is possible. Inflammatory conditions of the nose and nasopharynx are common in children. Antrochoanal polyps typically orig-

inate in the maxillary sinus and exit through the maxillary ostia, ultimately growing posteriorly into the nasopharynx. Similarly, sphenochoanal polyps arising from the sphenoid sinus extend through the sphenoid ostia into the sphenoethmoid recess and posterior choana. Nasal polyps, caused by inflammation or allergy, are not uncommon in children. Children with aspirin-sensitive allergies, cystic fibrosis, Woakes' syndrome, and Kartagener's syndrome (primary ciliary dyskinesia) are most likely to have nasal polyps. There is no evidence that this patient had any of these disorders. Nasal polyps in children are sometimes the initial manifestation of cystic fibrosis and a sweat chloride test should be performed whenever nasal polyps are discovered.

3. In the pediatric age group, the possibility of a foreign body as a cause for nasal obstruction should always be considered. Nasal foreign bodies usually present with unilateral purulent malodorous drainage.

4. Rhinoscopy in this child revealed a unilateral firm mass. The differential diagnosis should include both congenital lesions as well as neoplastic disorders, either benign or malignant.

5. Most nasal tumors in children are benign and include the juvenile angiofibroma in addition to schwannomas, fibromatosis, angiomatous polyps, and hemangiomas. Angiofibroma is the most common benign tumor in the nasal cavity in children. It usually presents in ado-

lescent males and spontaneous epistaxis is common. A CT scan of an angiofibroma will show irregular borders with intense vascular enhancement. Neither the clinical history nor the appearance of the lesion on radiologic studies in this case was compatible with this diagnosis. Malignant nasal tumors are rare in children. Rhabdomyosarcoma is the most common, while lymphoma, squamous cell carcinoma, and esthesioneuroblastoma occur less often. The duration of symptoms caused by malignant tumors is usually weeks or months rather than years as in this case. A definite diagnosis of a neoplasm can be made only by biopsy.

6. The most common congenital nasal masses in infants and children are encephaloceles, gliomas, and dermoids. Other lesions include teratomas and nasolacrimal duct cysts. Encephaloceles and gliomas may occur externally, intranasally, or as a combination of the two. The most important distinction of an encephalocele from a glioma is its patent intracranial connection. Therefore, an encephalocele is more often associated with previous meningitis. On physical examination, the mass is distinguished by its usually pulsatile nature and by its increase in size with compression of the jugular vein, thus reflecting connection with cerebrospinal fluid (CSF). CT and MRI are helpful in the differentiation between the two lesions.

Nasal dermoids often are accompanied by a widened nasal dorsum. They present as either cysts, sinus tracts (with or without fistulae), or as a combination of the two. Cysts may be located anywhere along the nasal dorsum and the floor of the frontal cranial fossa. The fistula often contains hair and most commonly occurs along the nasal dorsum but may be present even in the columella. Teratomas are uncommon tumors of the nasopharynx but may present intranasally and may be confused initially with an encephalocele. They are usually present at birth and, depending on the size, may cause nasal obstruction and respiratory distress.

Nasolacrimal duct cysts are quite rare. Such a cyst may protrude through the inferior meatus causing nasal obstruction. The patient usually presents with epiphora, dacryocystitis, and re-

spiratory distress. Intranasal examination reveals a cystic mass beneath the inferior turbinates, frequently bilaterally.

TEST INTERPRETATION

When a congenital nasal mass is suspected, a radiographic study is mandatory prior to biopsy or treatment. This determines, as best possible, whether an intracranial connection exists. Blind surgery with the presence of an intracranial component may result in a CSF leak or meningitis. MRI and CT are the two best diagnostic measures available. The MRI study is able to show intracranial extension if the skull base defect is not too small. It also better delineates the character of the soft tissue mass and is capable of presenting the anatomy in a multiplanar manner. Because of the limitation of MRI in evaluation of bone, CT is used to demonstrate the defect in the skull base. Thus, in combination, CT and MRI are the radiographic studies of choice.

A CT scan revealed a soft mass in the right nasal cavity with extension into the anterior cranial fossa through a bony defect (Fig. 69–1). MRI revealed brain tissue, which was actually herniating through the cribriform plate into the nasal cavity (Fig. 69–2). This brain tissue was surrounded by CSF and meninges.

DIAGNOSIS

Encephalocele.

MEDICAL MANAGEMENT

In cases where a bacterial meningitis develops, aggressive antimicrobial therapy according to CSF cultures is mandatory.

SURGICAL MANAGEMENT

Early surgical intervention is advised to alleviate the increased risk of meningitis. Also, the size of the lesion may increase with time and this increases the risk for a cosmetic deformity and the amount of herniated brain tissue that needs to be excised. A careful resection of the

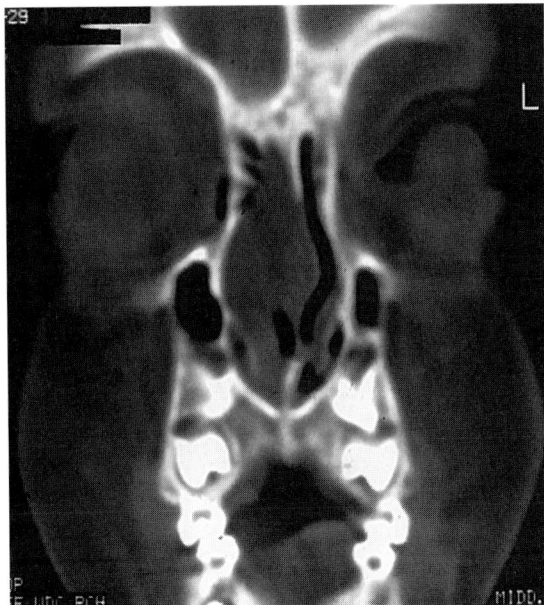

FIGURE 69–1 Coronal CT shows soft tissue mass in the right nasal cavity.

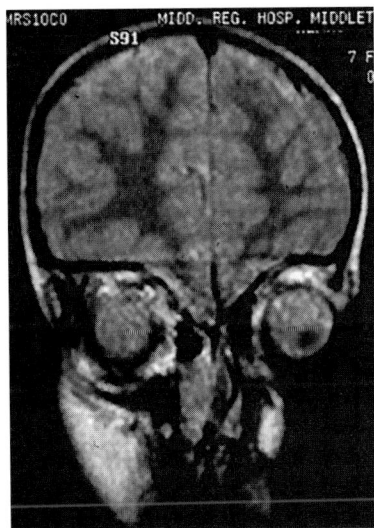

FIGURE 69–2 Coronal MRI shows brain tissue herniating through the cribriform plate.

encephalocele requires an intracranial exploration with a CSF-leakproof closure of the dural defect. These are almost impossible to achieve through subcranial approach. Therefore, a combined otolaryngologic and neurologic approach is required. A frontal craniotomy allows accurate identification of the intracranial extension as well as excellent visualization of the dural defect. Extracranial repair can be performed simultaneously or deferred to a later date. Surgical routes for extracranial excision include lateral rhinotomy, osteoplastic flap, or sagittal approach over the roof of the nose.

REHABILITATION AND FOLLOW-UP

In the immediate postoperative period, any sign of a CSF leak should be evaluated carefully and addressed as necessary. Once healed, the patient will be evaluated periodically in the clinic and imaging studies will be ordered if there is a suspicion of recurrence or CSF leak. A high incidence of other central nervous system anomalies exists with encephalocele. Therefore, a brain CT scan to look for other abnormalities, including absence of the corpus callosum and ventricular dilatation, is worthwhile.

SUGGESTED READINGS

HALEY EH. Pediatric congenital nasal masses. *ENT J.* 1991;70:28–32.

KENNARD CD, RASMUSSEN TE. Congenital midline nasal masses: diagnosis and management. *J Dermatol Surg Oncol.* 1990;16:1025–1036.

MORGAN DW, EVANS JNG. Developmental nasal anomalies. *J Laryngol.* 1990;104:394–403.

PALLER AS, PENSLER JM, TOMIT T. Nasal midline masses in infants and children: dermoids, enceophaloceles and gliomas. *Arch Dermatol.* 1991;127:362–366.

PROMINAURIS AND OTOPLASTY

J. Scott McMurray, M.D.
Glenn O. Bratcher, M.D.

HISTORY

A 3-year-old boy presents with parental complaints that his ears are too prominent. In the past, an uncle was teased throughout his school years because of his ears. He has strongly urged his sister to seek help for his nephew to prevent this from happening to him. The grandparents are upset with his persistent urging, because his ears are like many others in the family. Further history reveals that both maternal and paternal family members have had some form of prominent ears. The grandparents' generations had prominent ears in about half of the family members.

Physical examination is unremarkable except for mildly prominent ears (Fig. 70–1). There is underdevelopment of the antihelical fold causing furling of the helix. The conchal bowl is also prominent, cupping the ear. The auriculocephalic angle is approximately 45 degrees.

DIFFERENTIAL DIAGNOSIS— KEY POINTS

1. The diagnosis of prominauris or prominent ears relies on the clinician's ability to recognize the normal ear. Normal ears can be asymmetric in size, position, and protrusion. The cosmetically ideal auriculocephalic angle is 30 degrees (Fig. 70–2). Ninety-eight percent of normal ears show an auriculocephalic angle between 25 and 35 degrees. Angulation exceeding 40 to 45 degrees is generally considered abnormal. The fossa triangularis should face laterally rather than anteriorly. The long axis of the pinna averages 55 mm from lobule to the dome. The short axis averages 34 mm from the tragus to the helix.

2. Simple observation is generally used for the diagnosis of the prominent ear. Auricular deformity occurs in approximately 5% of whites. The most common cause of prominauris is unfurling or lack of development of the antihelical and superior crural folds. This causes anterior projection of the upper half of the auricle. The second most common deformity is related to a wide, broad, and thickened conchal bowl. This may occur alone or in combination with helical unfurling. Differential treatment plans require proper recognition of the abnormal portion of the pinna.

3. Many descriptive terms have been used to designate the several, sometimes overlapping types of auricular deformities. *Microtia* refers to underdevelopment and distinctive malformation of the pinna. The lobule and the vestigial remnants of the hillocks are the only recognizable structures. An arrest in development at the sixth to eighth week of of gestation is responsible for the auricular abnormality and is frequently associated with atresia of the external auditory canal. Other abnormalities of the first and second branchial arches should be ruled out.

The *lop ear* has cartilage that is soft and lacks strength. The ear hangs limp, folding forward at the upper pole due to faulty development of the helix, scapha, and antihelix. The ear appears to be smaller than normal.

The *cup ear* may display characteristics of both the lop and protruding ear. Overdevelopment of a deep concave concha is the main deformity. A poorly developed upper pole and antihelix are combined with a short helix and cupped lobule to give the characteristic deformity. The vertical height of the auricle is usually smaller than normal. The auric-

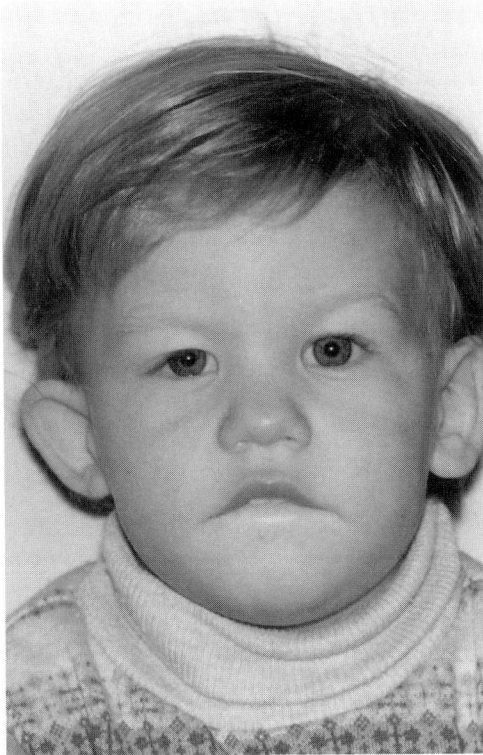

FIGURE 70-1 Mildly prominent ears in 3-year-old boy.

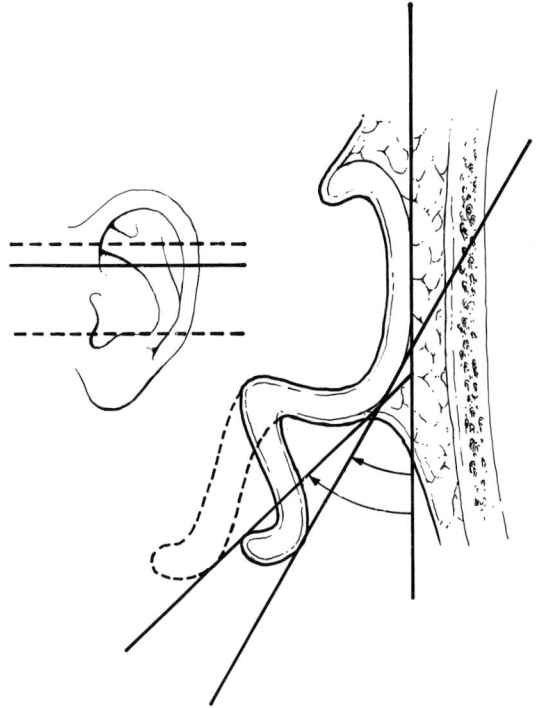

FIGURE 70-2 Auriculocephalic angle.

ular cartilage is usually thick and resilient, making surgical correction more difficult.

The *protruding ear* has a normally shaped and sized ear but with unfurling of the superior crus and antihelix. These abnormalities are usually present at birth but become more conspicuous with age.

4. The otic placode begins to develop during the third week of gestation. The pinna begins to develop during the sixth week of gestation as a series of swellings known as the auricular hillocks of His. These six growth centers surround the dorsal end of the first branchial (mandibular) arch and the caudal end of the second branchial (hyoid) arch. Most commonly accepted is that the six hillocks correlate directly with the tragus, helix, cymbum, scapha, antihelix, and antitragus. Near complete growth of the auricle occurs by the age of 5 to 6. Restoration of normal anatomic relations can be performed at this time before the child enters school.

5. Deformity criteria have been established to aid in the decision making for reconstruction. The auriculocephalic angle should be less than 35 degrees. The normal auricle has a vertical axis directed approximately 20 degrees posteriorly. The average vertical height of the auricle is 6 cm. The width is approximately 55% of the length. The helical rim should protrude approximately 1 to 2 cm from the skull. The superior aspect of the auricle is usually level with the brow. Other significant auricular landmark deformities include a poor antihelical fold, an overdeveloped concha, an abnormally formed scapha, and an obvious lack of superior and inferior crus surrounding the fossa triangularis. If the anatomic relationships of the ear are found to be outside these criteria, surgical intervention may be contemplated.

TEST INTERPRETATION

No specific tests are indicated in the evaluation of patients with simple prominauris. Evaluation should include photographic documentation of the deformity.

DIAGNOSIS

Prominauris, or prominent ears.

MEDICAL MANAGEMENT

There is no effective medical therapy for this problem. Psychosocial support and intervention are occasionally necessary in cases accompanied by the emotional consequences of teasing and harassment.

SURGICAL MANAGEMENT

Approximation of the normal parameters of the aesthetic ear is the goal of otoplasty. There are many surgical techniques that may be used depending on the abnormality encountered. The technique chosen should allow restoration of the normal auriculocephalic angle of 30 degrees, while maintaining the normal appearance and curvature of the auricular components. The helical curve should remain gentle without pinching or unusual breaks. Reduction of an enlarged conchal bowl may also be necessary.

Many surgical techniques have been created to correct the prominent ear. The development of each technique centers around correcting the anatomic abnormality identified. The basic steps in each technique attempt to recreate the antihelical fold and/or to correct the auriculocephalic angle. The main differences between the different techniques lie in those that incise or resect cartilage and those that do not. As stated earlier, the main goals of operative intervention are to recreate the normal folds of the auricle and to decrease the auriculocephalic angle.

Otoplasty techniques date back to the 10th century in India by Sushruta and the 16th century by Tagliacozzi from Bologna. The first surgical references, however, are attributed to Dieffenbach in 1845. He described postauricular skin excision and suturing of the auricular cartilage to the mastoid periosteum to set the ear back. Many modifications of this technique have been created including incisions in the auricular cartilage to relax its resilience. Some techniques, especially with anterior incisions and cartilaginous cuts, have left irregular anterior contours and were unacceptable.

Becker, in 1952, modified the cartilage incision and used buried mattress sutures to create the normal curve of the antihelix without an irregular contour. Converse continued on this theme but made two parallel cartilage incisions and used a wire brush to thin the cartilage giving an even, natural curve to the antihelix. He used buried sutures and advocated excision of excessive conchal cartilage to set the ear back. Farrior, in 1959, described a method of excision of longitudinal wedges of cartilage to weaken the cartilaginous resiliency and allow for adequate convexity of the antihelix secured with horizontal mattress sutures.

It is known that cartilage will bend away from the side on which it is scored. Attempts at anterior scoring of the cartilage to take advantage of this fact were investigated by Stenstrom in 1963 but these created irregular anterior abnormalities.

Mustarde, in 1963, eliminated the cartilaginous incision, avoiding anterior irregularities, and incorporated permanent scapha–conchal and scapha–fossa triangularis horizontal sutures. This gave a pleasing curve of the antihelix without anterior irregularities. It incorporated the stiff conchal bowl into the scapha and antihelix. Accurate placement of the sutures is required, however, to prevent pinching and abnormal auricular folds.

Furnas, in 1968, incorporated Mustarde's horizontal mattress sutures with a conchal–mastoid and a fossa triangularis–temporalis fascia suture to help decrease the auriculocephalic angle and decrease cupping and anterosuperior displacement of the pinna. Care must be taken, however, to avoid narrowing the external auditory canal with the conchal–mastoid sutures.

This child has prominauris on physical examination. He also has an auriculocephalic angle of 45 degrees and antihelical unfurling, adding to the appearance of his prominent ears. At the age of 3 years, however, his auricle is still growing and so surgical correction should be delayed until the age of 5.

The technique should as always be tailored to the abnormalities at hand. This child will require Mustarde sutures along the scapha to recreate the normal antihelical fold. Fossa triangularis–temporalis fascia sutures described by Furnas will help to direct the fossa triangularis laterally. Also, concha–mastoid sutures will help set the ear back into the correct auriculocephalic angle.

Four major complications are associated with otoplasty: (1) chondritis, (2) inadequate correction of the abnormality, (3) hematoma, and (4) acute infection. Chondritis is the most feared complication and may be prevented with sterile technique and careful postoperative care. Acute infection and hematoma are the easiest to diagnosis. Hematoma may be treated with simple drainage and should leave no sequelae. Acute infection should be treated with the appropriate antibiotic and may lead to chondritis. The most common complication is undercorrection, which can be treated with revision surgery in approximately 1 year.

REHABILITATION AND FOLLOW-UP

During the immediate postoperative period, care should be taken to avoid undue trauma to the region of the pinna. Once the initial inflammation from surgery has abated, the cosmetic effect is usually long lasting. With Mustarde horizontal mattress sutures, however, long-term problems occasionally result if one of the permanent sutures breaks. In these cases, a recurrence of the original deformity can occur.

SUGGESTED READINGS

ADAMSON PA, MORROW TA. Otoplasty. *In:* Lucente FE, Lawson W, Novick NL, eds. *The Extended Ear.* Philadelphia, PA: WB Saunders; 1995:220–242.

BECKER OJ. Surgical correction of the abnormally protruding ears. *Arch Otol.* 1949;50:541.

BRENDA E, MARQUES A, et al. Otoplasty and its origins for the correction of prominent ears. *J Craniomaxillofac Surg.* 1995;23(2):99–104.

CONVERSE JM, NIGRO A, et al. A technique for surgical correction of lop ears. *Plast Reconstr Surg.* 1955;15:411.

ELLIOTT RA Jr. Otoplasty: a combined approach. *Clin Plast Surg.* 1990;17(2):373–381.

ELY JF. Small incision otoplasty for prominent ears. *Aesthetic Plast Surg.* 1988;12(2):63–69.

FARRIOR RT. A method of otoplasty. *Arch Otol.* 1959;69:400.

FURNAS DW. Correction of prominent ears with multiple sutures. *Clin Plast Surg.* 1978;5(3):491.

FURNAS DW. Complications of surgery of the external ear. *Clin Plast Surg.* 1990;17(2):305–318.

MUSTARDE JC. The correction of prominent ears using simple mattress sutures. *Br J Plast Surg.* 1963;16:170.

STENSTROM SJ. A "natural" technique for correction of congenitally prominent ears. *Plast Reconstr Surg.* 1959;32:509.

CLEFT PALATE

Dana Thompson Link, M.D.
Glenn O. Bratcher, M.D.

HISTORY

Full-term infant delivered by vaginal birth presented with respiratory distress. Upon admission to the nursery the child was noted to have a large U-shaped cleft of the palate. Additional findings included mandibular hypoplasia and glossoptosis. Oral feedings were attempted but not tolerated, and the child developed moderate respiratory distress when placed in the supine position. A diagnosis of Pierre Robin sequence was established. Desaturations and breathing pauses were noted by nurses and family. Polysomnography was performed that showed numerous obstructive episodes and O_2 desaturations to 60%. The child was intubated and a tongue–lip adhesion was performed. Postoperative feedings were resumed after recovery from anesthesia. The tongue–lip adhesion was maintained until 18 months of age when growth of the child and mandible made airway obstruction unlikely. The adhesion was taken down and the cleft palate was repaired shortly thereafter (Figs. 71–1A and B).

DIFFERENTIAL DIAGNOSIS— KEY POINTS

1. The finding of a cleft palate should alert the clinician to the possibility of other anomalies or associated syndromes as was the case in this patient. Careful attention to potential airway compromise is essential. A genetics consultation is advisable.

2. The incidence of clefts of the lip, palate, or both represent one of the most frequently occurring congenital deformities. The frequency is higher in whites (1.34 per 1,000 births) than African-Americans (0.41 per 1,000). The chances for a future offspring to have a cleft palate, without cleft lip, are (1) one sibling has cleft, no parent cleft, 2%, (2) and one sibling has cleft, one parent, 17%, and (3) no sibling has cleft, one parent, 7%.

3. Children with cleft deformities are best managed by a team approach with a speech pathologist, orthodontist, prosthodontist, psychologist, geneticist, and dietitian, in addition to the surgeon.

4. The embryologic sequence involved in the normal closure of the palate includes (1) an intrinsic force that enables the palatal shelves to change from a vertical to a horizontal orientation, (2) migration of the tongue in an anterior–inferior direction away from the shelves, and (3) palatal fusion. The configuration of the skull base, size and migration of the tongue, mandible, or both, and many other factors may be responsible for the development of an isolated cleft of the palate.

5. Cleft palate can be associated with Pierre Robin sequence as was the case in this patient. The sequence consists of (1) mandibular hypoplasia, commonly but less properly termed micrognathia; (2) glossoptosis; (3) midline cleft of the palate. The sequence usually occurs as an isolated triad of abnormalities but occasionally constitutes part of more complex entities such as Trisomy 18 or Stickler's syndrome. Airway obstruction in patients with Pierre Robin sequence may be life threatening and should be addressed prior to palatal repair. Tracheostomy or tongue–lip adhesion are options for airway management. The etiology of cleft palate in Pierre Robin sequence is thought to be from retropositioning or underdevelopment of the mandible, leading to upward displacement of the tongue causing arrest of the developing palatal shelves eventually leading to cleft palate. Repair of the palate in a child with Pierre Robin sequence can be done at the usual age, provided that mandibular growth has occurred.

6. Feeding difficulties exist in nearly all infants with cleft palate especially during the first few weeks of life. The cleft defect prevents sealing of the oral cavity from the nasophar-

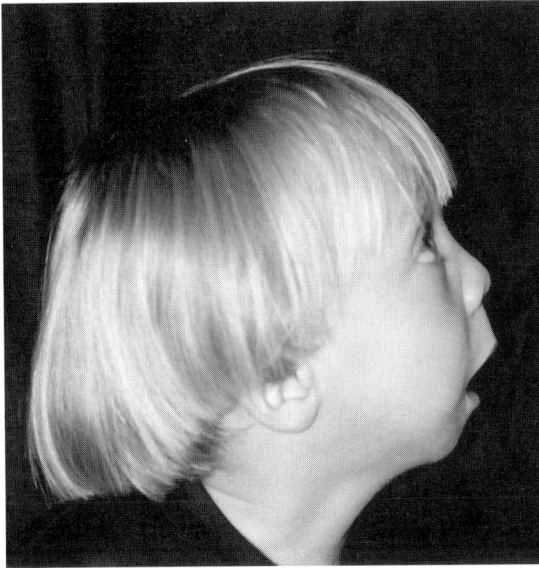

A

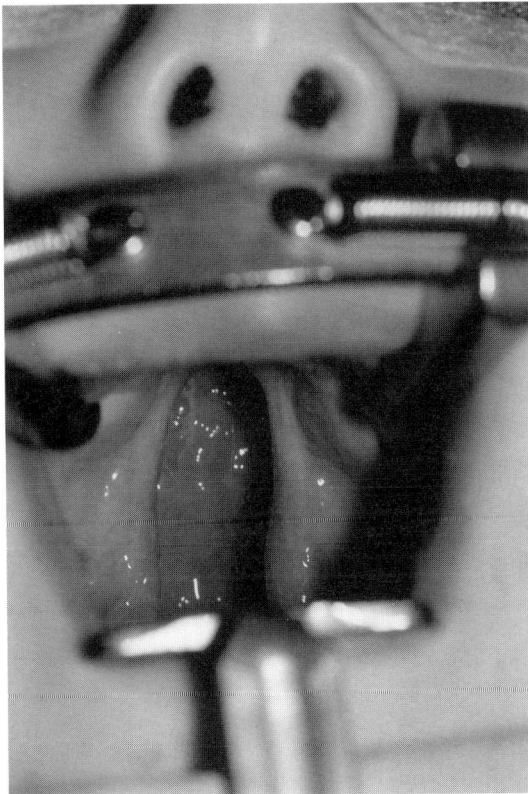

B

FIGURE 71-1 The patient presented with the typical features of Pierre Robin sequence. Note the (A) severely retrodisplaced mandible and (B) the palatal clefting.

ynx, resulting in an inability of the infant to develop adequate negative pressure required for sucking. Feeding in these infants is laborious and time consuming. Unless specific intervention through the use of adaptable feeding devices is done, these infants will fail to gain weight and develop.

7. More than 80% of patients with cleft palate will develop otitis media with middle ear effusion prior to cleft repair. Eustachian tube dysfunction is the etiology of middle ear effusions in this patient population.

TEST INTERPRETATION

Other than a careful physical examination, no specific laboratory or other diagnostic tests are needed to make this diagnosis.

DIAGNOSIS

Pierre Robin sequence with cleft palate.

MEDICAL MANAGEMENT

1. Feeding is an immediate concern following the birth of an infant with a cleft deformity. It is essential that the parents be taught how to feed the infant. It is necessary to deliver the food to the posterior surface of the tongue and allow the infant to initiate swallowing at that time. Many commercially available nipples of various shapes and sizes can be used to accomplish this goal. Breast-feeding is nearly impossible without the use of a prosthetic feeding devices. The primary caregiver is taught to feed the child slowly and allow for frequent burping throughout the feeding.

2. Other congenital anomalies are likely in a child born with a cleft palate. It is important for the physician to evaluate all organ systems or refer the child to a pediatrician with an interest or background in genetics.

3. Hearing and middle ear status should be addressed in all infants with cleft palate because of the high incidence of middle ear disease. Anticipatory care of middle ear effusion should be addressed early to aid in speech and language development.

4. Parental counseling in the preoperative period is essential. Parents need guidance and support regarding the potential medical and psychological ramifications.

5. Speech evaluation and training should start prior to the time of repair to maximize the benefit in the postoperative period.

6. Primary dental care should be undertaken prior to repair for assessment of the primary dentition and maximization of oral hygiene prior to repair. Children with cleft palate have a higher incidence of developing supernumerary teeth, dystrophied teeth, and congenitally missed teeth than the noncleft population.

7. Orthodontic evaluation is helpful in the evaluation of occlusion. Orthodontic care in these children is longitudinal and should be evaluated early.

SURGICAL MANAGEMENT

The timing of cleft palate surgery is as important as the particular surgical approach chosen to repair the defect. Early repair and establishment of velopharyngeal competency aid in speech development. Some surgeons advocate closure of the palate when the child is 12 to 18 months old. However, surgery before the deciduous molar teeth have erupted is believed to facilitate maxillary segment collapse and potentiate orthodontic abnormalities. Timing is left to the individual preference and experience of the surgeon and is individualized with each case. The case presented here, the cleft palate was not repaired until airway obstruction had resolved.

A variety of different types of surgical approaches can be undertaken to repair a cleft palate. The V-Y pushback and Langenbeck are the most commonly used. The reader is referred to a standard textbook on palate repair for details.

Early management of otitis media in children with cleft palate is advisable. Early myringotomy with aspiration of the effusion and insertion of tympanostomy tubes followed by repeat tube insertion as needed to maintain middle ear ventilation is advocated. This approach offers maintenance of an especially effusion-free state and normal hearing acuity with favorable development of hearing, language, and speech.

REHABILITATION AND FOLLOW-UP

Postoperative management in children with cleft palate deformities focuses around development of communication skills. Hearing should be followed closely in these children and middle ear effusions should be treated appropriately as discussed. Tubal dysfunction in these children appears to be a self-limiting problem for the majority over time.

Postoperative guidance by a speech pathologist is important. The efficacy of speech therapy has been demonstrated to produce objective improvement in language skills for preschool children with cleft palate. Additionally, a speech pathologist can aid in the evaluation of postoperative velopharyngeal competence. The assessment can include oral manometric pressure readings, lateral soft tissue roentgenograms during phonation, cineradiographic studies, and direct visualization of palatal motion using a fiber optic scope. These data provide assessment of the effectiveness of palatal closure and also permit an assessment of the role an oronasal fistula can play in speech problems if it occurs postoperatively.

Continued dental, orthodontic, and prosthodontic care is often needed to ensure proper development of occlusion.

SUGGESTED READINGS

GRABB WC, ROSENSTEIN SW, BZOCH KR, eds. Cleft Lip and Palate: Surgical, Dental and Speech Aspects. Boston: Little Brown; 1971.

MILLARD DR. Cleft Craft: The Evolution of Its Surgery, Vol. 1. Boston: Little Brown; 1976.

STOOL SE, RANDALL P. Unexpected ear disease in infants with cleft palate. Cleft Palate J. 1967;4:99.

Facial Cosmetic Surgery

POSTRHINOPLASTY NASAL OBSTRUCTION

Kevin A. Shumrick, M.D.

HISTORY

A 25-year-old male presents with complaints of nasal obstruction and external nasal deformity. He gives a history of having previously seen a surgeon with complaints of nasal obstruction and had a nasal procedure performed 1 year ago. The patient's physician had informed him that the septum and outer nose were "twisted" and needed to be fixed. The surgical procedure was described to the patient as an "internal and external reconstruction" and dictated on the operative report as a "nasal/septal reconstruction." The operative report describes an extensive submucous resection of the posterior cartilaginous septum, resection of the cephalic (superior) border of the lower lateral cartilages, resection of the cartilaginous and bony dorsum, and low to high osteotomies.

Examination of the external nose shows a very narrow dorsum with a pinched nasal tip. The tip appears very rotated, but did not project above the septal angle (Figs. 72–1A, B, and C). Intranasal examination shows a straight septum, which when palpated was found to be deficient of the posterior two-thirds of the cartilage and bone. The turbinates were moderately enlarged and shrunk considerably with topical decongestants. When the patient was asked to breathe through his nose there was significant collapse of the alar sidewalls. With external stabilization of the sidewall the patient reported significant improvement in nasal breathing.

DIFFERENTIAL DIAGNOSIS— KEY POINTS

1. The fact that this patient has nasal obstruction and an external nasal deformity following previous nasal septal surgery considerably narrows the differential diagnosis. The major consideration here is nasal airway obstruction caused by a fixed, anatomic obstruction versus a reactive mucosal condition.

2. The fact that there was some improvement in the nasal airway with topical decongestants should not be construed as diagnostic of a mucosal abnormality causing his obstruction. Even with normal noses there will be a decrease in nasal airway resistance, and improvement in nasal breathing, with topical decongestants.

3. The most likely cause of this patient's nasal airway obstruction is a combination of mucosal hypertrophy and loss of structural integrity of the nose due to surgical resection.

TEST INTERPRETATION

The diagnosis is made almost exclusively on the basis of the history and physical exam. Laboratory or radiologic testing is of little benefit.

DIAGNOSIS

Nasal airway obstruction from loss of structural support due to an overly aggressive septorhi-

263

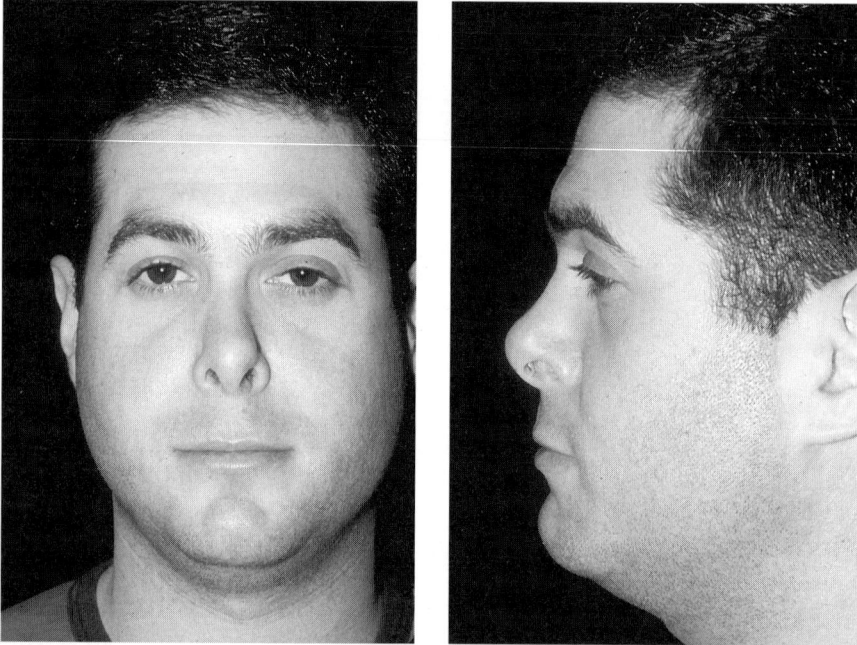

A

B

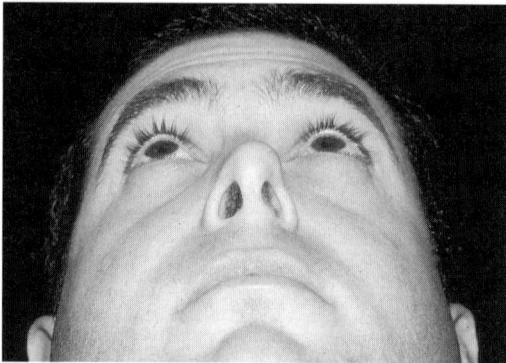

C

FIGURE 72–1 The typical "pinched tip" deformity that can occur following an aggressive septorhinoplasty can be observed in these three views of this patient. (A) Frontal; (B) lateral; (C) submental vertex.

noplasty. Moderate inferior turbinate hypertrophy contributing to the overall nasal airway obstruction.

MEDICAL MANAGEMENT

It is reasonable to try a course of medical management in order to treat any component of reactive nasal mucosal disease. In fact, for any chance at having this surgery for nasal airway obstruction covered by a third party there must be documentation in the chart that medical man-

agement was given a reasonable trial. A topical nasal steroid may be instituted and tried for at least 3 weeks to allow maximum effect. Additionally, a course of second-generation antihistamines (with decongestant) can also be tried.

SURGICAL MANAGEMENT

The primary cause of this patient's nasal airway obstruction is loss of structural integrity of the nose with resultant collapse of the nasal sidewalls in the region of the upper lateral and lower lateral cartilages on inspiration. In addition, the nasal vault is narrowed in the region of the upper lateral cartilages, which compromises the functioning of the internal nasal valve. This loss of structural components is also reflected in the external appearance of the nose—the pinched and overly rotated tip and scooped out dorsum. Correction of the airway and external appearance in a nose such as this requires replacement of the missing nasal components through bone and cartilage grafting. The first choice for grafting material would be septal cartilage and bone. Even though this patient has had a previous submucous resection of the septum performed, it is reasonable to examine closely the septum and even raise a unilateral mucosal and perichondrial flap. Usable cartilage or bone will often be found posteriorly and inferiorly. The remaining anterior and superior cartilage should be left undisturbed to avoid further external collapse. If sufficient septal cartilage and bone are not available, then the next source to consider would be auricular cartilage harvested from the conchal bowl. An alternative consideration for grafting material would be rib cartilage, but harvesting rib cartilage entails significantly more morbidity and the cartilage is often unsuitable in patients over 40 years of age due to calcification.

Finally, the question of alloplastic implants must be addressed. For many years alloplastic implants were felt to be contraindicated in secondary rhinoplasties because of the high incidence of infection and extrusion. However, with the newer materials available alloplastic implants are becoming more popular. In particular, expanded polytetrafluorethylene (ePTFE) (Gore-Tex, W. L. Gore and Associates, Flagstaff, AZ) for augmentation of the nasal dorsum is showing promise as a reliable, relatively complication-free material for nasal augmentation.

In a complicated revision case such as this most authorities would agree that the most reliable method of exposing the nasal skeleton would be with a open rhinoplasty approach. Once the nasal skeleton has been exposed the missing elements are replaced as completely and anatomically as possible. The missing portions of the lower lateral cartilages are reconstructed with auricular cartilage grafts. The narrowed nasal vault is expanded by placing cartilage spreader grafts between the upper lateral cartilages and the nasal septum. The missing nasal dorsum is reconstructed with either cartilage grafts (if available) or alloplastic implant material such as Gore-Tex.

At the end of the procedure the nose is packed with rolled telfa and the open rhinoplasty incision is closed with 7-0 prolene. If lateral osteotomies have not been performed then the nose is simply taped over the dorsum to help keep the dorsal cartilage grafts in position.

REHABILITATION AND FOLLOW-UP

Postoperative care is relatively straightforward and treated like any intranasal surgical procedure. Nasal packing is removed on the first postoperative day. If an open rhinoplasty approach has been used the sutures are removed on postoperative day 5. The dorsal tape is left in place until it begins to loosen and is then removed.

SUGGESTED READINGS

CAMPBELL A, SHUMRICK KA. The use of expanded polytetrafluorethylene in facial reconstruction and facial cosmetic surgery. *Curr Opin Otolaryngol Head Neck Surg.* 1996;4:249–252.

GODIN M, WALDMAN R, JOHNSON C. The use of expanded polytetrafluoroethylene (Gore-Tex) in rhinoplasty: a 6 year experience. *Arch Otolaryngol Head Neck Surg.* 1995;121:1131–1136.

JOHNSON CM, TORIUMI DM. *Open Structure Rhinoplasty.* Philadelphia, PA: WB Saunders; 1990:516.

OWSLEY T. TAYLOR C. The use of Gore-Tex for nasal augmentation: a retrospective analysis of 106 patients. *Plast Reconstr Surg.* 1994;94:241–248.

SHEEN JH, SHEEN AP. Problems in secondary rhinoplasty. In: Sheen JH, ed. *Aesthetic Rhinoplasty.* 2nd ed. St. Louis, MO: Mosby-Year Book; 1987:1135–1407.

EYELID REJUVENATION

Kevin A. Shumrick, M.D.
Robert C. Kersten, M.D.

HISTORY

A 54-year-old female presents with complaints of being told by her friends that she looks "tired and angry" and often being asked if she is getting enough sleep. She states that she looks just like her mother who was considered to have had "premature aging." She wants "eyelid" surgery and has been told by another physician that all she needs is to have the extra skin of the upper eyelid removed. She is seeing you for a second opinion.

The patient is otherwise healthy with a negative review of systems with the exception that she complains of frontal headaches that occur later in the day. She complains of tired feeling eyes, which she thinks may be related to an inappropriate eyeglass prescription. Also, she reports that her eyes are often red and itchy.

The patient is shown in Figures 73–1A and B. Examination shows that she is generally in good health, but does appear older than her stated age. With regard to examination of the periorbital region her upper lid margin was found to sit approximately 4 mm below the superior edge of the iris. The eyebrows were positioned below the orbital rim and there were deep vertical creases in the glabellar region.

DIFFERENTIAL DIAGNOSIS— KEY POINTS

1. Individuals presenting for elective cosmetic surgery of the eyelids are a special group of patients because what is assumed to be simply "sagging eyelids," which can be corrected by tightening procedures, may in fact represent systemic conditions or functional disorders. It is important to assess and diagnose accurately the cause of the patient's complaint in order to avoid missing an occult medical condition or performing inappropriate surgery that may actually cause harm to the patient.

2. Before discussing this patient's exam and diagnosis, a brief review of the confusing terminology used to describe various conditions of the eyelids may be helpful:
   - *Blepharochalasis* is a term that has been used as a generic description for any amount of excess skin of the upper eyelid. However, blepharochalasis should be reserved for a relatively uncommon variant of angioneurotic edema, which occurs in young women and is manifested by swelling and edema of the lids, which eventually leads to progressive tissue breakdown.
   - *Dermatochalasis* refers to relaxation of the skin and probably best describes the changes commonly associated with the aging process.
   - *Blepharoptosis* (or simply ptosis of the upper lid) refers to an inferior positioning of the eyelid margin over the iris due to levator muscle dysfunction and is not caused by excess tissue or fat herniation.
   - *Pseudoptosis* occurs when the lid margin remains in the proper position relative to the iris, but excess lid skin hangs down below the lid margin giving the appearance of ptosis (see Figs. 73–2A and B).
   - *Lid retraction* occurs when the lid margin is positioned above (or below in the case of the lower eyelid) the iris, and the white of the sclera is seen between the lid and the iris. Ptosis of the upper eyelid gives an individual the appearance of being sleepy, tired, or inattentive. Lid retraction gives the appearance of intense staring, anger, or surprise.

3. There are several systemic conditions that can present with eyelid manifestations:

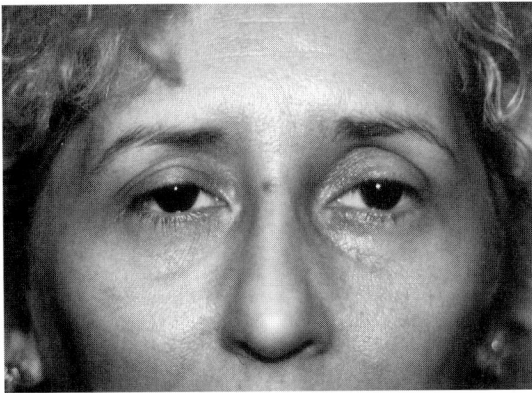
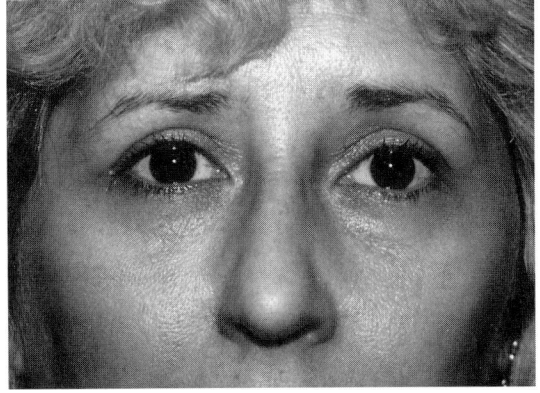

A   B

FIGURE 73–1   Patient presenting for upper lid blepharoplasty with complaints of "tired-looking eyes." Note that her real problem is upper lid ptosis with descent of the upper lid margin over the iris. (B) Same patient following ptosis repair as described in the text with out any skin excision. Note how much more alert she appears and how much more youthful her eyes look.

- Thyroid disease may present with several manifestations in the periorbital region. Hyperthyroidism due to Graves' disease often manifests with upper and lower lid retraction with globe proptosis. Hypothyroidism commonly presents with prominent symptoms of periorbital edema, particularly of the lower eyelid, with marked formation of lower eyelid bags often referred to as *festoons*.

- Various allergies may cause intermittent swelling and dermatitis of the eyelid skin in addition to periorbital edema.

- A variety of conditions can cause ptosis of the upper eyelid, which may be mistaken for aging changes. Congenital ptosis of the upper eyelid is due to abnormal development of the levator muscle. Acquired ptosis may be caused by muscular abnormalities such as ophthalmoplegia, oculopharyngeal dystrophy, and myasthenia gravis. Neurologic conditions such as oculomotor palsy,

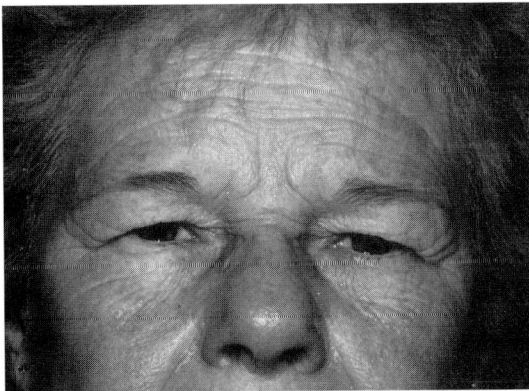
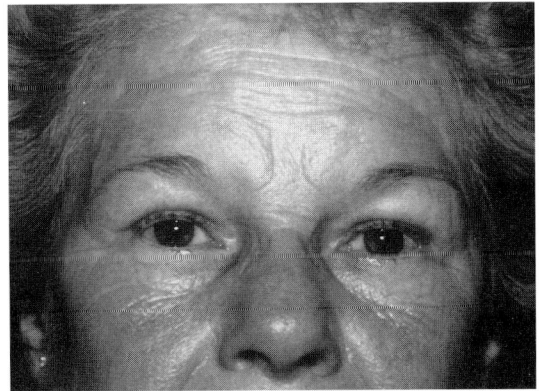

A   B

FIGURE 73–2   Patient with severe pseudoptosis of the upper eyelid skin. This is not true ptosis because if the upper lid skin is elevated the lid margin will be seen to be in the correct position at the margin of the iris. This patient also has severe brow ptosis contributing to her upper lid excess skin. (B) Same patient following upper lid blepharoplasty and brow lift.

Horner's syndrome, and other central nervous system diseases may cause ptosis. Increased weight of the upper lid from tumor or edema may cause a mechanical ptosis.

The most common cause of ptosis is involutional or senile ptosis as a result of dehiscence or disinsertion of the levator aponeurosis. Characteristic findings of senile ptosis include a high or absent lid crease, thinning of the upper lid tissue, and normal levator muscle function.

- An often overlooked cause of tired-looking eyes and what appears to be upper eyelid skin laxity, as well as frontal headaches and a constantly angry appearance, is brow ptosis. Brow ptosis results from a loss of skin elasticity, decreased bulk of subcutaneous tissue, and increased skull bone resorption. Due to the effects of gravity, there is sagging or ptosis of the forehead, glabella, temple, and eyebrows. Brow ptosis usually presents in the region of the lateral third of the eyebrow causing skin redundancy of the infrabrow region and upper eyelid with resultant hooding of the skin onto the upper lid. The skin hooding may be severe enough to cause a superolateral visual field defect. A common finding associated with brow ptosis is that patients tend to increase frontalis muscle activity in order to elevate the brows and remove the excess skin from the upper lid. With time this increased muscle activity can cause headaches and deep furrowing of the forehead as well as glabellar creases.

4. This patient also reports symptoms of eye irritation manifested by itching and redness. These symptoms may be caused by allergies, but it is important to consider the possibility of an undiagnosed dry eye syndrome. If the patient has a dry eye, blepharoplasty may lead to serious corneal problems due to exposure keratitis.

TEST INTERPRETATION

The major diagnostic considerations in this patient are related to careful physical exam and assessment. In general, any patient undergoing eyelid surgery should have a thorough ophthal-mologic evaluation including visual acuity and retinal exam. However, this discussion will focus on aspects of the physical exam pertinent to planning this particular patient's surgery. If there is any indication of a possible systemic disorder, it should be evaluated with the appropriate medical or neurologic consultation.

1. A major issue to be resolved with this patient is whether she has simple excess tissue of the upper lid or upper eyelid ptosis. The presence of ptosis may be documented in several ways. The easiest method of assessing ptosis is to have the patient visually fixate on a penlight held at arm's length in front of the patient and then you measure the distance between the corneal light reflex (which is centered over the pupil) and the height of the eyelid margin. Any measurement of the distance between the lid margin and the corneal light reflex of less than 3 mm is abnormal. In the case where upper eyelid skin is draping over the lid and causing pseudoptosis it is important to gently manually distract the excess lid skin upward so that the lid margin and lashes can be viewed directly. Note that patients will subconsciously attempt to fire the frontalis muscle and elevate the brow in order to compensate for ptosis; therefore, it is important to manually fix the brow with a thumb or finger in order to measure objectively the true extent of a suspected ptosis.

2. Function of the levator muscle of the upper lid should be documented by examining the range of motion of the upper lid. This is performed by placing a thumb or forefinger above the brow of the eye to be examined so as to prevent eyelid elevation due to raising the forehead and brow. With the brow fixed, the patient is asked to look in extreme downward than upward gaze. The distance traveled by the upper lid approximates the levator muscle function. With normal levator muscle function the lid should travel approximately 15 mm; 12 mm would be considered the lower limit of normal.

3. Positioning of the eyebrows should be evaluated in order to determine whether brow ptosis is contributing to the tissue redundancy of

the upper lid. Although there is considerable debate regarding the optimum aesthetic configuration of the eyebrow (it varies between men and women), it is generally agreed that the position of the eyebrow, with the forehead at rest, should be at or above the orbital rims.

4. This patient should also be evaluated for adequacy of tear production, which may be accomplished by examining the tear meniscus with a slit lamp or measuring tear production using Schirmer's strips. Schirmer's strips are commercially prepared strips of filter paper that function as a wick to allow measurement of tear production. The strips are drapped from the inferior lid fornix over the lower eyelid margin. As the tears are absorbed by the strips the rate at which the strips are wetted can be assessed and a rough approximation of tear production noted. With normal tearing at least 10 mm of the Schirmer's strip should be wetted within 5 minutes time. Additionally, if there is any question of chronic corneal irritation a slit lamp examination with fluorescein should be performed to look for the presence of corneal staining, which would indicate corneal irritation and keratinization. Finally corneal sensation can be tested with a cotton wisp or tissue paper to ensure an adequate corneal blink reflux.

As part of the necessary history in a blepharoplasty candidate, it is important to inquire about rheumatologic disorders because these are oftentimes associated with pathologic dry eyes and a condition known as keratoconjunctivitis sicca.

In this patient, the following measurements and interpretations were made: *Eyelid position:* Measurement of the upper eyelid position showed that the upper eyelid margin rested 2 mm above the corneal light reflex. This indicates that ptosis of the upper eyelid is present. *Brow position:* Both eyebrows were noted to sit just inferior to the orbital rims. As noted, the eyebrows should sit at the level of the orbital rims; therefore, this patient also has brow ptosis contributing to her upper lid problem. *Tear production:* With the Schimer's test wetting of 5 mm of the Schirmer's strips was seen within 5 minutes.

There should have been wetting of at least 10 mm of the strip, which indicates that this patient also has some degree of compromised tear production.

DIAGNOSIS

Senile ptosis of the upper lid, brow ptosis, and lower than optimum tear production.

MEDICAL MANAGEMENT

The only role medical management has in this patient would be with eye lubrication. The extent to which she would require additional lubrication depends on the changes found on exam of the cornea. A variety of methods is available for increasing eye lubrication. The simplest and most often used is the use of commercial artificial tear supplements in drop form during the day and lubricating ointment at bedtime. Occlusion of the lacrimal drainage puncta either with temporary silicone plugs or permanently with the use of thermal cautery is helpful in patients with documented keratoconjunctivitis sicca. Wrap-around glasses or eye shields are helpful to decrease evaporative drying of the tear film, and a moisture chamber goggle may be necessary in severe cases. Certainly, if surgery is to be performed careful attention to keeping the eye properly lubricated during the operative and postoperative period will be a major concern.

SURGICAL MANAGEMENT

While this patient presented with what she thought was primarily upper eyelid skin redundancy she, in fact, has senile ptosis of the upper lid, brow ptosis, and lower than optimum tear production. None of these conditions would have been improved by a conventional blepharoplasty and, in fact, there may be significant complications from trying to correct lid ptosis with simple upper lid skin excision.

The most effective method of managing this patient's condition is surgery directed at correcting the changes brought about by aging with relaxation of the upper lid levator aponeurosis and forehead skin.

A variety of surgical procedures have been described for treatment of the levator dehiscence or disinsertion found in senile ptosis. A basic approach is to expose the levator aponeurosis through a standard blepharoplasty incision at the upper lid crease. The aponeurosis is then tightened with permanent mattress sutures between the muscle and tarsal plate. This is performed with the patient under local anesthesia so that the results can be assessed at the time of surgery. Overcorrection and lid notching from uneven suture placement are the most common complications of ptosis repair.

There are many possible choices for correction of the brow ptosis including a direct brow lift, mid-forehead brow lift, pretracheal brow lift, and coronal brow lift. These procedures all have in common the necessity for skin or scalp excision (with resulting external scars, changes in hairline, and forehead numbness) in order to achieve brow elevation. Recently, endoscopic forehead lifting has become popular and is performed by completely elevating the forehead periosteum and releasing the periosteal attachments of the brows to the orbital rims. The entire brow forehead complex is then repositioned superiorly and held there until the periosteum reattaches at the new more superior position. The endoscopic forehead lift has the advantage of avoiding long scars and the need to excise skin or scalp. There have been some concerns about the longevity of results with endoscopic forehead lifting, particularly in patients with severe or functional brow ptosis. Long-term results are pending, but at present endoscopic forehead lifts appear to be a viable alternative to conventional forehead lifts.

The major potential complications with any type of forehead lift are forehead numbness for variable amount of time (it is rarely permanent), asymmetry of the brow position, and the possibility of injury to the frontalis branch of the facial nerve with forehead paralysis.

REHABILITATION AND FOLLOW-UP

Postoperatively, the patients are followed for adequacy of eye lubrication and lid and brow position. Generally, recovery is complete within 7 to 10 days.

SUGGESTED READINGS

ADAMSON PA. The aging forehead. In: Tardy ME, ed. *Head and Neck Surgery—Otolaryngology.* Philadelphia, PA: JB Lippincott; 1993;2258–2275.

BECKER FF, JHONSON CM. Surgical treatment of the upper third of the aging face. In: Cummings CW, Krause CJ, ed. *Otolaryngology—Head and Neck Surgery.* St. Louis, MO: Mosby Year Book; 1993:551–565.

COLTON JJ, BEEKHUIS GJ. Blepharoplasty. In: Cummings CW, Krause CJ, eds. *Otolaryngology—Head and Neck Surgery.* 2nd ed. St. Louis, MO: Mosby-Year Book; 1993:566–587.

DANIEL RK, TIRKANITS B. Endoscopic forehead lift: an operative technique. *Plast Reconstr Surg.* 1996; 98(7):1148–1157.

JONES LT, QUICKERT NH, WOBIG JL. The cure of ptosis by aponeurotic repair. *Arch Ophthalmol.* 1975; 93:629–634.

VASCONEZ LO, CORE GB, GAMBOA-BOBDILLA M, GUZMAN G, ASKREN C, YAMAMOTO Y. Endoscopic techniques in coronal brow lifting. *Plast Reconst Surg.* 1994;94(6):788–793.

EYELID SURGERY: POSTOPERATIVE COMPLICATION

Kevin A. Shumrick, M.D.
Robert C. Kersten, M.D.

HISTORY

Shortly after arriving in the recovery room a patient who had just undergone bilateral upper and lower blepharoplasties had a prolonged coughing episode and suddenly began complaining of severe bilateral eye pain.

The patient is a 55-year-old man who has a history of hypertension and smokes one pack of cigarettes per day. When questioned about medications, he recalled taking several aspirins the day before surgery for a headache. He was taking oral antihypertensive medications (which he did not take on the day of surgery) and had no known allergies.

Physical exam showed an anxious, uncomfortable male with bilateral periorbital ecchymosis and gross proptosis (Fig. 74–1). His blood pressure was 160/100 and his pulse was 115. Both eyes were ecchymotic and proptotic and the range of motion for both eyes was severely restricted. The patient stated that he felt as though he could not see as well as usual from either eye although he was able to count fingers.

DIFFERENTIAL DIAGNOSIS— KEY POINTS

1. The history of eyelid surgery with bilateral eye pain, ecchymosis, diminished vision, and proptosis is virtually diagnostic for an orbital hemorrhage. An acute glaucoma attack may present with pain and decreased vision, but will not have the proptosis and ecchymosis. A detached retina will have decreased vision, but no pain, ecchymosis, or proptosis. A corneal abrasion will present with pain, but without the rest of the symptom complex.

2. Two other additional physical exam findings would be important in this patient: (1) intraocular pressure and (2) fundoscopic exam looking at the retina and retinal artery. However, these are specialized exams that usually require an ophthalmologist to perform them accurately and reliably and due to the acuity of this situation definitive therapy should not be delayed until a consultation is available.

3. It should be realized that this is an acute vision-threatening situation that requires immediate and definitive management to avoid a devastating complication (loss of vision).

TEST INTERPRETATION

Other than the ophthalmologic physical examination, other stenting is not indicated in this acute emergent situation.

DIAGNOSIS

Postoperative orbital hemorrhage with bilateral orbital hematomas.

MEDICAL MANAGEMENT

Management of an orbital hemorrhage requires an awareness of the entity, a clear understanding of the problem, and a systematic approach to its resolution. Although the literature has traditionally emphasized an initial medical management similar to that employed for the treatment of acute glaucoma, it has subsequently been appreciated that the increased intraocular pressure in this situation reflects an increased orbital pressure and that standard glaucoma treatment (which is directed at intraglobe pressure) is not particularly relevant. Emphasis has subsequently been placed on the immediate expansion of the intraorbital volume. Although

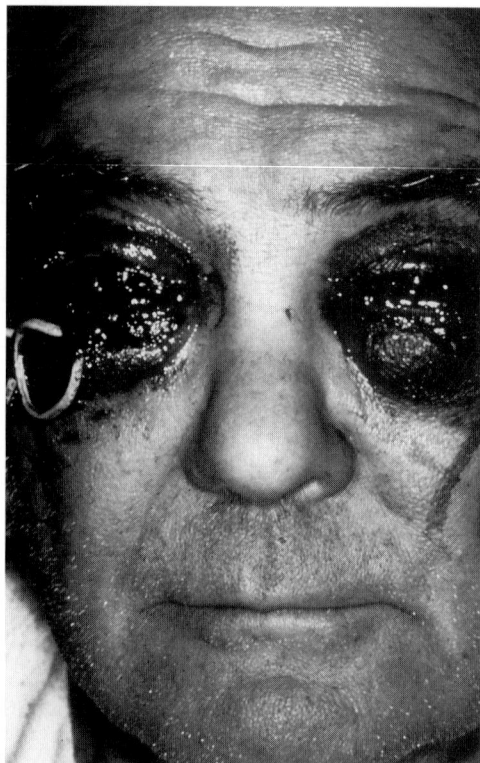

FIGURE 74-1 Bilateral periorbital ecchymosis and gross proptosis.

several methods are available for increasing orbital volume, the most expedient one is by surgically disinserting the eyelids from the lateral bony rim by performing a canthotomy and inferior cantholysis. However, in the specific setting of postblepharoplasty orbital hemorrhage the treating physician should proceed as follows:

1. Call for ophthalmologic consultation.

2. If a tarsorrhaphy suture is in place remove it.

3. Obtain a determination of visual acuity. If a handheld eye chart is available this would be excellent; however, in this emergency situation any print would be acceptable. At the very least recognition of finger movement should be documented.

4. Elevate the head of the patient's bed and remove sutures from the upper and lower eyelid incisions. Any obvious clots should be evacuated.

5. Palpate the globe to see if the orbital pressure has been reduced.

6. Recheck visual acuity to see if it has returned.

7. Dexamethasone (0.1 to 0.5 mg/kg) may be given in an attempt to reduce optic nerve edema.

8. In the past acetazolamide and mannitol have been given intravenously in an attempt to induce a diuresis and decrease intraorbital pressure (as is done with glaucoma), but it is now generally accepted that this approach will have little benefit in this situation.

9. If there is associated hypertension this should be brought under control with intravenous antihypertensives.

SURGICAL MANAGEMENT

Following the above-mentioned medical steps the status of the affected eye should continue to be monitored by patient assessment, external exam, ocular pressure, and fundoscopic evaluation. If significant improvement in all parameters is not seen, then surgical intervention is warranted. The initial step would consist of opening the surgical wounds and gently spreading the deep tissues in an attempt to allow a hematoma to decompress itself (Fig. 74–2). However, most orbital hematomas do not occur as discrete, drainable entities. Instead, the most common finding is that of diffusely infiltrated hemorrhage, and an attempt at simple drainage will not decompress the orbit.

What is required for a vision threatening orbital hemorrhage is a method of increasing the orbital volume to relieve pressure on the globe. One method of increasing orbital volume is to remove the inferior or medial bony walls and allow the orbital contents to expand into the periorbital sinuses. While removal of the orbital floor and/or medial wall is undoubtedly effective in decompressing the orbit, this is a somewhat involved procedure requiring a return to the operating room, general anesthesia, and at least 45 to 60 minutes to perform.

An alternative method for decompressing the orbit that is quick and can be performed in the recovery room is a lateral canthotomy and inferior cantholysis. By releasing the attachments of the lower lid to the lateral orbital wall the globe can expand 4 to 5 mm anteriorly. The canthotomy is performed by inserting one blade

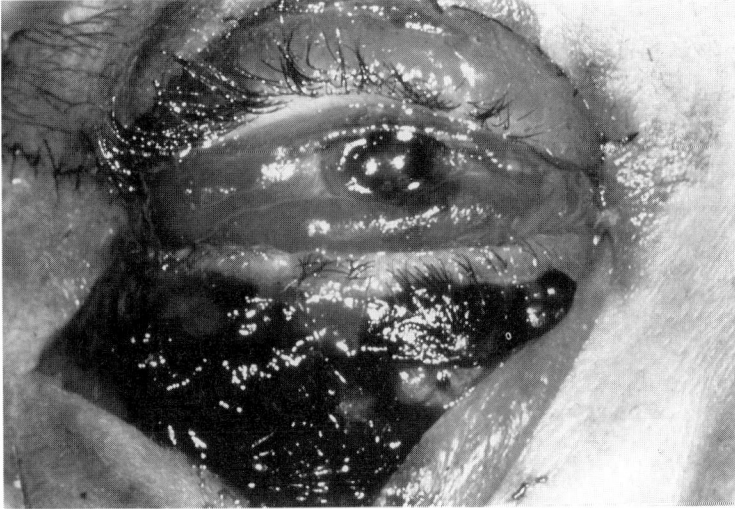

FIGURE 74-2 Opening the surgical wounds and gently spreading the deep tissues in an attempt to allow the hematoma to decompress itself.

of a pair of scissors on the conjunctival side of the lateral canthus and one blade on the skin side and then cutting to the marginal tubercle of the zygoma. The inferior cantholysis is performed by turning the scissors 90 degrees and dividing the inferior attachments of the lateral canthal tendon. This incision should continue through the orbital septum to completely detach the lower lid.

There have been reports of decompressing the globe through anterior chamber paracentesis, but it is now generally felt that this procedure's morbidity outweighs the expected benefits.

REHABILITATION AND FOLLOW-UP

The patient should be followed closely until the orbital exam stabilizes and begins to improve. Local measures such as iced saline soaks and head elevation may be of some benefit. If there is significant proptosis, then the patient should be followed for corneal exposure and chemosis and appropriate lubrication and corneal protection instituted. The lateral canthal tendon should be repaired when the orbital swelling and ecchymoses have resolved.

SUGGESTED READINGS

HARTLEY JH, LESTER JC, SCHATTEN WE. Acute retrobulbar hemorrhage during elective blepharoplasty: its pathophysiology and management. *Plast Reconstr Surg.* 1973;52:8–12.

HEINZE JB, HUESTON JT. Blindness after blepharoplasty: mechanism and early reversal. *Plast Reconstr Surg.* 1978;61:347–354.

SACHS SH, LAWSON W, EDELSTEIN D, GREEN RP. Surgical treatment of blindness secondary to introrbital hemorrhage. *Arch Otolaryngol Head Neck Surg.* 1988;114:801–803.

THOMPSON RF, GLUCKMAN JL, KULWIN D, SAVOURY L. Orbital hemorrhage suring ethmoid sinus surgery. *Otolaryngol Head Neck Surg.* 1990;102(1):45–50.

Case 75

MANDIBULAR FRACTURE

Kevin A. Shumrick, M.D.
Eve Cornell, D.D.S.

HISTORY

A 43-year-old male, unrestrained driver was stabilized and transported to the emergency department following a high-speed motor vehicle accident. While extracting the patient from the vehicle, the paramedic noted that the steering column was grossly distorted, suggesting the possibility of a high-impact injury to the cervicofacial region. The patient exhibited gross facial deformities with obvious mandibular symphyseal retrusion, increased interangle width, and severe malocclusion of the teeth. Closer examination revealed gross mobility and lingual tilting of the mandibular bodies. The patient had difficulty handling his oral secretions as well as speaking. He also complained of shortness of breath when lying flat on his back.

DIFFERENTIAL DIAGNOSIS— KEY POINTS

By history and exam this patient has suffered a significant traumatic event with injuries to the cervical facial region. A number of distinct clinical entities must be considered in a patient with this history and clinical presentation.

1. Any patient with a history of significant cervicofacial trauma should be considered to have a cervical spine injury until proven otherwise. This means restricting cervical motion with a neck collar until the appropriate radiologic films have ruled out a cervical-spine injury. Note that a patient with cervical facial injuries who is wearing a rigid cervical collar may have a very difficult time lying flat on his back. Therefore, the patient should not be left unattended and oral suction may be helpful in controlling secretions. If lying prone/supine causes significant dyspnea then elevating the head of the bed may be of some benefit.

2. Any patient with significant cervicofacial trauma and dyspnea should also be considered for a possible laryngotracheal injury. The two most serious types of laryngotracheal injuries are fractures of the laryngeal or cricoid cartilages and laryngotracheal separation. Laryngeal fractures classically present with ecchymosis of the anterior neck with loss of the thyroid cartilage prominence. Often there is subcutaneous crepitance (from air dissecting out into the soft tissue) or crepitance with palpation of the laryngeal skeleton (from the edges of the cartilages rubbing on each other). Examination of the larynx with a flexible scope will show ecchymosis and/or internal derangement of the internal anatomy. Patients will invariably have hoarseness and often hemoptysis. With laryngotracheal separation the trachea is avulsed from the larynx usually at the first couple of tracheal rings. The patient may initially have a good airway with only hoarseness (due to disruption of one or both the recurrent laryngeal nerves), but the airway will progressively worsen and eventually require intervention.

3. Another consideration in a patient with cervico-facial trauma and malocclusion would

be some variant of a LeFort fracture with separation of the teeth-bearing maxilla from the remaining portion of the facial skeleton.

4. Patients with significant cervical trauma from a deceleration-type injury should be considered for possible vascular involvement. The two major types of vascular injuries seen in blunt trauma to the face and neck are aortic transections and intimal disruptions of the carotid, both of which can result in serious morbidity and tend to present in a delayed fashion, catching the unwary clinician off guard.

5. The physical findings of retrognathia, malocclusion and widened intermandibular angle width suggest a comminuted mandibular fraction. A true flail mandible involves multiple fractures, most commonly, a symphyseal and bilateral subcondylar fractures. Variations may include bilateral subcondylar and two parasymphyseal or body fractures.

6. With disruption of the mandibular arch at two or more points, the ability of the mandible to maintain its anterior projection is lost and the bone is drawn posteriorly by the attached musculature. The tongue loses its anterior anchor and the lingual surface of the mandible and falls posteriorly. The suprahyoid muscles also lose a portion of their stabilizing insertion points. The net effect of this loss of a stable mandibular arch is collapse of the tongue and soft tissue posteriorly with airway encroachment and greatly diminished effectiveness of swallowing. The combination of a narrowed airway and inability to clear secretions puts these patients at tremendous risk for airway obstruction and airway maintenance should be the primary concern in the early hours of this patient's treatment.

TEST INTERPRETATION

The primary diagnostic testing in a trauma patient such as this patient will be radiologic. The initial tests should be directed toward ruling out acute life-threatening injuries. The primary condition to be concerned about in a patient with cervico-facial trauma would be a cervical spine injury, which may be imaged with anterior/posterior and lateral plain films of the cervical spine. However, if the radiologist is unable to clear the cervical spine the neck collar should be left in place until a spinal injury has been ruled out. Plain films of the neck may also give some clues to possible laryngeal or tracheal injuries by showing air in the neck soft tissues or disruption of the tracheal air column. If plain films are not definitive enough to rule out a cervical spine injury, then an axial computed tomography (CT) scan of the cervical spine may be required.

A chest x-ray should be reviewed to rule out a pneumothorax or even a tension pneumothorax. Additionally, the chest x-ray should be carefully examined for possible mediastinal widening, which would be a possible indicator of an aortic transection. If there is any question of an aortic transection, an arteriogram should be ordered.

After the potential life-threatening injuries (spinal, laryngotracheal, and vascular) have been ruled out, attention may be turned to evaluating the facial injuries. The physical exam of this patient is highly suggestive of a complicated mandibular fracture. The fractures should be visualized in at least two dimensions to assess accurately displacement of the segments. A Panorex, posterior–anterior, right and left lateral obliques, and a reverse Townes are the most diagnostic and inexpensive methods for obtaining an accurate assessment. However, obtaining these films may be difficult in the trauma patient whose cervical spine is not cleared. In addition, many emergency rooms do not have a Panorex machine. A CT scan including axial cuts and coronal cuts (if the cervical spine is cleared) can provide a good alternative to plain and panoramic films and can often be performed in conjunction with a CT scan of the head and cervical spine (Figure 75–1). Three-dimensional reconstruction images may also be helpful in determining displacement of subcondylar fractures.

DIAGNOSIS

Flail mandible secondary to bilateral mandibular body fractures.

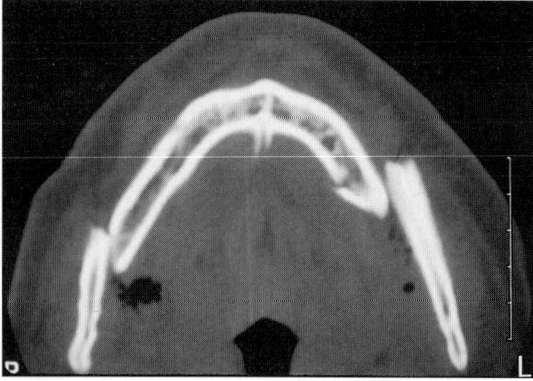

FIGURE 75-1 This axial CT scan through the mandibular arch clearly displays the bilateral mandibular body fracture, allowing posterior displacement of the entire anterior segment.

MEDICAL MANAGEMENT

Medical management is directed toward four goals: (1) maintenance of oxygenation and ventilation, (2) prevention of infection, (3) pain control, and (4) nutritional support. Airway patency and administering supplemental oxygen are of primary importance. Continuous pulse oximetry is a useful adjunct for monitoring the airway. Patient positioning, removal of grossly mobile teeth and debris, and the availability of a Yankauer-type suction device are key. Some authors recommend IV steroids to help control soft tissue swelling. Prevention of infection involves early initiation of IV antibiotics that provide coverage for intraoral microorganisms as well as normal skin flora if fracture segments have penetrated the skin. Chlorhexidine mouth rinse may also be of some benefit. Pain is often severe in the patient with a flail mandible. Moderate to heavy doses of narcotic analgesics are often required to control pain adequately, but narcotic use must be tempered by the potential for air compromise; pulse oximetry and close observation are essential. Finally, consideration should be given to providing nutritional supplementation because patients may have markedly decreased oral intake for a significant period postoperatively.

SURGICAL MANAGEMENT

Early surgical intervention may include emergent cricothyroidotomy (or tracheostomy) if the airway is thought to be unstable and it is not possible to secure the airway via tracheal intubation or mask ventilation. Definitive treatment of the flail mandible requires surgical intervention. Both treatment planning and surgery may prove to be both complex and challenging and depend on the location and complexity of the fractures, degree of segmental displacement, size of the mandible, presence and condition of dentition, and associated facial fractures. Treatment goals include accurate restoration of form in three planes of space (anteroposterior, vertical, medial–lateral), restoration of preinjury occlusion, and accurate condylar repositioning to facilitate optimal mandibular rotation and translation. Typically, this is accomplished by reestablishing the dental occlusion with arch bars and intermaxillary fixation. Next the fractures are exposed through either intraoral or external incisions; the segments are realigned and rigidly fixated with reconstruction plates and screws. It is not uncommon for the patient to be left in intermaxillary fixation for 3 to 6 weeks postoperatively to maximize the opportunity for primary bone healing. An important point to be made regarding the diagnosis of a flail mandible has to do with the long-term prognosis of satisfactory mandibular healing and restoration of proper occlusion. These are complicated, inherently unstable fractures with significant potential for nonunions and mandibular segment malalignment. These fractures should be handled by experienced personnel in a setting with the appropriate resources.

REHABILITATION AND FOLLOW-UP

Meticulous follow-up and rehabilitation are necessary for a maximally successful outcome. Initial follow-up should include radiographs to confirm accurate reduction and stabilization of segments. Maintenance of the planned occlusion should be verified initially and at regular intervals (weekly, then biweekly, then monthly) until healing is complete. Changes in occlusion should be treated when first identified. Rehabilitation should include initiation of staged range of motion exercises once the mandible is mobilized.

SUGGESTED READINGS

BUCCI MN, HOFF JT. Neurologic evaluation and management. In: Fonseca RJ, Walker RV, eds. *Oral and Maxillofacial Trauma*. Philadelphia, PA: WB Saunders; 1991:137–156.

GERLOCK A. The flared mandible sign of the flail mandible. *Radiology*. 1976;119(2):299–300.

GLUCKMAN JL, MANGAL AK. Laryngeal trauma. In: Paparella MM, Shumrick DA, Gluckman, JL, Meyerhoff WL, eds. *Otolaryngology*. 3rd. ed. Philadelphia, PA: WB Saunders; 1991:2231–2241.

KELLMAN R. The cervical spine in maxillofacial trauma: assessment and airway management. *Otolaryngol Clin North Am*. 1991;24:1–13.

SNOW JB. Diagnosis and therapy for acute laryngeal and tracheal trauma. *Otolaryngol Clin North Am*. 1984;17:101–106.

ORBITAL TRAUMA

Kevin A. Shumrick, M.D.
Robert C. Kersten, M.D.

HISTORY

A 22-year-old male was struck on the right periorbital region with a fist during an altercation 12 hours prior to being seen. The patient reports that he had been drinking, but feels there was no loss of consciousness. His eye swelled shut almost immediately so that he could not tell what his exact visual status was, but he felt he could at least detect light with his right eye. He was otherwise healthy with no other complaints.

The physical exam revealed a well-developed, well-nourished white male with moderate swelling and ecchymosis of the right periorbital region. The right eye was swollen shut and the patient was unable to open it without assistance. The pertinent physical findings were confined to the right periorbital region without evidence of other head and neck trauma. With retraction of the right upper and lower eyelids the globe could be visualized. The right globe appeared to be positioned somewhat more posteriorly and interiorly than the left globe; however, it was difficult to be certain about this due to amount of periorbital swelling. The pupil was round, reactive to light, and appeared to be the same size as the left pupil. Testing of visual acuity with a handheld card was grossly normal. When range of motion of the globes was tested the patient complained of pain in the right eye and was unable to elevate it (Figs. 76–1A and B). There was subjective diplopia on upward gaze.

DIFFERENTIAL DIAGNOSIS— KEY POINTS

1. When evaluating patients with head and neck trauma in general (and orbital trauma specifically), it is important to rule out the more serious concerns first and then focus on the problems that can be handled in a more elective fashion. In this patient the two most urgent concerns are the possibility of an intracranial injury and the possibility of a vision threatening injury to the globe. Because there was no loss of consciousness and the rest of the neurologic exam was intact, a significant neurologic injury would be extremely unlikely. The next major concern would then be ruling out an injury to the globe.

2. While the majority of the trauma appears to be centered around the right orbit, it is important to consider that other areas of the facial skeleton may have been injured through direct contact or transmission of forces. Specifically, the patient should be examined for the possibility of an associated zygomatic complex fracture (commonly referred to as a tripod fracture) or LeFort-type fracture. The infraorbital rim should be palpated and any step-offs or discontinuities noted. The zygomatic-frontal suture should also be palpated and step-offs or tenderness recorded. Additionally, note should be made of the position of the malar eminence and any malposition or depression.

3. Due to the fact that the infraorbital nerve runs across the floor of the orbit, it is frequently involved in significant orbital trauma with resultant numbness of the ipsilateral cheek and upper lip. Sensation of the cheek and upper lip on the side of trauma should be carefully examined and documented.

TEST INTERPRETATION

An important diagnostic test is a thorough ophthalmologic exam of the globe. Coincident injury to the globe is frequent with orbital or periorbital fractures, and failure to diagnose a significant globe injury in a timely fashion may be sight threatening. Specific injuries to rule out are corneal abrasion, ruptured globe, detached retina, hyphema (blood in the vitreous), and lens dislocation.

A high-resolution coronal and axial computed tomography (CT) scan provides the most

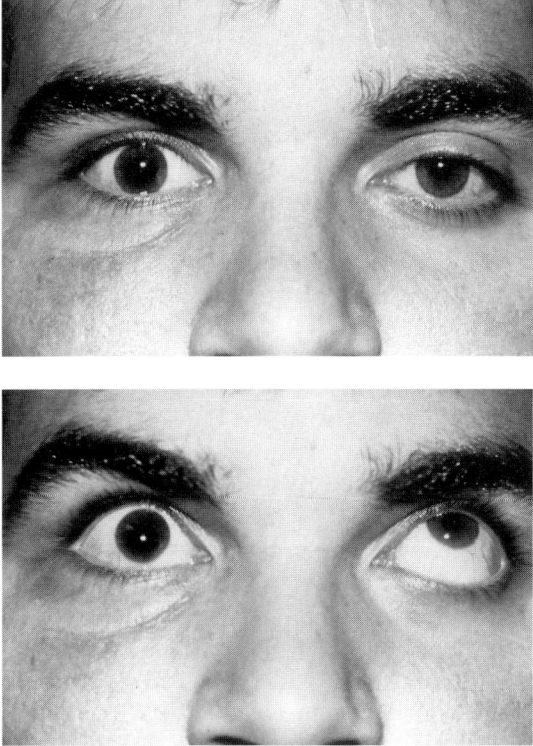

FIGURE 76–1 Range of motion of the globes. (A) normal vision with forward gaze, however, (B) subjective diplopia on upward gaze due to entrapment of right inferior rectus muscle.

useful radiologic information with regard to the status of the orbital floor and periorbital bones. Specific areas of interest are the condition of the orbital floor and whether or not there is evidence of orbital floor disruption. In addition, the orbital floor should be examined for signs of orbital content herniation through the orbital floor into the underlying maxillary sinus. Radiographic exam in this case showed that the zygoma and maxilla were intact with no displacement. However, the orbital floor was moderately disrupted with evidence of herniation of orbital contents into the maxillary sinus (Fig. 76–2).

A key physical exam is the "forced duction test," which is performed by grasping the insertion of the inferior rectus on the globe and moving the globe through a range of motion. This is then compared to the ease of moving the non-traumatized eye through a similar range of motion test.

An additional exam that may provide useful information regarding the position of the globe is with a Hertel exophthalmometer, which measures the position of the globe with regard to the orbital rim. It is most useful for gauging whether or not there is enophthalmos (movement of the eye posteriorly) rather than hypopthalmos (movement of the eye inferiorly). Note that the Hertel exophthalmometer relies on taking measurements of the globe position relative to the lateral orbital rim. Therefore, if there is displacement of the periorbital bones due to trauma accurate measurement of the globe position may be compromised. Forced duction testing revealed a significant restriction when moving the right globe as compared to the left globe. Measurement of globe position relative to the lateral orbital rim with the Hertel exophthalmometer showed that the right had 4 mm of enophthalmos.

The combination of physical findings of periorbital swelling and ecchymosis with restricted upward gaze, positive forced duction testing, and enophthalmos in combination with the radiologic findings of orbital floor disruption and herniation of orbital contents into the maxillary sinus fulfills the criteria for diagnosing an orbital blowout fracture. This fracture occurs as a result of sudden compression of the orbital contents with pressure on the thin orbital floor which fractures. There is then extrusion of orbital contents through the fracture into the maxillary sinus. The loss of orbital volume (due to fat herniation) causes the enophthalmos. However, the restriction of upward gaze is due to entrapment of the inferior rectus in the fracture line.

It is important to document that the cause of upward gaze limitation is due to actual muscle entrapment (which will not improve) rather than swelling or edema, which may well improve.

Although the majority of blowout fractures involve the inferior orbital floor with fat herniation and inferior rectus entrapment, there is a distinct entity in which there is a blowout fracture of the medial orbital wall with fat herniation and entrapment of the medial rectus. In the case of a medial wall blowout fracture, the physical findings are similar to inferior wall fractures with the exception that instead of restriction of upward gaze there is restriction of lateral gaze.

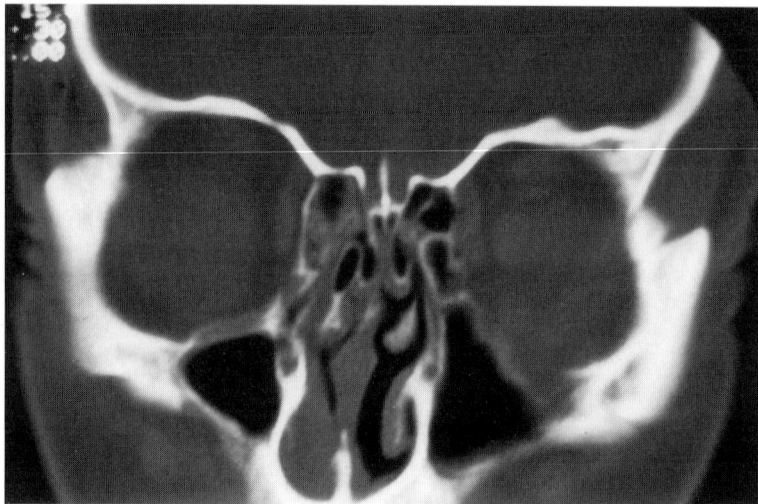

FIGURE 76-2 CT scan reveals evidence of herniation of orbital contents into the maxillary sinus.

DIAGNOSIS

Right orbital blow-out fracture with entrapment.

MEDICAL MANAGEMENT

It is well documented that not all orbital floor fractures require surgery. If surgery is required, it is almost never necessary on an emergent basis. The one exception to this is orbital floor fractures typically occurring in children under the age of 12 in which there is complete herniation and entrapment of the inferior rectus muscle into the maxillary sinus. Children with these severe floor fractures have extreme eye pain and nausea with attempted upward excursions of the globe and are generally unable to open or move the eye. Entrapment of the muscle through a "trapdoor fracture" can cause a laceration of the muscle belly and/or pressure ischemia with eventual muscle scarring, contracture, and diplopia. Therefore, early operative intervention with freeing of the entrapped muscle is recommended.

With the above exception noted, all other patients with orbital floor fractures are initially observed for resolution of motility restriction prior to proceeding with surgical intervention. Initial management is directed toward obtaining ophthalmologic consultation to rule out globe injury and warning the patient not to blow his or her nose (to prevent periorbital emphysema). Additionally, the patient is warned not to take aspirin or other platelet affecting drugs in case surgical intervention is required. If there is significant limitation of extraocular motility, prednisone 1 mg/kg/day for 1 week has been shown to speed its resolution and also to diminish long-term morbidity to the entrapped muscle. Patients are then subsequently followed serially for approximately 10 to 14 days to observe for improvement in extraocular motility and the development of enophthalmosis. If extraocular muscle restriction and diplopia persist during this time it is then appropriate to perform forced duction testing in order to differentiate extraocular muscle entrapment from paresis or contusion.

If the only positive findings are radiologic evidence of orbital floor disruption with some soft tissue herniation, without enophthalmos or muscle entrapment, then a conservative approach may be taken and the patient observed. Even if there is some limitation of globe motion this may be due to soft tissue contusion and edema rather than actual muscle entrapment. Therefore, forced duction testing to determine if muscle entrapment has occurred is very important for deciding if surgery is necessary.

With observation and the resolution of edema, enophthalmos that was not initially apparent may develop and require surgical management. However, most authors feel that a delayed orbital floor repair can still achieve an acceptable result with regard to globe position.

SURGICAL MANAGEMENT

If there is evidence of enophthalmos or muscle entrapment, then surgical exploration of the orbital floor is indicated. The orbital floor is exposed and the soft tissues carefully elevated out of the fracture. Typically the orbital floor is too comminuted for a primary repair and the integrity of the floor is restored with an onlay graft. The selection of material for onlay grafting is considerable and somewhat controversial. Although many authors advocate only autogenous bone grafts for floor reconstruction, we have had excellent results with several different alloplastic materials (porous polyethylene and Teflon plates). The development of these biocompatible materials, which have been used in numerous clinical series with excellent results and low morbidity, has rendered bone grafts, with their variable reabsorption and donor site morbidity, virtually obsolete for orbital floor reconstruction. Disimpaction of the muscle entrapment is fairly straightforward, but augmentation of the orbital floor for globe position may require considerable surgical judgment.

With regard to perioperative complications the major concern is orbital hemorrhage, which can occur up to 24 hours postoperatively. An orbital hemorrhage is heralded by increasing pain and proptosis of the affected eye. This is a true emergency due to the pressure that is put on the globe and the potential for shutting off blood flow to the retina and causing blindness. Treatment of an orbital hemorrhage consists of immediately opening the surgical incisions (at the bedside if necessary), a lateral canthotomy and inferior cantholysis, and return to the operating room for hematoma evacuation and control of bleeding if still active.

The major long-term complications are failure to return the globe to its exact pretrauma position with residual enophthalmos or exophthalmos (from to large a floor implant) or residual limitation of globe movement. Persistent limitation of globe motion may be due to continued muscle entrapment or muscle fibrosis and scarring due to the trauma. A high-resolution CT scan may be very useful in trying to distinguish between scarring and residual entrapment.

REHABILITATION AND FOLLOW-UP

Long-term follow-up shows that the upper lip numbness usually resolves over 2 to 3 months. Residual enophthalmos or exophthalmos may be treated with reexploration of the orbit and modification of the floor implant, but this should be delayed for at least 6 months in order to allow all edema to resolve. If there is evidence for continued muscle entrapment, then exploration and extraction of the muscle are indicated. If it appears that the limitation of motion is due to muscle dysfunction then surgical correction can be performed after a suitable time (6 months to a year).

SUGGESTED READINGS

CULLEN G, LUCE CM, SHANNON GM. Blindness following blow-out fractures. *Ophthalmic Surg Lasers.* 1977;8:60–62.

GILBARD S, MAFEE M, LAGOURDS P, LANGER B. Orbital blow-out fractures: the prognostic significance of computed tomography. *Ophthalmology.* 1985;92: 1523–1528.

HAWES MJ, DORTZBACH RK. Surgery on orbital floor fractures: influence of time on repair and fracture size. *Ophthalmology.* 1983;90:1066–1070.

LEDERMAN IR. Loss of vision associated with surgical treatment of zygomatic and orbital floor fracture. *Plast Reconstr Surg.* 1981;68:94–98.

LYON DB, NEWMAN SA. Evidence of direct damage to extraocular muscles as a cause of diplopia following orbital trauma. *Adv Ophthalmic Plast Reconstr Surg.* 1989;5:81–83.

MARKOWITZ BL, MANSON PN. Panfacial fractures: organization of treatment. *Clin Plast Surg.* 1989; 16:105–114.

MILLMAN AL, ROCCA RCD, SPECTOR S, et al. Steroids and orbital blow-out fractures—a new systematic concept in medical management and surgical decision-making. *Adv Ophthalmic Plast Reconstr Surg.* 1987;6:291–294.

Putterman AM, Stevens T, Urist MJ. Nonsurgical management of blow-out fractures of the orbital floor. *Am J Ophthalmol.* 1974;77:232–239.

Shumrick KA, Kersten RC, Kulwin DR, Smith CP. Criteria for selective management of the orbital rim and floor in zygomatic complex and midface fractures. *Arch Otolaryngol. Head Neck Surg.* 1997;123(4):378–384.

Thompson RF, Gluckman JL, Kulwin D, Savoury L. Orbital hemorrhage suring ethmoid sinus surgery. *Otolaryngol Head Neck Surg.* 1990;102(1):45–50.

MIDFACE FRACTURES

James Clemens, M.D.
Kevin A. Shumrick, M.D.

HISTORY

A 16-year-old white male was involved in a two-car, head-on motor vehicle accident as the restrained driver. Both the steering wheel and windshield were broken. There was extensive damage to his vehicle. He was transported by ambulance to the emergency room.

Physical exam revealed a mildly confused, but cooperative male. Vital signs were stable. He was in a C-collar and on a backboard. IV access was in place. There was a 2-cm laceration over the dorsum of the nose. The nasal dorsum was depressed with a "pig-nose" deformity (Fig. 77–1). Nasal bones were visible through the laceration and the nasal pyramid was mobile with crepitations. The septum was without hematoma. Mild epistaxis was present. Ocular exam revealed normal and equal pupils, extraocular motion, and intact vision. The intercanthal distance was 38 mm. The orbital rims, maxilla, and mandible were stable. Tympanic membranes were clear.

The remainder of his exam was significant for a fracture of the transverse process of T_1 and right lower extremity contusion. Chest radiograph was clear. Abdomen was benign.

An axial and coronal computed tomography (CT) scan of the facial bones was obtained (Fig. 77–2).

DIFFERENTIAL DIAGNOSIS— KEY POINTS

1. While this patient has obviously suffered severe trauma to the midface in the naso-orbital-ethmoid region, a complete trauma evaluation is necessary with stabilization of vitals and IV access.

2. A thorough exam of the face to gauge the extent of the fractures and damage to surrounding structures including the orbits and globe, the frontal lobe, the frontal sinus, the medial canthi, and the lacrimal system is necessary. The possibility of a cerebrospinal fluid (CSF) leak must also be considered and worked up appropriately.

3. If the frontal sinus is fractured the injury must have been caused by substantial force. Patients presenting with fractures of the frontal sinus have the following associated findings:
   - 75% have other serious associated injuries
   - 50% present in shock
   - 40% are comatose
   - 25% die of their injuries
   - 24% are conscious on presentation

4. Up to 67% of patients with naso-orbito-ethmoid (NOE) fractures have ocular trauma; 20 to 25% of these are considered serious and 3% result in blindness. Classic ocular findings include:
   - Telecanthus: >35 mm, suggestive of NOE; >40 mm, diagnostic of NOE
   - Normally the intercanthal distance is one-half the interpupillary distance
   - Rounding of the medial canthus
   - Epiphora, either from fractures involving the nasolacrimal duct or a displaced punctum and lacrimal sack due to avulsion of the medial canthus and lacrimal bone
   - Enophthalmus
   - Dystopia

5. Classic nasal findings include a loss of height of the nasal dorsum with superior rotation of the nasal tip (the pig-nose deformity).

6. Initial exam may be limited due to patient discomfort, bleeding, or swelling. NOE fractures are among the most difficult and challenging of facial fractures. The nasal appearance and structure are rarely returned to the pretraumatic state. Patients should be counseled prior to surgery to ensure that their expectations are realistic.

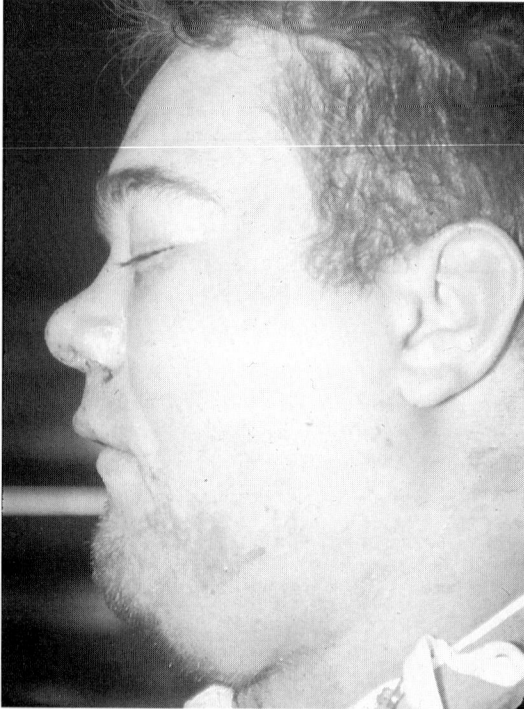

FIGURE 77–1 "Pig-nose" deformity.

TEST INTERPRETATION

Coronal and axial CT scan of the face should be obtained when the patient is stabilized (Fig. 77–2). This cut shows the nasal bones impacted into the ethmoid sinuses with nondisplaced fractures of the orbital rims. The nasolacrimal duct on the left has been involved in the fracture. CT scanning will not only highlight the NOE, but enable the evaluation of the orbits and remainder of the facial skeleton and mandible. CT of the brain may be indicated to rule out frontal contusion/bleeding or subarachnoid hemorrhage.

DIAGNOSIS

Naso-orbital-ethmoid fracture.

MEDICAL MANAGEMENT

There is no role for medical management in the care of NOE fractures. Unless the patient absolutely refuses repair, surgical intervention is indicated. CSF leaks are managed expectantly by elevating the head of bed, avoiding valsalva maneuvers, employing stool softeners and antitussives, avoiding nose blowing, and watching for spontaneous closure of the leak. Antibiotic coverage is debatable during this time period. Indications for surgical intervention include recurrent meningitis, pneumocephalus, and failure of spontaneous resolution. Fracture reduction is often accompanied by near immediate resolution of CSF leaks.

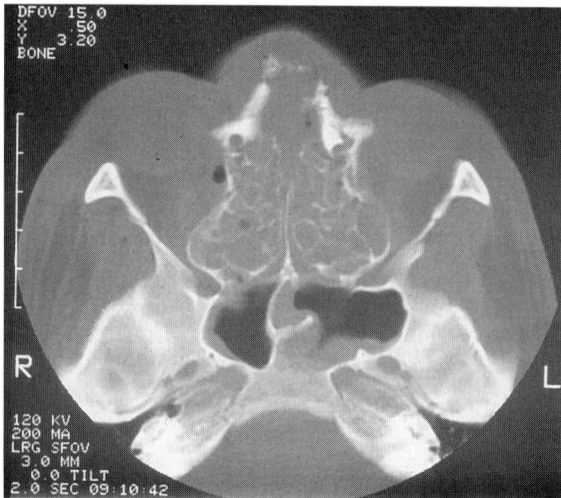

FIGURE 77–2 CT scan of the face shows the nasal bones impacted in the ethmoid sinuses with nondisplaced fractures of the orbital rims.

Ocular trauma often can be managed expectantly. Hyphema, corneal abrasions, and subconjunctival hemorrhage require no surgical intervention. Orbital trauma with nondisplaced fractures that do not involve the extraocular muscles also require no surgical intervention. Retrobulbar hemorrhage may result in blindness if not treated emergently (usually within 90 minutes of loss of vision). Initial management should consist of lateral cantholysis and administration of mannitol and acetazolamide to reduce intraocular pressure. Ophthalmologic consultation should be obtained to test formally and follow visual status.

SURGICAL MANAGEMENT

After delineating the extent of the fractures and the involved surrounding structures, planning the approach is next. The many options include

• Open sky or butterfly approach
• H-type incision
• Through the traumatic laceration (if present)
• Bicoronal
• Facial degloving

The open sky and H-approach have lost popularity secondary to obvious scarring postoperatively and numbness to the forehead and scalp.

Working through the wound is a viable option, although it is often limiting without significant extension of the wound. Combining this approach with a bicoronal and/or a facial degloving provides the most extensive exposure with the best cosmetic result.

In this case, the bicoronal approach was used. This approach has the advantage of exposing the area of the frontal sinus should it have fractures. There is also excellent exposure of the glabella, rhinion, medial canthal tendons, and nasal bones. An incision is carried from the helical root across the scalp to the contralateral helical root. The scalp is lifted off the galea in a broad front to 2 cm above the supraorbital rim. At this point the periosteum is incised and the elevation is carried out subperiosteally to protect the supraorbital and supratrochlear nerves. The periosteum must be severed from the temporal lines laterally. After identifying the supraorbital nerve and releasing them from their foramen (or notch) the same is done for the supratrochlear nerves. The periosteum of the orbit is then elevated. The elevation can be carried down to expose the lacrimal sack and medial canthal tendons. This allows adequate exposure for reduction and plating of these fractures and attachment of the canthi if they are avulsed. Most often the canthi are avulsed still attached to the lacrimal bone. With the advent of miniplating systems it is often possible to reposition the canthus using rigid fixation. The canthus must be positioned accurately or this will result in an obvious disparity in the canthal heights. If both canthii are avulsed, this can be quite difficult. Other options include transnasal intercanthal wiring over plates (usually lead) to maintain canthal position and support the comminuted nasal bones while healing.

The sublabial facial degloving will provide access to the lower aspect of the nasal framework, infraorbital rims, and the maxilla. This approach is basically an extended, bilateral sublabial incision in which the nasal skin is released from the nasal frame-work by a circumferential incision around the nasal vestibule. A significant complication is vestibular stenosis.

REHABILITATION AND FOLLOW-UP

Postoperatively, patients rarely regain their pretraumatic nasal contour and dorsal height. A septorhinoplasty with cartilage grafting is often needed to better restore this defect. Patients must also be followed for frontal sinus mucocele if the fractures involve the frontal sinus or nasofrontal duct.

SUGGESTED READINGS

ELLIS E. Sequencing treatment for naso-orbito-ethmoid fractures. *J Oral Maxillofacial Surg.* 1993; 51:543–558.

ROHRICH RJ et al. Management of frontal sinus fractures, changing concepts. *Clin Plast Surg.* 1992; 19(1):219–232.

SHUMRICK KA et al. Extended access/internal approaches for the management of facial trauma. *Arch Otolaryngol Head Neck Surg.* 1992;118:1105–1112.

AURICULAR AVULSION

James Clemens, M.D.
Kevin A. Shumrick, M.D.

HISTORY

A 21-year-old male involved in a motor vehicle accident presents to the emergency room 1 hour after the injury with a nearly complete avulsion at the left ear. The ear had been protected with moist gauze and an ice pack (Fig. 78–1).

The patient demonstrates no evidence of other serious injuries and the C-spine has been cleared.

DIFFERENTIAL DIAGNOSIS— KEY POINTS

1. In all trauma victims, the C-spine must be cleared and any life-threatening injuries to the head, thorax, or abdomen, and any limb-threatening injuries must be identified and treated immediately.

2. A pressure dressing should be applied (mastoid-type) to the wound to control bleeding. Avoid extensive cautery or clamping and ligation of vessels that may serve as vascular reanastomoses.

3. The auricle should be examined, cleaned, and any large vessels noted.

4. If the auricle was incompletely avulsed, the ear will often survive on even a very small pedicle.

5. A thorough exam of the tympanic membrane and external auditory canal should be performed. Depending on the mechanism of injury, the possibility of temporal bone fracture and damage to the facial nerve must be entertained. Auditory testing should be obtained when convenient.

TEST INTERPRETATION

The diagnosis is evident in this case. Most testing should be directed at ruling out any other injury and obtaining a hematocrit to rule out excessive blood loss.

DIAGNOSIS

Traumatic near-total auricular avulsion.

MEDICAL MANAGEMENT

There is no role for medical therapy of this injury. Medical management can be directed at educating the population about safe operation of motor vehicles, avoiding alcohol consumption while driving, and wearing seat belts.

SURGICAL MANAGEMENT

If, as in this case, the auricle remains attached by a pedicle—even if small—the ear will often survive. Meticulous reapproximation is carried out and broad-spectrum antibiotics are administered (Fig. 78–2). If venous congestion becomes a problem, medical grade leeches (*Hirudo medicinalis*) can be employed. Because leeches not only remove blood, but have an anticoagulant effect in the surrounding local tissues from a substance they secrete called hirudin, the patient should be monitored for dropping hematocrit if leeches are employed. In addition, leeches may transmit *Aeromons hydrophile*, a recognized pathogen that is susceptible to trimethoprim–sulfamethoxazole or ciprofloxacin.

If the auricle is completely avulsed, three options remain:

1. Microvascular anastomosis

2. Burying or covering the cartilage

3. Osseointegrated alloplastic reconstruction

Microvascular anastomosis is performed by locating an adequate vessel on the recipient bed

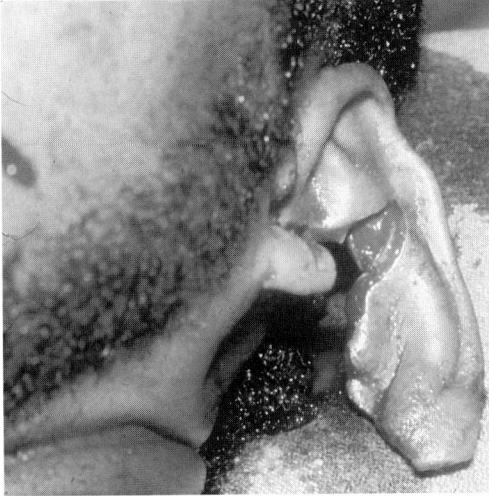

FIGURE 78–1 Near-complete avulsion of the left ear.

and on the auricle. Anastomosis is performed on arterial and venous vessels if possible. If a venous anastomosis is not possible, leeches may again be employed. If the auricle survives, this provides a superior result requiring limited revisions.

Many other methods have been described for preserving auricular cartilage. Postauricular skin and local scalp advancement flaps are the easiest and most direct. To employ these flaps, the auricular cartilage is either separated from

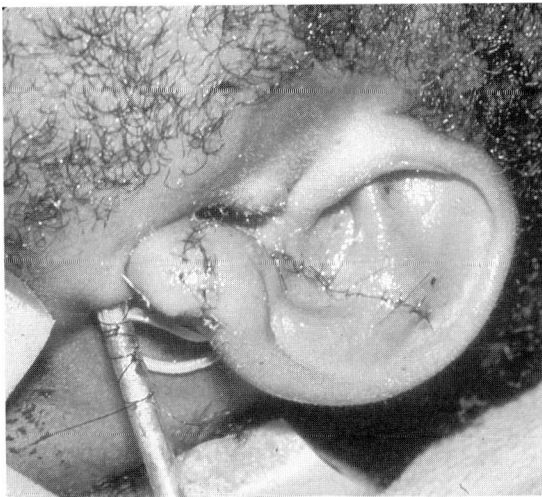

FIGURE 78–2 Meticulous reapproximation will save the ear.

the overlying skin or the skin is dermabraded to remove the epidermis. The cartilage is then placed in its anatomic position and meticulously reattached to the remaining intact cartilage and skin anteriorly. The cartilage is then buried by creating a subcutaneous pocket and advancing postauricular skin and/or scalp over the auricle. Depending on the amount of postauricular skin available and its elasticity, hair-bearing scalp may be advanced. After several months, the ear is usually revascularized. It is freed from the postauricular skin and covered using skin grafts. Any cartilage that did not survive can be restored using rib, septal, or contralateral conchal cartilage. Antibiotics are generally given during the postoperative period.

If there is damaged, inadequate, or missing postauricular skin, a temporoparietal fascial (TPF) flap may be used to cover the cartilage. The auricular skin is removed from the cartilage and the cartilage is placed in its normal anatomic position. The thin, flexible TPF flap is draped over the cartilagenous frame and covered with a skin graft. Some authors advocate creating "bur holes" in the cartilage to increase the amount of surface area in contact with the vascular supply. A suction drain will aid in seating the flap to the cartilage also. The TPF and skin grafts will shrink and conform to the cartilage over the next several weeks to months. Alternately, if the ipsilateral TPF is damaged in the trauma, the contralateral TPF may be harvested and used as a free flap. The radioulnar free flap may also be employed, although it is not as thin and induces more donor site morbidity.

Most surgeons employing microvascular anastomosis or free flaps use systemic anticoagulation in the operative and postoperative period with some combination of dextran, heparin, or aspirin being employed most commonly. The doses, combinations, and duration of use of these drugs varies with the physician and institution; however, their use should be considered. The role of hyperbaric oxygen (HBO) is controversial. While HBO may help survival of amputated body parts during the initial phases of revascularization, it does not take the place of meticulous surgical technique and will not rescue devitalized tissue. Its use should be considered, but must be weighed against its potential complications.

Finally, an often quite acceptable option for auricular reconstruction is osseointegrated implants for mounting a prosthetic ear. A prosthetic ear is fashioned around clips that attach to the abutments of the implants.

During reconstruction attention must also be directed to the external ear canal (EAC). If the EAC is transected or nearly transected, packing must be placed to prevent stenosis during the healing process.

REHABILITATION AND FOLLOW-UP

Many of the options for reattaching an auricle require multiple stages and prolonged follow-up. Realistically, the final result will never approach the untraumatized ear, and both the physician and patient must confront the problem with this in mind. However, once successful reimplantation is completed, little follow-up is necessary.

SUGGESTED READINGS

BRENT B. Secondary ear reconstruction with cartilage grafts covered by axial, random, and free flaps of the temporoparietal fascia. *Plast Reconstr Surg.* 1983;72:141–151.

BRENT B. The correction of microtia with autogenous cartilage grafts: I. the classic deformity. *Plast Reconstr Surg.* 1980;66:1–12.

DECHALAIN T, JONES G. Replantation of the avulsed pinna, 100% survival with a single arterial anastomosis and substitution of letters for a venous anastomosis. *Plast Reconstr Surg.* 1995;95:1275–1279.

DESTRO M, SPERANZINI MB. Total reconstruction of the auricle after traumatic amputation. *Plast Reconstr Surg.* 1994;94:859–864.

ERIKSSON E, VOGT PM. Ear reconstruction. *Clin Plast Surg.* 1992;19(3):637–643.

MUTIMER KL, BANIS JC, UPTON J. Microsurgical reattachment of totally amputated ears. *Plast Reconstr Surg.* 1987;79:535–540.

PARK C, LEE CH, SHIN KS. An improved burying method for salvaging an amputated auricular cartilage. *Plast Reconstr Surg.* 1995;96:207–210.

WILKES GH, WOLFAARDT JF. Osseointegrated alloplastic verous autogenous ear reconstruction: criteria for treatment selection. *Plast Reconstr Surg.* 1994;93:967–979.

Case 79

FACIAL BURNS

Mark J. Abrams, M.D.
Kevin A. Shumrick, M.D.

HISTORY

A 27-year-old male victim of a house fire presents to the emergency department with burns to the face and right upper extremity. He was pulled from the burning house before losing consciousness and is now lying in the trauma bay and is in significant pain.

He denies significant medical problems and reports no drug allergies or prescribed medications. He is also a nonsmoker and nondrinker.

Physical exam reveals a well-nourished, well-developed white male in moderate distress. He is being administered 100% O_2 by face mask and has an oxygen saturation of 100%. His vital signs include a respiratory rate of 30 to 35 per minute with mild inspiratory stridor, a pulse of 110, and a blood pressure of 120/70; he is afebrile. His face reveals the findings shown in Fig. 79–1. He also has burns of the majority of his right forearm and hand with remnants of his burnt shirt sleeve still present. Head and neck exam reveals areas of erythema and edema of his oral mucous membranes and his soft palate is discolored from soot. Otherwise his head and neck exam is unremarkable. His pulmonary exam is clear to auscultation except for the aforementioned mild stridor. Otherwise, the remainder of his exam is unremarkable.

DIFFERENTIAL DIAGNOSIS— KEY POINTS

1. While this patient presents with facial burns, a more serious overall condition may be developing. First of all, the signs of injury to the oral mucosa and discoloration from carbonaceous material are suggestive of a possible thermal airway injury as well as a possible inhalational pulmonary injury. The spectrum of this patient's problems may include carbon

monoxide intoxication, inhalational asphyxia from noxious gases, thermal injury with significant possible upper airway obstruction, and inhalational bronchopulmonary injury. The evaluation of these conditions is discussed in the next section.

2. The systemic cardiovascular effects of a burn injury are also important to consider. The so-called "rule of 9's" may aid in approximating the extent of the burn injury. Significant fluid shifts from extracellular extravasation may occur with burns of greater than 15% body surface area (BSA) in children and greater than 20% BSA in adults and will require aggressive IV rehydration with isotonic fluids to avoid shock. Often sodium bicarbonate is added to the fluids to counteract the often accompanied metabolic acidosis, and colloid may be used to help preserve intravascular volume. These patients and those with serious functional or airway injuries should be admitted to the intensive care unit (ICU) for close monitoring of the airway, cardiovascular status, and respiratory status. Invasive monitoring with Foley catheters and central lines (CVP or Swan–Ganz) may be prudent in these patients to monitor for signs of renal insufficiency and cardiovascular decompensation. In this case, the patient has less than a 15% BSA burn injury, but the airway findings warrant ICU monitoring.

3. The estimation of burn depth and size is aided by using the size of the patient's palm as an estimate of 1% of the patient's body surface area. Partial thickness burns can be distinguished from full thickness burns as being red, moist with blisters and severe pain, while full thickness burns are usually characterized by a charred dry appearance and the area is often insensate. As can be seen in Fig. 79-1, it is apparent that this patient has a mixture of partial and full thickness burns.

289

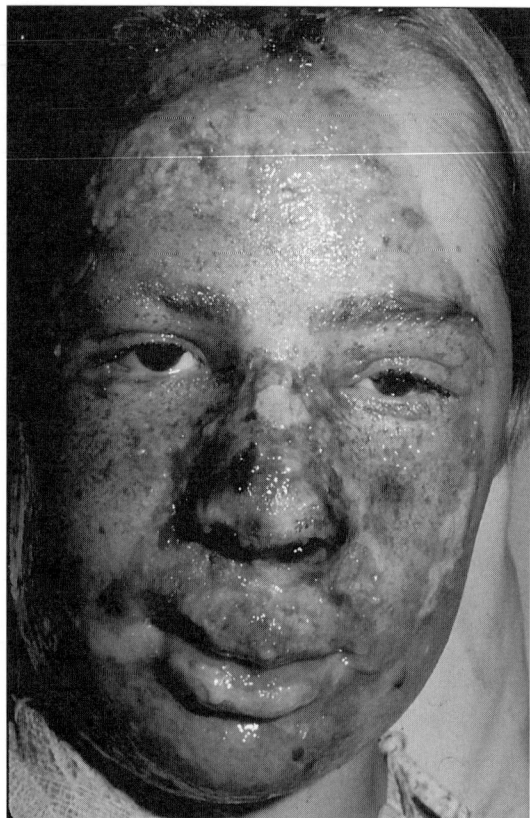

FIGURE 79–1 This patient has facial burns of varying depths. Note the perinasal and lip burns. This should raise the possibility of an inhalation injury.

TEST INTERPRETATION

Tests should include a baseline oxygen saturation, ABG, and a carboxyhemoglobin level. In addition, a baseline body weight, complete blood count (CBC), renal panel, and urine analysis should be obtained along with hourly vital signs. A chest x-ray should be obtained to document the extent of lung injury and a xenon-133 perfusion scan should be considered if significant inhalation injury is apparent. (A delay of clearance of xenon greater than 90 seconds correlates to a significant injury.)

In this particular case the following results were found:

- Room air saturation: 92%
- Room air ABG: PaO_2—62, $PaCO_2$—45, pH—7.45
- COHb—5%

- CBC, renal, UA are all normal
- Weight—76 kg
- Chest x-ray—clear with signs of mild pulmonary edema
- Xe-133 scan—60 seconds (within normal limits)

In this case, a significant thermal airway injury is suspected and bronchoscopy with possible intubation or tracheotomy to manage the airway is recommended.

The patient is taken to the operating room for flexible bronchoscopy with preparation made for possible intubation over the bronchoscope or an emergent tracheotomy given a sudden decompensation in his airway. In the case of severe inhalational injury, a tracheotomy may be prefered over placing a tube through a thermally injured larynx in order to prevent scarring sequelae. Endoscopy revealed mild to moderate edema and erythema of the vocal cords and the epiglottis but the airway was adequate. The distal airway revealed no significant mucosal injury but some scant carbonaceous material.

DIAGNOSIS

1. Mild thermal inhalational airway injury with possible pulmonary inhalational injury of mild extent.
2. Partial and full thickness burns involving the face and the right upper extremity.

MEDICAL MANAGEMENT

1. *Inhalation injury.* Given the findings described, observation in the ICU with 100% oxygen with warm, humidified air administered is warranted. A more severe injury would require intubation and possible invasive airway intervention as tracheotomy or cricothyrotomy. The use of steroids and antibiotics is controversial in the setting of thermal airway injury because no significant beneficial effect has been demonstrated in studies.

The carboxyhemoglobin level of 5% is reassuring but serial COHb and ABG levels should be followed during the ICU stay to rule out carbon monoxide poisoning. In addition 100% oxygen use should be used for this problem and other noxious gas injury.

To aid in the early detection of pulmonary edema secondary to inhalational injury, shock, or fluid overload, serial chest x-rays should also be ordered.

2. *Burn injury.* By the "rule of 9's," injury in this particular patient is less than 15%. Therefore, only routine IV rehydration is necessary. If the extent of burn injury exceeds 15 or 20% in children or adults, respectively, a more aggressive fluid rehydration regimen is recommended. The Duke method and modified Brooke formula are well-documented strategies for rehydration in these severe cases.

3. *Limb injuries.* The right upper extremity should be observed for vascular compromise secondary to significant circumferential edema. Therefore, frequent examinations should be performed by the nursing staff, which includes checking of capillary refill and distal limb pulses including vascular doppler evaluations, if necessary. Cyanosis, decreased capillary refill, and increased pain may signify limb ischemia. An escharotomy may be necessary. Limb elevation and active exercises for 2 to 3 minutes every 2 hours in the first 24 to 48 hours after injury may reduce edema.

4. *Wound considerations.* Generally, gentle cleansing with a nonalcohol containing soap and gentle daily debridement following cleansing is recommended. Ample narcotic analgesia is often required. Application of a topical antimicrobial ointment such as sulfamylon or silvidine is recommended. The use of systemic antibiotics is controversial. However, tetanus prophylaxis is generally recommended in these patients.

SURGICAL TREATMENT

There are three phases of treatment in facial burn injuries: early, intermediate, and late. The key to effective treatment in facial burns is the early prevention of functional deformities such as lid, ectropion, microstomia, and nasal stenosis. Early intervention is focused on preventing these functional problems and the more severe

cosmetic issues are addressed next, especially those requiring multiple stages.

1. *Early reconstruction.* Eyelid reconstruction should be considered early for both functional and cosmetic reasons. Full thickness skin grafts or high-quality partial thickness skin grafts should be used. Also at this point, large scalp injuries should be addressed with excision and skin grafting along with the use of tissue expanders for later scalp reconstruction. The treatment of significant neck contracture should also be considered early to prevent scarring to an extent that would prohibit intubation for general anesthetics required for later reconstructions. Another important early treatment strategy is to use oral splints and nasal stents to prevent oral and nasal stenosis. Finally, areas of exposed bone and cartilage should be grafted with local or vascularized free flaps.

2. *Intermediate reconstruction.* This group includes cheek scars and deformities of the lip, mouth, and nasolabial fold. Aesthetic skin unit grafts or tissue expansion of adjacent skin for local reconstruction is recommended. Oral reconstruction is delayed until this point to allow for scar maturation and correction by splinting. Vestibular or full nasal reconstruction should also be entertained at this point as these are often multistaged operations.

3. *Late reconstruction.* Full scar maturation is recommended for chin and lower lip reconstruction and for partial nasal deformity reconstruction. Reconstruction of ears and eyebrows is delayed until late because these are less important functional or cosmetic deformities that can often be hidden by makeup or hairstyle.

REHABILITATION AND FOLLOW-UP

Burn patients in general require extensive follow-up and a multiteam approach, often coordinated by a burn specialist. This team often includes pulmonologists, respiratory therapists, physical therapists, occu ational therapists, facial plastic surgeons, and other specialized plastic surgeons in order to rehabilitate and reconstruct the many deformities that burns create. Specifically relating to facial burn injuries, oculoplastic surgeons and ophthalmologists may also need to be involved. Finally, psychiatric counselors and social workers may also be required to aid with the emotional and social challenges that the long and often difficult rehabilitation process requires.

SUGGESTED READINGS

Achauer B. Reconstructing the burn face. *Clin Plast Surg.* 1992;19(3)623–36.

Housinger T, Hills J, Warden G. Management of pediatric facial burns. *J Burn Care Rehabil.* 1994; 15(5)408–411.

Pruitt S. Burns. In: Lyerly H, ed. *Handbook of Surgical Intensive Care: Practices of the Surgery Residents at the Duke University Medical Center.* 2nd ed. Year Book Medical Publishers; 1989:Chapter 18.

Rose E. Aesthetic restoration of the severely disfigured face and burn victims: a comprehensive strategy. *Plas Reconstr Surg.* 1995;96(7)1573–85.

FRONTAL SINUS TRAUMA

Thomas A. Tami, M.D.

HISTORY

A 22-year-old man was involved in a motor vehicle accident. Because he was not using his seatbelt, his face and head were thrown forward into the steering wheel. He lost consciousness at the time of the accident and was somewhat confused and mildly disoriented during his evaluation in a community hospital emergency department.

No gross focal neurologic deficits were described during the initial assessment. He had several lacerations on the forehead and in the periorbital region, which were easily repaired in the emergency department. Exploration of the wounds revealed depressed fractures of the forehead, so a lateral cervical spine film and a computed tomography (CT) scan of the head were ordered (Figs. 80–1 and 80–2).

When the patient was returning from radiology, he became hypotensive and had abdominal distention. An immediate peritoneal lavage was performed, which was positive for blood. His hemodynamic status was stabilized and he was taken immediately to the surgical suite for exploratory laparotomy.

During surgery, a ruptured spleen was identified and repaired. Since the CT scan revealed abnormalities in the frontal sinuses, surgical management of this problem was undertaken simultaneously.

When the patient was awakened from anesthesia, he appeared to be awake and alert, but could not be weaned from ventilatory support. Over the ensuing 12 hours it became obvious that he was quadriplegic.

DIFFERENTIAL DIAGNOSIS— KEY POINTS

1. This multiple trauma victim presenting to an emergency department must be treated and managed as a trauma patient. Although there are always obvious injuries that tend to focus the evaluation to a limited anatomic region, a full assessment must nevertheless be performed. In small community emergency departments where major trauma is encountered only occasionally, strict routines for trauma assessment are often not in place or adhered to, thus allowing major traumatic injuries to be overlooked.

2. This patient had obvious facial and forehead injuries, and these were addressed early on in the management of this patient. While records reveal that a brief neurologic examination was performed, it is also noteworthy that the patient was confused and mildly disoriented. In such a situation, a complete physical assessment is even more important, since the patient is often unaware of or unable to relay clinical signs and symptoms suggesting major injuries in other anatomic areas.

3. While it was appropriate to obtain a CT of the head and sinuses in this patient with significant head trauma and loss of consciousness, a complete exam appears not to have been performed prior to sending him to the radiology department. The abdominal injury would probably have been noted earlier had this been closely examined, and the need to rapidly recussitate this patient and subsequent rush to the operating room could have been accomplished in a more orderly fashion.

4. The incidence of concurrent cervical spine injury in patients with maxillofacial trauma is very high. Not obtaining complete cervical spine films to clear the spine prior to manipulation such as surgery on the frontal sinuses is an unforgivable omission. Even if the emergent nature of the clinical situation dictates against complete cervical spine radiography,

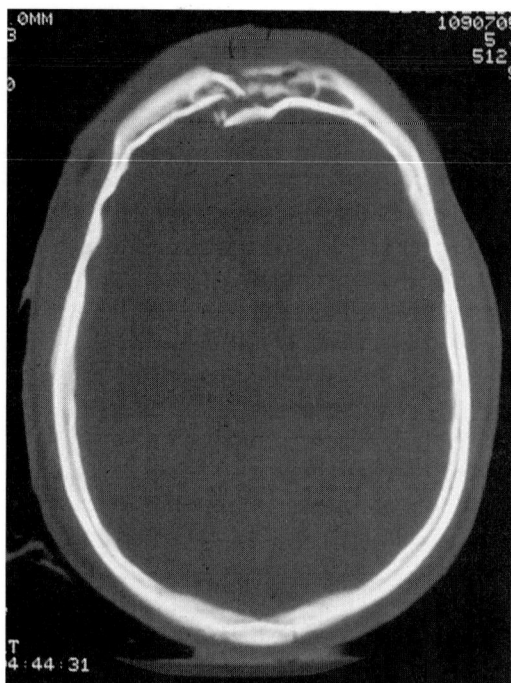

FIGURE 80–1 CT scan of the head reveals a severely comminuted frontal sinus fracture.

the neck must be immobilized and protected from any out-of-axis movements until appropriate imaging has ruled out an accompanying injury.

TEST INTERPRETATION

The CT (Fig. 80–1) image through the anterior skull and frontal sinus shows a severely comminuted frontal sinus fracture, which involves both the anterior and posterior tables. The injury appears to include both right and left frontal sinuses. The posterior table appears displaced posteriorly into dura and brain.

The lateral cervical spine x-ray (Fig. 80-2) failed to reveal any significant injury; however, it was an incomplete study. As is often the case in an emergency situation, the lower cervical vertebrae were not visible on this single lateral neck view.

DIAGNOSIS

1. Multiple facial lacerations
2. Frontal sinus fracture—anterior and posterior table, displaced

3. Cervical spine fracture with spinal cord injury and quadriplegia

MEDICAL MANAGEMENT

This patient has primarily surgical problems. He is young and otherwise healthy, so he should not have factors confounding his ultimate management.

Prophylactic antibiotics should be considered prior to surgery. The facial and forehead wounds as well as the lacerations and sinus fractures are contaminated injuries. Coverage should include an antibiotic active against *Staphylococcus aureus*.

Given the severity of the fracture and the posterior displacement of the back wall of the frontal sinus, a dural tear with subsequent cerebrospinal fluid leak is highly likely. This consideration must be kept in mind during the initial management of the patient as well as during the surgical exploration.

SURGICAL MANAGEMENT

As noted earlier, this patient must be managed from initial presentation as a multiple trauma victim. Had the primary principles or trauma management been adhered to, the occult cervical spine fracture would have been identified, the cervical spine stabilized, and the neurologic disaster avoided. Every patient presenting with maxillofacial trauma must be thoroughly evaluated. Manipulation of the cervical spine must be avoided until a complete evaluation has been accomplished. Many cases of low cervical spine injury are missed, even when an evaluation has been performed, due to the difficulty often encountered in radiographically imaging this area. Patience and persistence are important in these cases so that a thorough assessment can be undertaken.

The management of frontal sinus fractures depends on the type of fracture. If only the anterior table is fractured, and the nasofrontal duct is not affected, the repair is primarily done to preserve the cosmetic contour of the forehead. In these instances, elevation of the depressed bony segment with fixation, often with one or two mini bone plates is appropriate. Occasion-

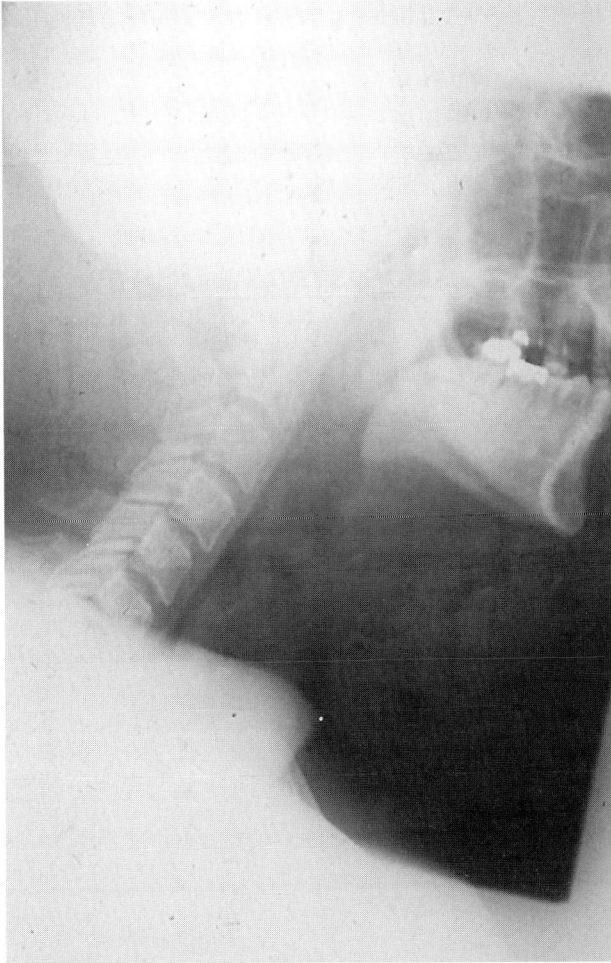

FIGURE 80-2 Lateral cervical spine film reveals no significant injury.

ally, fixation is not needed if the reduced bone segment can independently maintain its anatomic position.

When the posterior table is affected, most surgeons opt for obliteration of the sinus. The rationale behind this recommendation is the high incidence of frontal mucocele if left unattended. Mucosa can be trapped between the bony fracture edges and begin to grow, thereby resulting in a mucocele, usually many years later. An osteoplastic flap is utilized to visualize the frontal sinus. The mucosa is stripped from the sinus, the bony walls are polished with a diamond drill to assure that no mucosa remains, the frontal ducts are plugged with muscle or fascia, and the frontal sinus is obliterated. Abdominal fat is usually the graft material of

choice to obliterate the sinus. More recently, some experience with the use of cancellous bone from the iliac crest has proved a good alternative to fat obliteration.

In cases where the posterior table is not affected, but the nasofrontal outflow region is involved by the fracture, obliteration is also generally considered the most effective treatment option. Although a drainage procedure, such as a Lynch procedure, is an enticing alternative, long-term frontal duct patency rates following this approach are generally low.

Finally, when the posterior table is severely comminuted, consideration should be given to a cranialization procedure. In this technique, the posterior table of the sinus is removed in its entirety, the mucosa is eliminated and the frontal duct plugged. While this approach is occasionally used, it must usually be performed in conjunction with neurosurgery since there is often accompanying frontal lobe and dural injury.

In this case, an obliteration would probably be the best choice for this patient. The fairly severe displacement of the posterior table has most likely resulted in dural injury that will probably require the attention of a neurosurgeon. While fat could be used in this case, cancellous bone may be an ideal obliteration material because of the possible loss of segments of the bony wall of the frontal sinus.

REHABILITATION AND FOLLOW-UP

This patient will undoubtedly require long-term follow-up in a rehabilitation facility for his cervical spine injury.

With regard to the frontal sinus injury, if obliteration is successfully accomplished, no specific long-term follow-up should be necessary. However, even in cases of obliteration, subsequent mucocele formation has been reported. This fact should be part of the initial evaluation and consent process with this patient so that he can recognize potential problems as they may arise in the frontal sinus region many years into the future.

SUGGESTED READINGS

Davidson JS, Birdsell DC. Cervical spine injury in patients with facial skeletal trauma. *J Trauma.* 1989; 29:1276–1278.

Rohrich RJ, Hollier LH. Management of frontal sinus fractures. *Clin Plast Surg.* 1992;19:219–232.

Shockley WW, Stucker FF, Gage-White L, Anthony SO. Frontal sinus fractures: some problems—some solutions. *Laryngoscope.* 1988;98:18.

Shumrick KA, Smith CP. The use of cancellous bone for frontal sinus obliteration and reconstruction of frontal bony defects. *Arch Otolaryngol Head Neck Surg.* 1994;120:1003–1009.

Wallis A, Donald PJ. Frontal sinus fractures. A review of 72 cases. *Laryngoscope.* 1988;98:593–598.

PENETRATING NECK TRAUMA

Douglas B. Villaret, M.D.
Kevin A. Shumrick, M.D.

HISTORY

A 60-year-old male presented to the emergency department with a knife wound to the posterior right neck; the weapon had not been removed (Fig. 81–1). The patient was tachypneic and tachycardic but did not have any airway compromise. His only complaints were pain at the wound site and moderate dysphagia. Two 14-gauge IVs were started and oxygen was given via nasal cannulae. There was minimal bleeding from his wound. His blood pressure was 190/92 with a pulse rate of 105. No other injuries were found. A portable chest roentgenogram was obtained and trauma labs were sent.

A history of an altercation with his wife was obtained. The only preexisting medical history was mild hypertension.

A thorough physical exam revealed an anxious black male in no acute distress. He was alert and oriented. The carotid pulse could be palpated distal to the knife wound, and was symmetric to the contralateral side. All cranial nerves were intact. There were no motor or neurologic deficits. Oral exam and flexible nasopharyngoscopy failed to reveal any blood or mucosal tears. With the knife in place an emergent arteriogram was ordered, followed by a swallowing study.

DIFFERENTIAL DIAGNOSIS— KEY POINTS

1. All trauma patients arriving in the emergency room should be initially managed according to the ATLS protocol. The airway is managed first, and often includes tracheostomy under local anesthesia for laryngotracheal injuries. Large-bore IVs are then started and the patient's fluid resuscitated as needed.

2. The neck is divided into three zones for trauma evaluations.
   Zone 1: From bottom of cricoid cartilage to clavicles
   Zone 2: From angle of mandible to bottom of cricoid cartilage
   Zone 3: From skull base to angle of mandible

3. Most studies recommend immediate exploration for wounds presenting with obvious clinical signs: severe active bleeding, expanding hematoma, absent or diminished peripheral pulses, shock not responding to fluid resuscitation, increasing subcutaneous emphysema, air bubbling through the wound, major hemoptysis, and neurologic deficits.

4. A controversy exists over the appropriate management of patients who do not present with the above signs. Literature from the 1950s supported exploration of all wounds that traversed the platysma. With the advance of interventional radiology, all zone 1 and 3 injured patients received an arteriogram. Several recent studies have shown that in the absence of clinical signs (item 3 above), arteriography yields only a 1 to 2% diagnostic rate, beyond physical exam, of lesions significant enough to explore surgically. Some centers employ color-flow duplex ultrasonography to assist in the decision making. Although less invasive than arteriography, it offers a similarly low yield.

5. Gunshot wounds (GSW) result in a higher morbidity than stab wounds (SW). In one series, 16.5% of GSWs required a therapeutic operation compared to only 10% of SWs. This is mostly due to the kinetic energy of the bullet traumatizing the surrounding tissue. However, most of these injuries were managed nonoperatively based on the absence of clinical signs.

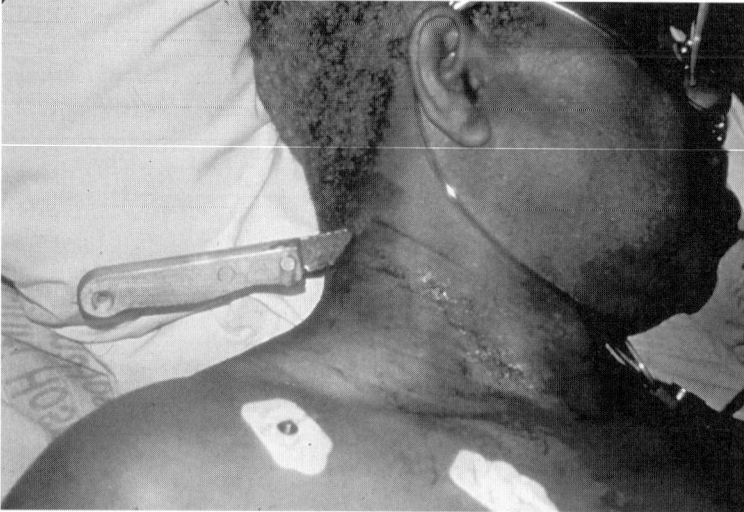

FIGURE 81-1 A knife wound to the posterior right neck.

6. The extent of zone 1 injuries is often difficult to diagnosis depending on the mental status of the patient. These are also the most lethal injuries. Bleeding into the chest or mediastinum may occur with few external signs. Arterial injuries may present with diminished peripheral pulses. Due to the difficulty in evaluating even significant injuries, many people recommend arteriogram, regardless of whether the patient exhibits symptoms. Depending on the proximity of the wound tract, a fluoroscopic or endoscopic evaluation of the esophagus may be required.

7. Penetrating injuries to zone II do not require an arteriogram. Physical exam alone is sufficient to evaluate the need for operative exploration. Neurologic status changes are very important to assess if observation is being advocated. (Remember, there are still some who advocate that all wounds which breach the platysma must be explored.)

8. Zone III trauma is fortunately the least common location in the neck for penetrating wounds. In asymptomatic patients, 24- to 48-hour observation is acceptable. Any *change* in the patient's status should prompt an immediate arteriogram followed by appropriate surgical intervention. Exposure of this area can be exceedingly difficult because the carotid follows its course medial to the mandible toward the skull base.

TEST INTERPRETATION

- Hgb/Hct—11/41.2
- Renal panel—WNC; PT/PTT 3.2/20
- CXR—no airspace disease, normal diaphragms
- Arteriogram—no extravasation or intimal injury (Fig. 81–2)
- Barium swallow—normal study

DIAGNOSIS

Zone II penetrating neck injury.

MEDICAL MANAGEMENT

All patients should be treated according to the principles put forth in the Advanced Trauma Life Support protocols. The airway must be secured first; 10% of victims of penetrating neck trauma have airway compromise. If the larynx is involved in the injury, a low tracheostomy under local anesthesia is recommended. Two large-bore IVs are started and fluid resuscitation is begun. These should not be on the same side as the injury due to the possibility of venous lacerations proximal to the IV. The patient is placed in the Trendelenburg position to minimize the potential of air embolism. The wounds

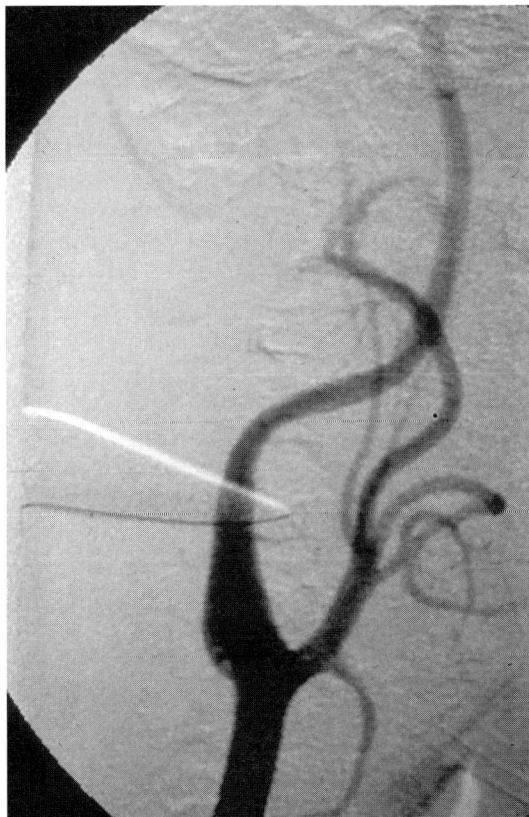

FIGURE 81–2   An arteriogram reveals no extravasation or intimal injury.

are tamponaded and the extent of the injuries evaluated.

SURGICAL MANAGEMENT

This patient was managed simply with removal of the knife. He was released 24 hours later and was without sequelae at his 2 month follow-up. Vascular injuries include the following:

1. *Carotid.* The carotid is the most commonly injured artery, occurring in about 6% of cases. Mortality may be as high as 60%, dropping to 10 to 20% for those that reach the hospital. Exposure may require a median sternotomy with or without a "book" thoracotomy for zone I injuries. Zone II is explored via an incision anterior to the sternocleidomastoid muscle. Exposure for zone III injuries is facilitated with anterior subluxation of the mandi-

ble or even a vertical osteotomy of the ramus of the mandible.

   The decision to ligate or repair the vessel is predicated on the ability to obtain retrograde flow (distal patency) and the concern of escalating an ischemic cerebral infarct into a hemorrhagic infarct. Most trauma centers now do not revascularize if the patient has been in a coma for more than 4 hours or if there is an established ischemic infarct.

   Minor anomalies picked up on arteriogram such as small intimal tears or false aneurysms may be followed periodically with ultrasound, obviating surgical intervention.

2. *Subclavian.* Occurs in 4% of cases. A median sternotomy with or without medial clavicular excision for right-sided injuries can be used versus a left thoracotomy with "book" or "trapdoor" extension for left-sided wounds. Primary repair should be performed to prevent the subclavian steal syndrome if the laceration is proximal to the vertebral artery.

3. *Vertebral artery.* This artery runs in a bony canal through the transverse processes of C_6–C_1. The incidence with routine four-vessel angiography approaches 20%; without angiography, the detection rate is around 2%. There is a low morbidity to observing minor injuries to the vertebral artery. Embolization can be used effectively. For severe bleeding, an anterior approach removing the costotransverse bar can be used for access. Occasionally, this may be the source of thromboembolic events.

4. *Internal jugular vein.* Occurs in 9% of penetrating trauma, increasing to 33% in cases where the common carotid is involved. Some advocate routine repair, especially if lacerated bilaterally. This can be a major cause of mortality from an air embolism.

5. *Laryngotracheal injuries.* These include a broad category from minor punctures of the lumen to laryngotracheal separations. Concomitant injuries must be sought, especially esophageal, vascular, and recurrent laryngeal nerves. Signs include dyspnea, stridor, dysphonia, subcutaneous emphysema, hemoptysis, and air bubbling through the wound.

   In severe cases, a low tracheostomy under local anesthesia is advocated. Tracheal injuries may be repaired primarily using 3-0 monofilament sutures that go through the cartilage rings but do not pass into the tracheal lumen. For minor, incomplete lacerations, tracheostomy may not be required. Suprahyoid releasing incisions may be required for additional length.

Laryngeal injuries are more complex and are covered elsewhere.

The cervical esophageal injuries are equally numerous with laryngotracheal injuries: around 10%. A high degree of suspicion must be held as they are the most commonly missed injury. Mortality rates soar to 67% for mid to lower esophageal injuries diagnosed after 24 hours from injury.

Odynophagia, subcutaneous emphysema, hematemesis (or blood from the nasogastric aspirate), and fever are the most common findings.

A gastrograffin fluoroscopic study followed (if negative) by a barium swallow is 92% sensitive. Some studies have found rigid esophagoscopy to be 96 to 100% sensitive.

Immediate repair with a two- or three-layered closure and drainage is the optimum management. Some authors recommend routine coverage with vascularized local muscle flaps. Debridement with a controlled fistula or exclusion operations may be performed, but there is a high mortality associated with the latter option.

REHABILITATION AND FOLLOW-UP

Zone I injuries are the most lethal; up to 66% if the common carotid artery is lacerated. Zone II are the most common. There seems to be no economic advantage of conservative management over surgical exploration.

Missed esophageal injuries carries a grave diagnosis. Although cervical esophageal injuries are less morbid than mid and lower injuries, there is still a 20% mortality associated with delayed diagnosis. A controlled fistula appears to be the best management option for infected esophageal trauma.

For carotid injuries that require ligation of the common or internal carotid system, there is a 30% stroke rate.

Rehabilitation is specific for the injury. Follow-up appointments should be at 1 week to remove sutures and assess any changes, then again at 1, 3, and 6 months to evaluate for any neurologic changes suggestive of vascular injury and thromboembolic events.

SELECTED READINGS

ARMSTRONG NB, DETAR TR, STANLEY RB. Diagnosis and management of external penetrating cervical esophageal injuries. *Ann Otol Rhinol Laryngol.* 1994;103:863–871.

ATTEBERRY LR, DENNIS JW, MENAWAT SS, FRYLCBERG LR. Physical examination alone is safe and accurate for evaluation of vascular injuries in penetrating zone II neck trauma. *J Am College Surg.* 1994;179:657–662.

BRENNAN JA, MYERS AO, JAFEK BW. Penetrating neck trauma: a five year review of the literature, 1983 to 1988. *Am J Otol.* 1990;11:191–197.

DEMETRIADES D, ASENSIO JA, VELMAHOS G, THAL E. Complex problems in penetrating neck trauma. *Surg Clin North Am.* 1996;76:661–683.

MCCONNELL DB, TRUNKEY DD. Management of penetrating trauma to the neck. *Adv Surg.* 1994;27:90–127.

MILLER RH, DUPLECHAIR JK. Penetrating wounds of the neck. *Otolaryngol Clin North Am.* 1991;24:15–21.

RAMADAN F, RUTLEDGE K, OLLER D, et al. Carotid artery trauma: a review of contemporary trauma center experiences. *J Vasc Surg.* 1995;21:46–55.

SELF-ASSESSMENT: QUESTIONS

1. In the evaluation of patients with maxillary sinus carcinoma, Ohngren's line can be drawn between
A. The lateral and medial vault of the maxillary sinus
B. The angle of the mandible and the medial canthus
C. The infraorbital foramen and the nasal spine
D. The maxillary tuberosity and the condyle of the mandible
E. The inferior turbinate and the lateral canthus

2. In patients with a cleft palate secondary to the Pierre Robin sequence, the palatal repair should be performed
A. Immediately following birth
B. At the same time as the tracheotomy
C. When the airway problem has finally resolved due to mandibular growth
D. At age 6
E. At any age

3. Of the following which does *not* constitute a common finding of transverse temporal bone fracture?
A. Anacusis
B. Debilitating vertigo
C. Facial paralysis
D. Involvement of foramen spinosum
E. Fracture of the stylomastoid foramen

4. A 48-year-old man presents with a post-traumatic subglottic stenosis. He has stridor with exertion. CT scan reveals an approximately 4-cm segment of stenotic trachea beginning in the immediate subcricoid region. The best treatment for this patient would be
A. CO_2 laser excision of the stenotic segment
B. Sequential dilation of the segment
C. Transoral placement of a Montgomery T-tube
D. An indwelling expandable intraluminal stent
E. Tracheal resection

5. A 48-year-old woman presents complaining of tired-looking eyes. On examination, her lid margins appear to be in the proper position relative to the iris, but excess lid skin hangs down below the lid margin. This condition is referred to as
A. Pseudoptosis
B. Blepharoptosis
C. Dermatochalasis
D. Blepharochalasis
E. Lid retraction

6. A common finding in patients with obstructive sleep apnea is
A. Clubbing of the fingers
B. Hypertension
C. Psychosis
D. Narcolepsy
E. Nasal obstruction

7. The most effective class of drugs that can be used to improve the symptoms of reflux laryngitis is
A. Systemic steroids
B. Topical inhaled steroids
C. Seratonin reuptake inhibitor
D. Calcium channel blockers
E. Proton pump inhibitors

8. Which of the following factors is most commonly associated with postoperative carotid artery rupture?
A. Previous radiation therapy
B. Patient older than age 70
C. The MacFee incision
D. Smoking
E. Diabetes

9. Most cases of obstructive anosmia can be successfully treated with
A. Steroid administration
B. Septoplasty
C. Phenylpropanolamine
D. Topical chromilyn sodium
E. Cryotherapy

10. The primary predisposing factor that results in stomal recurrence following laryngectomy is
A. Preoperative emergency tracheotomy
B. Poor histopathologic differentiation of the tumor
C. Advanced laryngeal tumor with subglottic extent
D. Poor nutritional status
E. Bilateral cervical nodal metastasis

11. A typical CT scan finding in a patient with surgical necrotizing fasciitis is
A. Free air is almost always seen within the fascial plains
B. Multiple distinct abscesses are usually seen within the soft tissues of the neck
C. The appearance of fluid collections that conform to the fascial plains of the neck is typical
D. Thrombosis of the internal and / or external jugular veins is almost universal
E. Extension to the prevertebral fascia is almost always present

12. Surgical excision of a first branchial arch cyst in an infant should be postponed until the child reaches the age of 2. The reason for this is
A. Because the cyst may degenerate and disappear
B. To allow the cyst to increase in size and thereby facilitate the dissection
C. To facilitate dissection of the facial nerve
D. To allow any associated tracts to involute and resorb
E. To allow infection to occur prior to recommending surgical removal

13. Which of the following surgical therapies have been used successfully for vasomotor rhinitis?
A. Endoscopic total sphenoethmoidectomy
B. Ablative surgery to the inferior turbinate
C. Tympanic neurectomy
D. Stellate ganglion block
E. Young's procedure

14. A 29-year-old man presents with evidence of a parapharyngeal space abscess. The most likely microbiologic flora responsible for this infection is
A. Group A and non-Group A streptococcus
B. Anaerobic organisms
C. Gram-negative organisms
D. Polymicrobial flora with both aerobic and anaerobic organisms
E. *Staphylococcus aureus*

15. All of the following tumors would commonly be included in the differential diagnosis of facial palsy except
A. Neuroma
B. Meningioma
C. Adenoma
D. Glomus tumor
E. Clival chordoma

16. The most common benign tumor of the submandibular gland is
A. Monomorphic adenoma
B. Lymphoepithelial cyst
C. Warthin's tumor
D. Schwannoma
E. Pleomorphic adenoma

17. The term *Carhart's notch* refers to which of the following?
A. The maximal airborne gap demonstrated on audiogram
B. The narrowest airbone gap demonstrated on audiogram
C. A low-frequency sensorineural trough
D. A shallow sensorineural loss noted at 2,000 Hz
E. The high-frequency sensorineural peak noted on audiogram

18. Following a total thyroidectomy you are called to see a patient complaining of severe anxiety and paresthesias of the face and hands. During your evaluation she has a seizure. Following establishment of an airway and stabilization of this patient, the next therapeutic modality should be
A. Immediate IV administration of potassium chloride
B. Immediate intramuscular injection of magnesium
C. To start oral calcium carbonate supplementation

D. Immediate institution of intravenous calcium gluconate

E. To draw ionized calcium level and base further therapy on this lab test

19. Suppurative labyrinthitis may occur when bacteria invade the otic capsule. Which of the following symptom complexes reflects invasion of the petrous apex?

A. Severe vertigo with profound sensorineural hearing loss

B. Facial paralysis with sensorineural loss

C. Facial paresthesias with retro-orbital pain

D. Suppurative otorrhea and facial paralysis

E. Retro-orbital pain and sixth nerve palsy

20. Patients with advanced laryngeal carcinoma (stage III or stage IV)

A. Always require surgery as part of their therapeutic regimen

B. Can be treated in an organ preservation program only if they do not respond to chemotherapy

C. Are only candidates for organ preservation therapy if they respond favorably to chemotherapy

D. Can usually be treated with radiation therapy alone

E. Rarely require concomitant therapy of the neck

21. In an elderly patient with poor hearing and ongoing debilitating vertigo the treatment would be

A. Cochleosacculotomy

B. Labyrinthectomy

C. Vestibular neurectomy

D. Transtympanic gentamicin

E. Ventilation tube placement

22. Foreign bodies of the aerodigestive tract are associated with the highest mortality when the site of impaction is the

A. Oropharynx

B. Larynx

C. Trachea

D. Main stem bronchus

E. Esophagus

23. Elective radical neck dissection should be considered in cases of malignant melanoma with

A. A thickness of less than 0.75 mm

B. A thickness greater than 4 mm

C. Lesions between 0.75 and 4 mm in thickness

D. Any time the parotid gland is in the lymphatic drainage pathway

E. Any time distant metastases can be excluded

24. Radiotherapy in the treatment of juvenile nasopharyngeal angiofibroma is generally used

A. Following surgical excision to help prevent recurrence

B. Preoperatively to decrease blood supply

C. When there is extension into the nasal cavity

D. When there is extension into the ethmoid or maxillary sinus

E. When there is intracranial extension with involvement of vital structures

25. The most common congenital nasal masses are encephaloceles, gliomas, and dermoids. An encephalocele may be distinguished from a glioma based on a positive Furstenberg sign. This sign reflects

A. Venous engorgement

B. Arterial supply from both the internal and external carotid arteries

C. A patent intracranial communication with cerebrospinal fluid

D. Absence of a patent intracranial connection with cerebrospinal fluid

E. Connection to the skull base

26. A 61-year-old male undergoes Moh's excision of a large basal cell carcinoma involving the right nasal alar margin. The final defect includes 65% of the right ala along with the lower lateral cartilage; however, the nasal lining remains intact. The most appropriate method of reconstruction is

A. Allow to heal by secondary intention

B. A midline forehead flap

C. A free conchal cartilage graft with midline forehead flap

D. A free conchal cartilage graft with midline forehead flap after resecting the remaining alar skin

E. A full thickness skin graft

27. One of the easiest techniques currently available for identifying suspicious mucosa in patients with field cancerization is

A. Supravital staining with toluidine blue

B. Identification of fluorescence using a Wood's lamp

C. High-resolution MRI scanning

D. Cytologic evaluation of tissue surface scrapings

E. Contact surface microscopy

28. A 57-year-old male presents with an enlarging ulcerative lesion involving the floor of the mouth. Clinical findings that would suggest mandibular invasion include

A. Tenderness to palpation

B. Pain with eating

C. Decreased sensation along the tongue

D. Decreased sensation along the lower lip

E. Palpable submandibular lymph nodes

29. A 28-year-old woman presents with a granulomatous nasal condition. A microscopic vasculitis with fibrinoid vascular necrosis is identified histopathologically. Further evaluation of this patient should include

A. Serum angiotensin converting enzyme levels

B. Purified protein derivative (PPD)

C. Nasal culture

D. Antinuclear antibody (ANA)

E. Chest x-ray

30. A 30-year-old woman is diagnosed with ameloblastoma of the mandible. The most appropriate therapy of this lesion is

A. Simple enucleation or curretage

B. Radiation therapy

C. Curettage followed by radiation therapy

D. Complete excision, including marginal or segmental mandibulectomy if indicated, to obtain clear margins

E. Complete excision with radical neck dissection

31. In patients with papillary carcinoma of the thyroid with tumors greater than 1.5 cm, the best therapy is

A. Iodine-131 therapy

B. Total thyroidectomy followed by iodine-131 therapy

C. Hemithyroidectomy followed by close postoperative observation

D. Total thyroidectomy and bilateral anterior neck dissections

E. Total thyroidectomy followed by external beam radiation therapy

32. In an adult who presents with signs and symptoms consistent with acute epiglottis, the best initial clinical assessment tool is

A. Lateral soft tissue x-ray of the neck

B. Fiber optic laryngoscopy

C. Blood cultures

D. General anesthesia with direct laryngoscopy and possible tracheotomy

E. IV antibiotics and observation

33. The gradual onset of biphasic stridor in a previously healthy 6-month-old infant suggests which of the following diagnoses?

A. Epiglottis

B. Congenital bilateral vocal cord paralysis

C. Foreign body aspiration

D. Subglottic stenosis

E. Croup

34. Patients with Down syndrome are prone to recurrent episodes of croup. This is because of

A. Recurrent tonsillitis with tonsillar hypertrophy

B. Depressed immunity

C. Macroglossia

D. The high incidence of sleep apnea

E. Subglottic narrowing

35. The optimal age for surgical excision of a large congenital cervicofacial lymphangioma is

A. At the time of delivery due to the potential for airway compromise

B. At approximately 1 week of age, before the infant is discharged but otherwise has been stabilized

C. At several months of age, allowing time to determine whether the airway will be compromised

D. At several years of age, to allow the child time to grow

E. It should not be resected, because these lesions will always regress

36. Sudden sensorineural hearing loss occurs with what frequency in patients with acoustic neuroma?
A. 1%
B. 5%
C. 15%
D. 30%
E. 50%

37. The most appropriate first-line treatment for early laryngeal papillomatosis in a child is
A. CO_2 laser excision
B. Tracheostomy
C. Interferon
D. Photodynamic therapy
E. Acyclovir

38. The classic histologic appearance of a minor salivary gland in a patient with Sjögren's disease is
A. Charco–Leyden crystals throughout
B. Oncocytic proliferation in the acinar region
C. Multiple areas of cystic degeneration
D. Lymphocytic infiltration with ductal hyperplasia
E. Severe vasculitis

39. The most common cause of subglottic stenosis is
A. Esophageal reflux
B. Wegener's granulomatosis
C. Relapsing polychondritis
D. Endotracheal tube trauma to the airway
E. Scleroma

40. A 51-year-old woman presents with a stage I tonsillar squamous cell carcinoma. Treatment of this lesion can best be provided utilizing
A. Radiation therapy alone
B. Surgical therapy alone

C. The efficacy of both surgical and radiation therapy in this situation is approximately equal to that of chemotherapy

D. This patient will require surgical therapy followed by postoperative radiation therapy

E. Surgical or radiation therapy to the primary site followed by elective neck dissection

41. When evaluating a patient with hereditary hemorrhagic telangiectasial (HHT) the workup should include
A. Upper and lower GI endoscopy
B. Intravenous pyelogram
C. Chest CT scan
D. Serum clotting factors
E. Electrocardiogram

42. Confirmation of cerebrospinal fluid leakage is best made by which laboratory assessment?
A. Total protein
B. Testing blood glucose
C. β_2-transferrin
D. Amylase
E. Enolase

43. The most common audiologic pattern for children with congenital atresia would show
A. 50 to 60 dB conductive hearing loss with normal nerve function
B. 20 to 30 dB conductive hearing loss with normal nerve function
C. 10 to 20 dB conductive hearing loss with normal nerve function
D. 60 dB airbone gap with a mild to moderate nerve loss
E. 20 to 30 dB conductive hearing loss with moderate to severe nerve component

44. Characteristics of benign intracranial hypertension include the following except
A. Pulsatile tinnitus
B. Papilledema
C. Increased intracranial pressure
D. Visual field defect
E. Hearing loss

45. Allergic mucin is typically characterized by
A. Eosinophils and Charco–Leyden crystals
B. Periodic acid–Schiff positive intranuclear inclusions
C. Granulomatous inflammation
D. A thin watery consistency
E. Submucosal fungal invasion

46. Surgical resection of the recurrent laryngeal nerve is no longer recommended for spasmodic dysphonia because
A. Long-term results are poor despite good short-term improvement
B. There is a high incidence of breathiness following this procedure
C. If the opposite vocal cord becomes spasmodic, stridor will result
D. Both vocal cords are usually involved with spasmodic dysphonia
E. Spasmodic dysphonia is usually a multisystem disorder unaffected by treating the larynx alone

47. In a patient presenting with grade 5 laryngeal trauma
A. Conservative management is appropriate
B. Endotracheal intubation is the preferred technique for airway control
C. Chest tubes should be placed prophylactically on both the right and left sides
D. A nasogastric tube should be carefully passed into the stomach
E. Hoarseness may only be intermittent

48. When a patient presents with cervical necrotizing fasciitis, the best way to rule out mediastinal involvement is
A. A CT scan including the neck and mediastinum
B. Direct surgical exploration of the mediastinum
C. Findings of hypoesthesia and necrosis of the skin of the chest wall
D. Careful auscultation of the chest in the region of the superior mediastinum
E. Mediastinoscopy

49. An HIV-infected man has white pseudomembranous inflammatory patches throughout his oral cavity. He is also complaining of severe odynophagia and retrosternal discomfort. The next step in the evaluation of this patient should be
A. Esophagoscopy
B. Electrocardiogram
C. Esophageal manometry
D. Pulmonary function testing
E. Place a PPD

50. A common presenting symptom in patients with myasthenia gravis is
A. Vertigo
B. Ptosis and diplopia
C. Aphasia
D. Spasmodic dysphonia
E. Visual field defects

51. Malignant transformation of long-standing recurrent pleomorphic adenoma more commonly occurs
A. If the recurrence is a single nodule of tumor
B. If the recurrence is multiple small nodules
C. When the recurrence is in the deep lobe of the parotid
D. When the previous surgery was simply a lumpectomy
E. In patients with diabetes

52. A child awakens from a chronic ear procedure (tympanomastoidectomy) with a dense unilateral facial paralysis. The surgeon should
A. Assure the patients that the nerve will recover
B. Start the patient on antibiotics
C. Institute steroids and release the packing and dressing
D. Immediately take the patient to the operating room
E. Prepare the patient for a VII/XII anastomosis

53. A patient sustains severe frontal trauma during a motor vehicle accident. The cervical spine is cleared with a single lateral neck X-ray. Some injuries of the cervical spine will be missed from this single view because
A. Such patients are usually poorly cooperative, making for an inadequate study
B. It is difficult to position patients properly for these views

C. The upper cervical vertebrae are not well visualized on this film
D. The lower cervical vertebrae are not well visualized on this film
E. Such films are difficult to interpret because of soft tissue injury

A. Stop the bleeding
B. Decrease intraglobe pressure
C. Expand intraorbital volume
D. Maintain intraorbital volume
E. Decrease intraorbital volume

54. Up to 67% of patients with naso-orbitoethmoid fractures have associated ocular trauma. The incidence of blindness is
A. 2%
B. 3%
C. 4%
D. 5%
E. More than 5%

55. A 30-year-old male victim of a house fire presents to the Emergency room. He is alert and communicative, and no external burns of the skin are visible. His lips are erythematous with carbonatious discoloration around the mouth. No stridor is audible; however, the patient is slightly tachypneic, and O₂ saturation is 96%. The most appropriate treatment would be
A. Place some antibiotic ointment around the lips and discharge the patient to be followed up the next day as an outpatient
B. Administer 100% humidified oxygen and observe the patient for 4 to 6 hours
C. Administer 100% humidified oxygen and admit the patient to the intensive care unit overnight for observation
D. Place a central line for monitoring cardiovascular status and a Foley catheter for monitoring fluids, and admit the patient to the intensive care unit
E. Perform a tracheotomy

56. The following physical finding is suggestive of a naso-orbitoethmoid fracture
A. An intracanthal distance equal to half the interpupillary distance
B. Bilateral periorbital ecchymoses
C. Proptosis
D. Pig-nose deformity
E. Epistaxis

57. A blepharoplasty patient presents with postoperative orbital hemorrhage and secondary hematoma. The goal of therapy is to

58. Nine months following a total laryngectomy to remove a squamous cell carcinoma, a patient presents with a recurrence at the superior aspect of his stoma. CT scan reveals no evidence of extension to the esophagus or superior mediastinum. The chances of successful surgical management of this lesion are
A. Less than 5%
B. 20 to 30%
C. Greater than 80%
D. Dependent on the histopathologic grading of the tumor
E. Dependent on the patient's pulmonary function tests

59. A 56-year-old man presents with a maxillary sinus carcinoma confined primarily to the medial wall of the maxillary sinus. It extends into the bony alveolar ridge but does not extend up to the orbital floor. The best surgical therapeutic modality to manage this lesion might be
A. An infrastructure maxillectomy
B. Radical maxillectomy
C. A superstructure maxillectomy
D. A medial maxillectomy
E. A total maxillectomy with orbital exoneration

60. A 37-year-old man presents with a unilateral nasal mass, which on biopsy is diagnosed as esthesioneuroblastoma. The lesion appears to penetrate the skull base to the dura but it does not penetrate the dura. The best therapy for this patient is
A. Chemotherapy and palliative radiation therapy
B. Radiation therapy followed by surgery for salvage
C. Craniofacial resection followed by radiation therapy
D. Intranasal debulking followed by radiation therapy
E. Radiation using interstitial implants

61. The highest mortality and functional morbidity associated with basal cell carcinoma occurs in
A. The postauricular region
B. The nasal vestibule
C. The lower lip
D. The nasal tip
E. The medial canthus

62. The treatment for Wegener's granulomatosis includes all of the following except
A. Radiation therapy
B. Cyclophosphamide
C. Corticosteroids
D. Trimethoprim-sulfamethoxazole
E. Frequent debridement of crusts in the nasal cavity

63. In patients with facial nerve paralysis electroneuronographic degeneration greater than which percentile portends a potentially poor prognosis?
A. 25%
B. 50%
C. 75%
D. 80%
E. 95%

64. Which of the following statements best defines cholesteatoma?
A. Cholesteatoma is the presence of keratinizing squamous epithelium found to be invading the spaces of the temporal bone
B. Cholesteatoma is a skin cyst that forms at the site of PE tube placement
C. Cholesteatoma is a benign neoplasm commonly found in the temporal bone
D. Cholesteatoma is a cyst containing globules of fat formed in the temporal bone at the previous site of mastoid inflammation.
E. Cholesteatoma is a premalignant skin condition found in chronic otitis media

65. A 60-year-old man has undergone full-course radiation therapy for a tonsillar carcinoma. He is now complaining of dry mouth, burning tongue, and loss of taste. Examination of his oral cavity reveals generalized erythema of the tongue. It has a bald smooth appearance secondary to depapillation. The best treatment for this patient's problem is

A. Chlorhexidine gluconate
B. Pilocarpine
C. Clotrimazole oral lozenges
D. Topical steroid solution
E. Dental fluoride applications

66. The most important diagnostic test that should be performed in patients suspected of having postradiation chondronecrosis of the larynx is
A. A barium swallow
B. CT or MRI scan of the larynx
C. Chest x-ray
D. Pulmonary function tests
E. A laryngeal biopsy

67. A 55-year-old woman is evaluated for possible blepharoplasty. She is determined to have senile ptosis of the upper lid. The best therapeutic treatment for this would be
A. Upper lid blepharoplasty
B. Upper and lower lid blepharoplasty
C. Tightening of the apeurosis of the levator of the upper lid
D. A brow lift
E. Brow lift combined with upper lid blepharoplasty

68. A common physical finding in patients with laryngitis secondary to esophageal reflux is
A. Pooling of secretions in the pyriform sinus
B. Early penetration and aspiration of ingested liquids
C. Erythema and edema of the arytenoid mucosa and occasional granulomas in this same region
D. Leukoplakia of the anterior commissure
E. Laryngomalacia of the epiglottis

69. A pleomorphic adenoma of the parapharyngeal space has been diagnosed using imaging and fine-needle aspiration biopsy. It is determined that this tumor is probably of extraparotid origin. Treatment should include
A. Total parotidectomy and facial nerve dissection
B. Mandibular osteotomy for complete exposure
C. Preoperative angiography and embolization

D. Simple blunt dissection and removal through an external approach without parotidectomy
E. Partial pharyngectomy and intraoral tumor removal

70. The best time to perform an otoplasty for protruding ears is
A. Within the first 6 months of life
B. At age 5 or 6 prior to entering school
C. During the late teens following the growth spurt
D. When the child is old enough to decide if he or she wants to have the surgery
E. There is no ideal time for performing this surgery

71. Diagnosis of the perilymph fistula can be best made with
A. Hennebert's test
B. Tullio's test
C. Brown's test
D. Exploratory tympanotomy
E. Metrizomide CT scan

72. A 19-year-old woman presents with a temperature of 102°F. She has swelling at the angle of the jaw, swelling in the left peritonsillar region, and complains of trismus. In addition, she is noted to have Horner's syndrome. The most likely site of infection is
A. A peritonsillar abscess
B. An anterior compartment, lateral pharyngeal space abscess
C. A posterior compartment, lateral pharyngeal space abscess
D. A septic thrombosis of the internal jugular vein
E. A retropharyngeal space abscess

73. Speckled leukoplakia
A. Has the same incidence of malignant transformation as does erythroplakia
B. Has the same incidence of malignant transformation as does leukoplakia
C. Is more likely to become malignant than plain leukoplakia
D. Is caused by a viral infection and has no malignant transformation potential
E. Is another name for carcinoma *in situ*

74. Which of the following statements is false?
A. Of all children with sensorineural hearing loss, 75% have loss due to noncongenital causes, while 25% are due to congenital causes
B. Half of all congenital hearing impairment is due to nonhereditary causes
C. Fewer than 50 syndromes have actually been associated with hearing impairment
D. Eighty percent of genetic hearing loss is due to autosomal recessive transmission
E. Five percent of hearing loss is due to X-linked chromosomal disorders

75. A 68-year-old woman complains of nasal obstruction. She has undergone previous rhinoplasty and has a pinched overly rotated tip and a scooped-out dorsum. In repairing this defect, which of the following implant materials would not be suitable?
A. Rib cartilage
B. Auricular cartilage
C. Septal bone and cartilage
D. Polytetrafluorethylene
E. An implant material should never be used in this situation

76. Meniere's syndrome has been associated with all of the following except
A. Otosyphilis
B. Acoustic neuroma
C. Autoimmune disease
D. Viral labyrinthitis
E. Gardner's syndrome

77. When a patient presents with an acute postoperative carotid artery rupture following head and neck cancer surgery, the most common site of injury is the
A. External carotid artery
B. Internal carotid artery
C. Common carotid artery
D. Carotid bulb
E. All sites are equally likely to rupture

78. The classic audiometric findings in cupulolithiasis would be
A. A high-frequency sensorineural hearing loss

B. A low-frequency sensorineural hearing loss
C. A flat sensorineural hearing loss at 40 dB
D. Mixed hearing loss
E. Normal hearing

79. The primary limitation of a contrast cysternogram for localizing the site of a cerebrospinal fluid leak is
A. A high percentage of patients are allergic to the contrast material
B. Most patients develop aseptic meningitis following this study
C. The leak must be very brisk during the procedure for this technique to be useful
D. Surgery must be delayed for up to 2 weeks following this diagnostic test
E. A lumbar drain is often needed to relieve the severe headache that can accompany this test

80. A radiographic finding indicating possible subluxation of the stapes would include
A. Soft tissue in the mastoid
B. A fracture in the epitympanum
C. Pars flaccida retraction with scutal erosion
D. Pneumolabyrinth
E. Extended IAC

81. Following the excision of a medial canthal basal cell carcinoma with clear margins, it is elected to perform a full-thickness skin graft to this area. The best donor site for full-thickness skin to be placed in this anatomic region is
A. The inner thigh
B. Lower back
C. Supraclavicular region
D. Upper eye lid
E. Dorsum of the foot

82. Chronic sinusitis is a common problem in patients with cystic fibrosis. The incidence of nasal polyps in this population is
A. 0%
B. 25%
C. 50%
D. 75%
E. 100%

83. Hearing should be assessed in patients with Pierre Robin sequence because

A. This syndrome is often associated with middle ear ossicular deformities
B. Recurrent middle ear effusions are common
C. This condition is often associated with a Mondini deformity
D. Speech therapy will almost always be necessary
E. The sensorineural hearing loss associated with this syndrome is often progressive.

84. A 25-year-old male is diagnosed with cervical tuberculosis. He has an approximately 3-cm mass in the right neck from which a fine-needle aspiration biopsy was positive for tuberculosis. The primary treatment of this disease is
A. Medical therapy with multiple antituberculosis drugs
B. Surgical therapy consisting of the removal of the involved lymph node
C. Surgical therapy combined with antituberculosis antibiotic therapy
D. Currettage of the lymph node followed by antituberculosis chemotherapy
E. Combination of rifampin and alpha-interferon

85. For a patient with vocal cord paralysis the procedure that provides the best rotation of the vocal process of the arytenoid and therefore best glottic closure is the
A. Teflon injection
B. Thyroplasty type I
C. Arytenoid adduction procedure
D. Collagen or gelfoam injection
E. Vocal cord reinnervation procedure

86. The most definitive test for establishing the identification of a foreign body in the upper aerodigestive tract is
A. PA and lateral neck x-ray
B. PA and lateral chest x-ray
C. Lateral decubitus x-ray
D. Fluoroscopy
E. Direct endoscopy

87. Which of the following drugs should not be used in a patient with chronic sinusitis?
A. Systemic steroids
B. Guaifenesin
C. Phenylpropanolamine

D. Loratidine

E. Chlorpheniramine

88. A 2-cm parotid mass is found during examination of a 29-year-old HIV-infected man. Fine-needle aspiration reveals straw-colored cystic fluid. The best management of this parotid lesion is

A. Antituberculosis antibiotics

B. Superficial parotidectomy

C. Surgical enucleation of the mass

D. Radiation therapy

E. Repeated needle aspirations as needed

89. When performing a biopsy of a skin lesion, the following method should be avoided due to its failure to demonstrate tumor thickness

A. Excisional biopsy

B. Punch biopsy

C. Incisional biopsy

D. Shave biopsy

E. Skin lesions should not undergo a preliminary biopsy

90. If a lumpectomy is performed for a parotid pleomorphic adenoma, the incidence of recurrence is increased. The reason for this high incidence of recurrence is felt to be

A. Tumor spillage during the initial procedure

B. Inadequate resection by enucleation

C. Multicentric pleomorphic adenoma unrecognized at the time of initial surgery

D. A genetic predisposition to forming multiple tumors

E. Tumorigenic factors released during the surgical procedure

91. The Anti-SS-A and Anti-SS-B tests are often useful in making the diagnosis of Sjögren's syndrome. These tests measure:

A. Serum levels of Sjögrens factors

B. Circulating serum antibodies to specific nuclear antigens

C. The functional status of major and minor salivary glands

D. The functional status of circulating C-8 lymphocytes

E. The titre of circulating anti acinar cell antibodies

92. Cervical nodal metastasis in patients with tonsillar carcinoma are often

A. Primarily in the posterior cervical region

B. Cystic in appearance on CT or MRI

C. Difficult to palpate on physical examination

D. Extending into the parotid lymph chain

E. Difficult to remove surgically because of the sclerosis and fibrosis that is often associated with these lymph nodes

93. When healing does not occur in a postoperative fistula following major resection for head and neck squamous cell carcinoma, the first concern should be

A. Nutritional depletion

B. Persistent cancer

C. Electrolyte imbalance

D. Persistent infection

E. Poorly vascularized tissues

94. The Mustarde technique for repairing protruding ears consists of

A. Decreasing the cupping and displacement of the pinna by placing chondral mastoid sutures

B. Recreating the antihelix by incorporating permanent scapha chondral and scapha fossa triangularis horizontal sutures

C. Recreating the antihelix by incising the cartilage and placing buried mattress sutures

D. Making parallel cartilage incisions to weaken the cartilage

E. Scoring the anterior aspect of the auricular cartilage to create posterior bending

95. The Hertel exophthalmometer measures

A. Enophthalmus

B. Hypophthalmus

C. Entrapment

D. Proptosis

E. Intraocular pressure

96. The most likely diagnosis in a 4-year-old child with persistent hoarseness is

A. Laryngitis

B. Vocal cord nodule

C. Vocal cord papillomas

D. Vocal cord paralysis

E. Gastroesophageal reflux

97. The halo or ring sign seen on CT scan in a patient with otosclerosis is indicative of

A. Congenital otosclerosis
B. Paget's disease
C. Associated meningitis
D. Cochlear otosclerosis
E. Neural otosclerosis

98. Indications for open exploration of a laryngeal fracture include which of the following?
A. Subcutaneous emphysema
B. Ecchymosis of the anterior neck
C. Hoarseness
D. Displaced laryngeal skeletal fracture
E. Dysphagia

99. Following a total thyroidectomy a routine serum albumin level is obtained. A slight decrease in serum albumin is noted. This factor can probably be explained by
A. Serum albumin loss interoperatively
B. Urinary proteinuria
C. A dilutional effect due to overzealous intravenous fluid therapy during surgery
D. The effects of the release of ADH in the immediate postoperative period
E. Pending liver dysfunction, probably as a result of hypothyroidism

100. Vasomotor rhinitis can often be effectively treated with ipratropium bromide. This agent works by
A. Decreasing mucosal inflammation in the nasal cavity
B. Acting as a topical anticholinergic and inhibiting mucosal glandular secretion of the nasal cavity.
C. Inducing atrophic changes of the nasal cavity
D. Producing a strong vasoconstrictive effect through its sympathomimetic action
E. Causing the release and depletion of substance P in the nasal mucosa

101. WHO type III nasopharyngeal carcinoma is
A. Not associated with elevated Epstein–Barr virus titers
B. A keratinizing squamous cell carcinoma
C. The most common type of nasopharyngeal carcinoma encountered

D. Almost never associated with skull base invasion
E. Easily treated with surgery

102. Of the following studies, which would be most beneficial prior to surgical intervention in patients with temporal bone fracture?
A. Routine audiometrics
B. ABR
C. ENG
D. High-resolution CT scanning
E. MRI with gadolinium

103. A 49-year-old man presents with a 1-cm irregular variegated pigmented lesion of the right cheek. A shave biopsy should not be obtained of this lesion because
A. This will increase the rate of metastasis if it is malignant
B. This does not allow identification of cells at the basal layer that may be malignant
C. It is impossible to make a definitive diagnosis using this technique
D. The thickness of the lesion will be difficult to determine for tumor staging purposes
E. If this is a benign lesion, shaved biopsies often lead to malignant transformation

104. A 40-year-old woman presents with what appears to be a parapharyngeal space mass on the right. A CT scan is obtained and there appears to be a 2-cm poststyloid mass in the parapharyngeal space. At this point you should proceed with
A. A fine-needle aspiration biopsy
B. A transoral biopsy
C. Immediate surgical exploration and removal through an external approach
D. An MRI and possibly MRA
E. Angiography

105. The treatment of spasmodic dysphonia with the injection of botulinum toxin type A is effective because
A. The recurrent laryngeal nerve is paralyzed by this agent
B. This agent produces an immunologic response to the laryngeal muscles
C. By interfering with transmission at the neuromuscular junction this agent causes temporary vocal cord paralysis

D. This agent produces a central effect in the region of the basal ganglia

E. This agent causes an immediate improvement in voice, which lasts for up to 1 year

106. Following an extensive rhinoplasty a patient complains of nasal obstruction. Examination reveals collapse of the upper lateral cartilages, as well as retraction of the ala secondary to overzealous lower lateral cartilage resection. The best approach to manage this problem would be

A. An open rhinoplasty approach
B. Bilateral rhinotomies
C. Delivery of the lower lateral cartilages through a closed approach
D. To perform a transcartilagenous approach to the nasal tip
E. To perform a facial degloving

107. The easiest and most widely utilized test of olfactory function is the University of Pennsylvania smell identification test. This test allows the examiner to

A. Determine a threshold for odorant detection
B. Determine the precise etiology of an olfactory problem
C. Provide a sensitive test of olfactory loss
D. Differentiate between parosmia and phantosmia
E. Specifically identify the site of dysfunction along the olfactory tract

108. A 50-year-old man presents with a 2- × 2-cm mass in the left submandibular gland. Fine-needle aspiration biopsy confirms the diagnosis of adenoid cystic carcinoma. MRI scan reveals no involvement into the mandible and no pathologically involved neck nodes. Therapy should consist of

A. Surgical resection of the tumor followed by full-course radiation therapy
B. Concurrent chemotherapy and radiation therapy followed by surgical salvage
C. Surgical resection including a radical neck dissection followed by full-course radiation therapy
D. Full-course radiation therapy alone followed by close follow-up

E. Palliation therapy only since this is an incurable lesion

109. Neonatal audiometric screening is important to establish the early detection of hearing loss. Which of the following entities does *not* portend a specific risk factor for hearing impairment?

A. A family history of hearing loss
B. Craniofacial anomalies
C. Asphyxia
D. Birth weight under 2,500 grams
E. Mechanical ventilation for 5 days or longer

110. In Chandler's staging system of orbital complications of sinusitis, stage IV is characterized by

A. Proptosis ophthalmoplegia and occasionally visual loss
B. Lateral displacement of the globe with possible diplopia and decreased visual acuity
C. Edema and erythema of the periorbital region including the conjunctiva
D. Ophthalmoplegia, visual loss, and extension to the contralateral eye
E. Intracranial extension with meningitis, epidural abscess, subdural empyema, or brain abscess

111. Angular cheilitis, which is characterized by redness and cracking at the angles of the mouth, is most often secondary to

A. Herpes simplex
B. Herpes zoster
C. *Aspergillus*
D. Cytomegalovirus
E. *Candida albicans*

112. A 48-year-old woman presents with hoarseness following a hemithyroidectomy. She undergoes laryngeal EMG, which shows spontaneous activity with no voluntary motor units

A. Return of function is very likely in this situation
B. There is a 50% chance of return of normal function
C. Return of function is not likely
D. The laryngeal EMG should be repeated because this is probably a spurious result
E. These results are of no prognostic significance

113. Currently the most sensitive test available to diagnose multiple sclerosis is
A. ENG
B. CSF protein electrophoresis
C. Myelin specific protein (MSP)
D. MRI scanning
E. Auditory brain stem response audiometry

114. Due to its morphology, the type of lymphangioma most often associated with incomplete excision is
A. Cystic hygroma
B. Lymphangioma simplex
C. Cavernous lymphangioma
D. Capillary lymphangioma
E. Cervical lymphangioma

115. Following an MVA, a patient presents with a severe frontal sinus fracture involving extensive comminution of the anterior and posterior tables, with some moderate loss of bone. Radiologic study indicates no intracranial injury. The most appropriate method for repair includes
A. Open reduction with plate fixation through an osteoplastic flap
B. Open reduction with fat obliteration of the frontal sinuses through an osteoplastic approach
C. Open reduction with obliteration using cancellous bone, through an osteoplastic approach
D. Open reduction with obliteration of the frontal sinus using an alloplastic material such as methylmethacrolate, via an osteoplastic approach
E. A Lynch external frontoethmoidectomy

116. Risk factors associated with the development of congenital facial paralysis include all of the following except
A. Forceps delivery
B. Birth weight of greater than 3,500 grams
C. Primiparity
D. Multiparity
E. Traumatic delivery

117. To optimize surgical results from atresia repair, Jahrsdoerfer suggests all of the following be present except

A. Stapes suprastructure
B. Round window
C. Oval window
D. Malleus incus complex
E. Normal fallopian canal

118. In the absence of prior surgery or infection, the rate of recurrence after surgical resection of branchial anomalies is:
A. 5%
B. 10%
C. 15%
D. 20%
E. 25%

119. Secondary post-tonsillectomy hemorrhage generally occurs
A. Within the first 24 hours following surgery
B. 1 to 3 days postop
C. 3 to 5 days postop
D. 5 to 7 days postop
E. More than 10 days postop

120. A woman presents with a thyroid mass that is evaluated with a fine-needle aspiration biopsy. The cytopathologist returns a diagnosis of follicular cell carcinoma. At this point the appropriate therapy for this patient is
A. Total thyroidectomy
B. Hemithyroidectomy
C. Total thyroidectomy with neck dissection on the side of the lesion
D. Total thyroidectomy followed by iodine-131 therapy
E. A thorough discussion with the cytopathologist regarding his histopathologic diagnosis

121. A 63-year-old man presents with a unilateral nasal mass. He is also complaining trismus and hypoesthesia in the distribution of V2 on the side of the mass. Intranasal biopsy in the office reveals findings consistent with inverting papilloma. The next step in this patient's workup should be
A. Imaging studies to assess the extent of the underlying tumor
B. Intranasal polypectomy for palliation
C. Caldwell Luc operation to obtain more biopsy material

D. A complete metastatic workup
E. Referral to radiation oncology for consideration for therapy

122. The roentgenographic sign considered pathognomonic for juvenile nasopharyngeal angiofibroma is the Holman–Miller sign. This is
A. Anterior bowing of the posterior wall of the maxillary antrum
B. Erosion of the sphenoid bone
C. Erosion of the hard palate
D. Erosion of the medial maxillary sinus
E. Displacement of the nasal septum

123. The incidence of epiglottitis has decreased in children during the past 15 years. This decrease can probably be attributed to
A. Inherent decreased virulence of organisms responsible for epiglottitis
B. Improved public health conditions in the public schools
C. The *Haemophilus influenzae* type B vaccine
D. Widespread use of broad-spectrum antibiotics
E. A greater awareness of this disease on the part of pediatricians

124. When treating patients with chronic sinusitis, which of the following antibiotic regimens would be most appropriate?
A. Amoxicillin for 3 weeks
B. Cefuroxime axetil for 10 days
C. Ciprofloxacin for 3 weeks
D. Amoxicillin/clavulanate for 3 weeks
E. Clindamycin for 3 weeks

125. The fibula osteocutaneous flap is an ideal flap for reconstructing large mandibular defects. Its advantages include
A. Reliability of the skin paddle
B. Decreased donor site morbidity
C. Length of available bone for reconstruction
D. Easy plate fixation
E. Decreased operative time

126. A patient with obstructive sleep apnea is determined to have type III obstruction. The most effective treatment for this patient would be

A. Nasal continuous positive airway pressure (CPAP)
B. Uvulopalatal pharyngoplasty (UPPP)
C. Genioglossus advancement with hyoid myotomy (GAHM)
D. Maxillomandibular advancement
E. Nasal septoplasty

127. The initial management for cerebrospinal fluid otorhinorrhea associated with temporal bone fracture includes
A. Head elevation with bed rest
B. Antibiotic treatment
C. Lumbar drainage
D. Exploratory tympanotomy
E. Steroid utilization

128. Of the following viruses, which is most commonly associated with unilateral sensorineural hearing loss?
A. Cytomegalovirus
B. Mumps
C. Measles
D. Herpes
E. Rubella

129. Medical therapy for chronic sinusitis in patients with cystic fibrosis is often disappointing. It is particularly important that medical therapy in this population cover
A. *Aspergillus fumigatus*
B. *Candida albicans*
C. *Pseudomonas aeruginosa*
D. *Klebsiella*
E. *Mycoplasma pneumoniae*

130. The most common site of metastasis for esthesioneuroblastoma is
A. Lung
B. Liver
C. Cervical spine
D. Cervical lymph nodes
E. Bone marrow

131. The anatomic site most commonly associated with a naturally dehiscent facial nerve is
A. Vertical segment
B. Second genu
C. Tympanic segment
D. First genu
E. Geniculate ganglion

132. An 8-year-old girl presents with bilateral nasal polyps. The initial workup should include a test for
A. Aspirin sensitivity
B. Inhalant sensitivities
C. Cystic fibrosis
D. Kartagener's syndrome
E. Asthma

133. Which of the following is *not* indicative of an aberrant internal carotid artery?
A. Enlargement of the inferior tympanic canaliculus
B. Enhancing mass in the hypotympanum
C. Absence of the vertical segment of the internal carotid
D. Absence of the bony covering of the internal carotid
E. Transposed fallopian canal

134. The best test currently available to diagnose cerebrospinal fluid rhinorrhea is the
A. Chloride level in the fluid
B. Glucose level of the fluid
C. β-transferrin test
D. Radioimmunoassay for neuronal specific antigen (NSA)
E. Air contrast cysternogram

135. A 61-year-old male underwent a total laryngectomy and lateral pharyngectomy for a large pyriform sinus carcinoma. Reconstruction was performed with a pectoralis myocutaneous flap. On the fifth postoperative day, a foul-smelling discharge appeared through the lower end of the wound just lateral to the laryngostome. Further examination revealed a defect at the upper end of the closure adjacent to the pectoralis skin paddle and posterior tongue. Initial treatment should be
A. Open the wound more superiorly to establish direct drainage
B. Increase tube feedings to ensure adequate nutrition
C. Return the patient to the operating room for surgical debridement and closure
D. Schedule the patient for a gastrostomy placement and removal of the nasogastric tube
E. Place the patient on thyroid hormone supplements

136. Significant fluid shifts occur with total body surface area burn in adults exceeding
A. 10%
B. 20%
C. 30%
D. 40%
E. More than 50%

137. Facial paralysis secondary to developmental defects usually presents at birth. All of the following are commonly associated with the exception of
A. Cleft palate defect
B. Hypoplastic maxilla
C. Auricular atresia or microtia
D. Gait instability and unsteadiness
E. Sensorineural hearing loss

138. One of the primary reasons for the resurgence of tuberculosis in the United States is
A. Poor public health conditions in inner cities
B. Increased intravenous drug usage
C. Acquired immunodeficiency syndrome (AIDS)
D. The overuse of antituberculosis chemotherapy
E. Genetic mutations occurring in *mycobacterium* tuberculosis

139. The hallmark of nonsurgical management of cholesteatoma would be represented by which of the following?
A. Systemic antibiotic treatment
B. Topical drop application
C. Active otomicroscopic debridement
D. Aural antibiotics with aural douche
E. Radiation

140. The reliability of EEMG or ENoG is most dependable at
A. 24 hours
B. 48 hours
C. 1 week
D. 3 weeks
E. 6 months

141. Forced duction testing measures
A. Enophthalmus
B. Exophthalmos
C. Entrapment

D. Proptosis
E. Intraocular pressure

142. In penetrating neck trauma, the mortality approaches 66% when the common carotid artery is lacerated and the injury is in
A. Zone 1
B. Zone 2
C. Zone 3
D. The oral cavity
E. The region of the larynx

143. A 27-year-old male is involved in a high-speed motor vehicle accident. Preliminary examination reveals a possible LeFort II and mandible fracture. Preliminary cervical spine films and a chest x-ray are obtained. The cervical spine is cleared, and the chest x-ray is normal except for possible mediastinal widening. The next test should be
A. CT scan of the face to better define the facial injury
B. CT scan of the neck to more definitively rule out a cervical spine injury
C. CT scan of the chest
D. Arteriogram
E. A barium swallow

144. The most specific serologic test for evaluating Epstein–Barr virus titers in patients with nasopharyngeal carcinoma is the
A. Viral core antigen
B. Viral capsid antigen
C. The mono spot test
D. Antinuclear Epstein–Barr virus antigen
E. Short-chain anti-IgG antibody

145. Of the following diagnoses, which is made by radiographic finding?
A. Acute mastoiditis
B. Coalescent mastoiditis
C. Suppurative labyrinthitis
D. Petrous apicitis
E. Bezold's abscess

146. A 20-year-old male involved in a motor vehicle accident presents to the emergency room with near complete avulsion of his left ear. It remains attached only by a very small superior pedicle. The most appropriate method of reconstruction is

A. Simple reapproximation
B. Reapproximation with a microvascular anastomosis
C. Reapproximation and at the same time burying the cartilage under a postauricular skin flap
D. Reanastomosis with application of medical-grade leeches
E. If the ear does survive, the reconstructive result will be poor; it is best to cut the pedicle and plan reconstruction using osseointegrated implants

147. A patient has suffered a mandibular fracture. If the mandibular arch is disrupted at two or more points
A. The airway may become compromised
B. Restoring proper occlusion becomes very difficult
C. The patient will have great difficulty eating
D. The patient is best kept in a supine position
E. The patient is best kept in a prone position

148. A 39-year-old woman presents following a motor vehicle accident with almost complete avulsion of the left ear. The ear is reattached primarily. The most likely reason for failure would be
A. Infection
B. Inadequate arterial supply
C. Venous engorgement
D. Technically improper closure
E. Cartilage necrosis

149. In penetrating neck trauma, an arteriogram is not routinely indicated when the injury occurs in
A. Zone 1
B. Zone 2
C. Zone 3
D. The temporal bone
E. The region of the sphenoid sinus

150. A 4-month-old infant presents with increasing respiratory stridor, but as yet no respiratory compromise. Endoscopic examination reveals a large subglottic hemangioma encompassing close to 50% of the subglottic lumen. The most appropriate first step is
A. Administration of high-dose steroids
B. Tracheostomy

C. Surgical excision using the CO_2 laser
D. Cryotherapy
E. Embolization

151. Before starting medical therapy for a patient with allergic fungal sinusitis, the workup should include
A. A creatine clearance
B. A glucose tolerance test
C. A histopathologic review of silver stained biopsy specimens
D. A serum immunoglobulin electrophoresis
E. A chest CT scan

152. Hereditary hemorrhagic telangiectasia (HHT) is
A. An autosomal dominant disorder
B. An autosomal recessive disorder
C. A sex-linked disorder
D. Always sporadic in its appearance
E. Of unknown genetic etiology

153. A 37-year-old woman underwent bilateral upper and lower lid blepharoplasty. In the recovery room, she complains of severe left eye pain, and examination reveals ecchymosis, proptosis, and decreased range of motion. A gross test of visual acuity indicated only light perception. The next step should be to
A. Elevate the head of the bed and apply ice packs
B. IV mannitol
C. Place a tarsorrhaphy to prevent corneal injury
D. Incise and drain the orbital hematoma
E. A lateral canthotomy and inferior cantholysis

154. A 9-year-old Down syndrome patient presents with an acute peritonsillar abscess, high fever, and impending airway obstruction. The patient is taken to the operating room for emergent tonsillectomy and drainage of the abscess. Because of the history of Down syndrome
A. A tracheostomy should be performed
B. A large endotracheal tube should be utilized to secure the airway
C. The surgery should be performed with the patient in the neutral position
D. The abscess only should be drained and the tonsils not removed

E. An uvulopalatopharyngoplasty should be performed at the same time

155. A 65-year-old man has received 7,000 cGy of radiation for a T3 glottic squamous cell carcinoma. Approximately 1 year following therapy he presents with increasing pain upon swallowing and mild stridor. Physical examination reveals an ulcerative region on the laryngeal surface of the epiglottis, in addition to generalized laryngeal edema. The most likely etiology for this patient's laryngeal problem is
A. Invasive laryngeal candidiasis
B. Postradiation chondrosarcoma of the larynx
C. Recurrent squamous cell carcinoma of the larynx
D. Postradiation chondritis
E. Severe reflux esophagitis

156. The most reliable predictor for post-tonsillectomy hemorrhage is
A. Patient history
B. Physical examination
C. CBC
D. PT, PTT
E. Bleeding time

157. All of the following would be considered in the different diagnosis of Bell's palsy except
A. Herpes zoster oticus
B. Facial neuroma
C. Acoustic neuroma
D. Jugular foramen tumor
E. Otosclerosis

158. A patient presents with a T3N2 squamous cell carcinoma of the larynx. He has palpable nodes in the left neck, however, no palpable adenopathy on the right. His primary lesion crosses the midline. In managing the neck disease in this patient
A. He should undergo a radical neck dissection on both the right and left sides
B. No therapy is indicated for the right neck since it is clinically negative for tumor
C. If a right neck dissection is undertaken, the spinal accessory nerve can usually be preserved but the jugular vein should always be taken
D. Both necks should be treated

E.   The right neck dissection should be performed only if there is extra capsular spread in the left neck.

159.   If a patient presents with an orbital or periorbital infection secondary to acute sinusitis, an appropriate initial antibiotic regimen would be
A.   Cefuroxime and metronidazole
B.   Ampicillin
C.   Ciprofloxacin
D.   Clindamycin
E.   Erythromycin

160.   Nystagmus associated with benign paroxysmal positional vertigo is characterized by all of the following except
A.   Fatiguability
B.   Latency
C.   Geotropic nystagmus

D.   Ageotropic nystagmus
E.   Habituation

161.   Of the following clinical findings in a patient with an odontogenic tumor, which suggests a malignancy?
A.   Dysesthesia, pain, and loose dentition
B.   A bruit
C.   Radiographic evidence of sclerotic bony walls surrounding the lesion
D.   Occurrence of the tumor on the maxilla
E.   Occurrence of the tumor on the mandible

162.   The incidence of malignant transformation of inverting papilloma to squamous cell carcinoma is
A.   1%
B.   10 to 15%
C.   60 to 70%
D.   Unknown
E.   Highly dependent on the age of the patient

SELF-ASSESSMENT: ANSWERS

1. B (Case 28)	42. C (Case 8)	83. B (Case 71)	123. C (Case 35)
2. C (Case 71)	43. A (Case 2)	84. A (Case 38)	124. D (Case 42)
3. E (Case 7)	44. E (Case 10)	85. C (Case 49)	125. C (Case 66)
4. E (Case 52)	45. A (Case 44)	86. E (Case 57)	126. A (Case 54)
5. A (Case 73)	46. A (Case 50)	87. E (Case 42)	127. A (Case 7)
6. B (Case 54)	47. B (Case 53)	88. E (Case 39)	128. B (Case 9)
7. E (Case 51)	48. A (Case 40)	89. D (Case 68)	129. C (Case 63)
8. A (Case 20)	49. A (Case 39)	90. B (Case 31)	130. D (Case 27)
9. A (Case 47)	50. B (Case 55)	91. B (Case 56)	131. C (Case 16)
10. C (Case 17)	51. C (Case 31)	92. B (Case 22)	132. C (Case 69)
11. C (Case 40)	52. C (Case 16)	93. B (Case 67)	133. E (Case 10)
12. C (Case 58)	53. D (Case 80)	94. B (Case 70)	134. C (Case 45)
13. B (Case 48)	54. B (Case 77)	95. A (Case 76)	135. A (Case 67)
14. D (Case 36)	55. C (Case 79)	96. B (Case 65)	136. B (Case 79)
15. E (Case 14)	56. D (Case 77)	97. D (Case 6)	137. D (Case 4)
16. E (Case 32)	57. C (Case 74)	98. D (Case 53)	138. C (Case 38)
17. D (Case 6)	58. B (Case 17)	99. D (Case 25)	139. C (Case 5)
18. D (Case 25)	59. A (Case 28)	100. B (Case 48)	140. C (Case 14)
19. E (Case 3)	60. C (Case 27)	101. C (Case 19)	141. C (Case 76)
20. C (Case 23)	61. E (Case 33)	102. D (Case 8)	142. A (Case 81)
21. B (Case 11)	62. A (Case 43)	103. D (Case 34)	143. D (Case 75)
22. B (Case 57)	63. E (Case 15)	104. D (Case 30)	144. B (Case 19)
23. C (Case 34)	64. A (Case 5)	105. C (Case 50)	145. B (Case 3)
24. E (Case 60)	65. C (Case 37)	106. A (Case 72)	146. A (Case 78)
25. C (Case 69)	66. E (Case 24)	107. C (Case 47)	147. A (Case 75)
26. D (Case 68)	67. C (Case 73)	108. A (Case 32)	148. C (Case 78)
27. A (Case 18)	68. C (Case 51)	109. D (Case 1)	149. B (Case 81)
28. D (Case 66)	69. D (Case 30)	110. A (Case 41)	150. B (Case 62)
29. E (Case 43)	70. B (Case 70)	111. E (Case 37)	151. C (Case 44)
30. D (Case 21)	71. D (Case 13)	112. C (Case 49)	152. A (Case 46)
31. B (Case 26)	72. C (Case 36)	113. D (Case 55)	153. E (Case 74)
32. B (Case 35)	73. C (Case 18)	114. C (Case 59)	154. C (Case 64)
33. D (Case 62)	74. C (Case 1)	115. C (Case 80)	155. C (Case 24)
34. E (Case 64)	75. A (Case 72)	116. D (Case 4)	156. A (Case 61)
35. B (Case 59)	76. E (Case 11)	117. B (Case 2)	157. E (Case 15)
36. C (Case 9)	77. D (Case 20)	118. A (Case 58)	158. D (Case 23)
37. A (Case 65)	78. E (Case 12)	119. D (Case 61)	159. A (Case 41)
38. D (Case 56)	79. C (Case 45)	120. E (Case 26)	160. D (Case 12)
39. D (Case 52)	80. D (Case 13)	121. A (Case 29)	161. A (Case 21)
40. A (Case 22)	81. D (Case 33)	122. A (Case 60)	162. B (Case 29)
41. C (Case 46)	82. C (Case 63)		

Index

Note: "f" designates a figure.

Trauma. *See* specific types
Trismus
  deep neck space, 104, 130
  Down syndrome, 233
  maxillary sinus, 104
Tuberculosis
  Acquired Immunodeficiency Syndrome (AIDS)
    and, 139–141
  cervical. *See* Cervical tuberculosis
  pulmonary, 140
  resurgence of, 136
Tumors. *See* specific types
Turbinate hypertrophy, 153
Tympanic membrane
  bulging of, 11, 12 f
  laceration of, 27
Tympanomastoidectomy, 56
Tympanoplasty, 47

U
Unilateral hearing loss
  acoustic neuroma causing, 31
  CT scan of, 32
  diagnosis of, 32
  differential diagnosis of, 30
  endolymphatic hydrops causing, 31
  history of, 30
  labyrinthitis causing, 30
  medical management of, 32
  Mondini's deformity causing, 31 f
  mumps causing, 30
  neoplastic, 31
  otosclerosis causing, 31
  rehabilitation and follow-up, 32–33
  suggested readings, 33
  surgical management of, 32
  temporal bone fracture causing, 31
  test interpretation of, 31–32
  tinnitus, 30
  toxins causing, 31
  trauma causing, 31
Upper eyelids
  excess tissue, 268
  levator muscle of, 268
  rejuvenation. *See* Eyelid rejuvenation
Uvulopalatopharyngoplasty (UPPP), 193

V
Vasomotor rhinitis
  diagnosis of, 172
  differential diagnosis of, 170–172
  history of, 170
  medical management of, 172
  pregnant women, 173
  rehabilitation and follow-up, 173
  special situations, 173
  suggested readings, 173
  surgical management of, 173
  test interpretation of, 172
Venous hum tinnitus, 34
Vertebral injuries, 299
Vertigo
  benign paroxysmal positional. *See* Benign paroxysmal positional vertigo
  cholesteatoma, 17
  Meniere's disease causing, 39
  temporal bone fracture causing, 24
Vestibular neuritis, 43
Vocal cord paralysis
  acoustic analysis, 176
  diagnosis of, 176
  differential diagnosis of, 175
  history of, 175
  laryngeal electromyography, 176
  medical management of, 176
  nasolaryngoscopy, 176 f
  rehabilitation and follow-up, 177
  suggested readings, 177
  surgical management of, 176
  test interpretation of, 175–176
  videostroboscopy, 176
Vocal cords, subglottic mass of, 237
Vocal fold granulomas, 181

W
Wegener's granulomatosis, 31, 153–155
Wound healing, tobacco abuse preventing, 245

X
Xerostomia
  radiation-induced, 134
  Sjögren's syndrome, 200